The Johns Hopkins Guide
to Diabetes

A JOHNS HOPKINS PRESS
HEALTH BOOK

CHRISTOPHER D. SAUDEK, M.D., is Professor of Medicine at the Johns Hopkins University School of Medicine and Director of the Johns Hopkins Diabetes Center.

RICHARD R. RUBIN, Ph.D., CDE, is an instructor in medicine and pediatrics at the Johns Hopkins University School of Medicine and a staff member at the Johns Hopkins Diabetes Center and the Johns Hopkins Pediatric Diabetes Clinic. He also has a private practice specializing in counseling people with diabetes.

CYNTHIA S. SHUMP, R.N., M.S., CDE, is Diabetes Nurse Educator at the Johns Hopkins Diabetes Center.

THE JOHNS HOPKINS GUIDE TO DIABETES

For Today and Tomorrow

CHRISTOPHER D. SAUDEK, M.D.

RICHARD R. RUBIN, Ph.D., CDE

CYNTHIA S. SHUMP, R.N., CDE

THE JOHNS HOPKINS UNIVERSITY PRESS

Baltimore & London

Note to the reader:
This book is not meant to substitute for medical care of people with diabetes, and treatment should not
be based solely on its contents. Instead, treatment must be developed in a dialogue between
the individual and his or her physician. Our book has been
written to help with that dialogue.

© 1997 The Johns Hopkins University Press
All rights reserved. Published 1997
Printed in the United States of America on acid-free paper
4 5 6 7 8 9

The Johns Hopkins University Press
2715 North Charles Street
Baltimore, Maryland 21218-4363
www.press.jhu.edu

Library of Congress Cataloging-in-Publication Data will be found at the end of this book.
A catalog record for this book is available from the British Library.

ISBN 0-8018-5580-2
ISBN 0-8018-5581-0 (pbk.)

Illustrations by Cynthia S. Shump, R.N., CDE

We dedicate this book to people with diabetes. They fight the daily battles great and small. Their courage and perseverance inspire us and teach not just about diabetes but about the human spirit.

Contents

Part III. *Living with Diabetes*

Part IV. *Complications*

Part V. *Sexuality, Pregnancy, and Genetics*

Part VI. *The Future of Care*

Preface

This book grew out of our experiences in caring for people with diabetes, particularly at the self-management program of the Johns Hopkins Diabetes Center. Much that we discuss in this book is drawn from the material used in our teaching sessions—and indeed, from the material taught by diabetes educators throughout the country.

As we wrote *The Johns Hopkins Guide to Diabetes: For Today and Tomorrow,* we included stories we had heard from our patients and other people. These vignettes gradually became a central element of the book, and it dawned on us that, like many teachers, we learn far more from our students than we teach them.

We are sharing what we have learned, and we hope that it's helpful. We know, however, that your "truth" will come from many sources, not only this book. You may jump into the primary literature, reading original research articles. You will almost certainly talk with people, too: family members, people with diabetes, your health care professionals. We hope you read the diabetes magazines and keep your eyes open for information from many directions. You will need to sort through all these sources of information and figure out what works for you.

You know your own self best. You know how you feel, what you eat, how much you exercise, and how your blood sugar responds. No one else knows you in as much detail as you know yourself. But we provide another perspective, the perspective of professionals who have had lots of experience with diabetes. Actually, we provide three perspectives.

Chris Saudek is a clinically oriented academic physician. In addition to caring for people with diabetes on a daily basis, he is in charge of teaching medical students at Johns Hopkins about diabetes, has contributed to various treatment advances, and has held positions in professional diabetes organizations. It is his business to stay in touch with the literature. He has tried to be sure that the information provided here is factually correct and that current research findings are accurately integrated into the text. But mainly, with some 25 years invested in clinical care, he cares for and about people with diabetes.

Richard Rubin's professional life is also devoted to diabetes, but in a different way. He has an active private practice in mental health counseling and has written and lectured extensively. He too is active with several professional diabetes organizations. With a handful of others around the country, Richard has taught what should have been obvious all along: that psychological factors play a definitive role in the success of any treatment.

Finally, Cindy Shump exemplifies the burgeoning profession of diabetes nurse educator. She and her growing number of colleagues throughout America are often the first line of defense for people with diabetes, the ones who make sense of all the medical gibberish, put it in practical terms, and always offer support. Cindy has served this vital role at the Johns Hopkins Diabetes Center for many years now, teaching groups and individuals with skill and compassion.

So *The Johns Hopkins Guide to Diabetes: For Today and Tomorrow* provides not one but three perspectives, each essential: that of the physician, that of the mental health counselor, and that of the nurse educator. The different views are woven into the whole fabric of the book. The only perspective we have highlighted for special attention, though, is *yours*. The stories you tell and the concerns, frustrations, and triumphs that are repeated over and over again from day to day, person to person: these are the basis of all our understanding and all our teaching.

Acknowledgments

The authors are indebted to countless people who have taught us and encouraged us over the years. Foremost are our families. We are always grateful for their love and support as we have taken yet more time away to pursue the writing of this book.

We want specifically to acknowledge the help of the following colleagues: G. William Benedict, Charlene E. Freeman, Sherman M. Holvey, Robert H. Knopp, Maria Lim, Lynn D. Mahbubani, Simeon Margolis, David Marrero, Margaret O'Neil, Nancy Neville, Leslie Plotnick, Robert E. Ratner, Gayle E. Reiber, Catherine S. Sackett, Paul J. Scheel Jr., Kristi Silver, and Judith Wylie-Rosett. These experts reviewed portions of the manuscript.

Gloria Elfert not only contributed significantly to the dietary portions of the text but has been the model teacher of nutrition to generations of participants in the Johns Hopkins Diabetes Center. Likewise, the Center's programs, including much of what appears in this book, could not have been accomplished without the central contributions of Joseph Napora, Mark Peyrot, Samuel Zaccari, and the physician-educators from the Johns Hopkins faculty, Division of Endocrinology and Metabolism.

Finally, we especially want to thank our editor, Jacqueline Wehmueller, for having originated the project and guiding us through it with patience, good counsel, and unwavering support.

Part I

Understanding Diabetes

There are enough uncertainties in life without wondering whether you have diabetes. And if you do, you won't want to spend time worrying about what kind of diabetes. Nevertheless, a great many people are confused on these very basic issues. Part I will clear up the confusion. We will consistently reject such phrases as "a touch of sugar," "just in my blood, not in my urine," and "the sugar's just a little high," making it clear that either you have diabetes or you don't. And we will point out the misfortunes that can result from denial.

This is not because we are unsympathetic or like to beat people over the head with the fact that they have diabetes. Quite the opposite. We feel nothing but compassion for and solidarity with our patients, friends, and relatives with diabetes. It's perfectly clear why they would like to deny the disease, wish it away, wake up one morning without it.

But we also see on a daily basis the effects of living in long-term denial. We see people who for one reason or another didn't come to grips with their diabetes, didn't hear the diagnosis, and paid dearly.

So in Part I we lay out the fundamentals of making the diagnosis. We describe the types of diabetes and set a foundation for understanding what blood sugar measurement is all about. It would be terrific if we could also set out certainties, provide unambiguous criteria, and give definitions that will never change. Unfortunately, this isn't possible. The criteria, definitions, and even names do change from time to time, as scientific evidence evolves. But the basic facts remain: it is crucial to know when you have diabetes, to hear the diagnosis, and to pay attention to it.

Chapter 1

The Diagnosis of Diabetes
Making It and Hearing It

- *"It hit me like a ton of bricks. How could this be possible? I didn't know a thing about diabetes. Why me? It was never in my family."*

- *"I'm a doctor, so you would think I'd recognize the symptoms. But when my son started drinking all the time and losing weight, I thought it was just because of summer; and when he urinated it was just all the Cokes he was drinking. It didn't cross my mind that he had diabetes until he was really quite sick. Then it hit me."*

- *"I had a suspicion, since there is so much diabetes in my family. To tell the truth, I pretty much knew I had it, and told the doctor so."*

- *"It's strange, but when the doctor told me I had diabetes, I was actually relieved, because I was convinced I had cancer. I'd been losing weight for so long, feeling worse and worse. To my way of thinking, diabetes was a whole lot better than cancer."*

- *"Looking back, I'll bet I've had diabetes a long time. Sometimes when I'd go to the doctor, he would say something like, 'Your sugar's a little high' or 'You may have a touch of diabetes in your blood test.' But he never made much of it, and I felt pretty good, so I just forgot about it."*

As these statements illustrate, when a person first hears the diagnosis of diabetes, he or she may be devastated—or take it in stride. Some people ignore it altogether. For some people, however, the symptoms are impossible to ignore, which brings them to medical attention quickly. In other people the symptoms are mild or nonexistent, and these people may go years without even knowing they have the disease. In fact, about half of all the people with diabetes in America don't know that they have it.

Doctors may unintentionally encourage a person to deny the diabetes by using convenient phrases that minimize the problems—phrases like "a touch of sugar." We wish everyone would ask the doctor specifically, "Do you mean I have diabetes?" But, as is only natural, people usually don't want to hear the answer. Denial is a potent defense mechanism, and we've seen people deny their diabetes almost to the point of death.

A central theme of this book is that you can live a long and healthy life with diabetes, but it is a dangerous disease to ignore. The first step is to know whether you have diabetes, so that, if you do, you can begin taking care of it. In this chapter, we will emphasize that the diagnosis of diabetes can and should be clearly made: *either you have it or you don't.*

We've helped hundreds of people come to grips with the diagnosis of diabetes, and we have seen the shock that goes along with learning that diagnosis. So in this chapter we also consider how people cope personally when their diabetes is first discovered. Then we start the process of understanding what blood sugar values really mean and how they fluctuate in diabetes.

Diagnosing Diabetes

The name *diabetes mellitus* is a good description: the word *diabetes* comes from the Greek for "siphon." We recently saw a man who described such bad thirst and frequent urination that he would literally drink water while he urinated—as though he were, in fact, a siphon, the water just flowing in and flowing out. *Mellitus* is from the Latin for "sweet," referring to the sugar in the urine. (*Diabetes insipidus* is another disease altogether, characterized by excess urination but unrelated to blood sugar. It has nothing to do with diabetes mellitus, which is the subject of this book.)

Diabetes has many different causes and involves many different systems and organs in the body. But it is defined very specifically, and that definition depends on only one thing: high blood sugar.

The *blood sugar,* also called *blood glucose* or *plasma glucose,* refers to the amount, or concentration, of sugar in the blood. The units used in measuring the amount are milligrams per deciliter, or mg/dl; in most countries other than the United States, millimoles per liter, or mM, are used instead of mg/dl. (To convert mM to mg/dl, multiply the mM by 18; to convert from mg/dl to mM, divide by 18. For example, 100 mg/dl equals 5.5 mM.)

Everyone has some sugar in the blood, usually about 60–115 mg/dl in the person without diabetes. The brain needs glucose to function normally; this is why, when the sugar level in the blood drops too low *(hypoglycemia)*, a person's ability to reason is impaired and coma may even result. When the blood sugar is found to be too high *(hyperglycemia)*, the diagnosis of diabetes is made.

Usually, the diagnosis is obvious to doctors, because the symptoms are so characteristic. The most common (discussed more fully in Chapter 22) include excessive thirst, excessive urination, weight loss, persistent vaginal infections in women, and general fatigue. In the presence of these symptoms, the diagnosis of diabetes can be confirmed by a "random" test of blood sugar, meaning that the blood is drawn at any time during the day, rather than specifically before you eat breakfast. If the person is thirsty and urinating large amounts, the blood sugar will usually be well over 200 mg/dl, sometimes up in the 300s, 400s, or even higher.

Sometimes there are few or no symptoms, and the high blood sugar is found on a blood test done during a routine physical examination. In this case, the diagnosis can be tricky, and it is in this situation that people may not be told specifically that they have diabetes. So let's look more closely at the criteria for diagnosing diabetes when the classic symptoms aren't present and the random blood glucose isn't over 200.

First, a *fasting* blood glucose may be elevated. This means the blood glucose is drawn at least 10 hours after a meal, when it is usually at its lowest point in the day. In 1979, when an expert committee agreed upon the criteria for diagnosing diabetes, a fasting glucose (technically, plasma glucose measured twice) of 140 mg/dl or more made the diagnosis of diabetes. In June of 1997, this level was changed from the earlier criterion of 140 mg/dl down to the new criterion of 126 mg/dl.

If the random blood glucose isn't over 200 *and* the fasting glucose isn't over 126, then neither one confirms a diagnosis of diabetes. If there is a strong suspicion that you have diabetes or an important reason to screen for it (such as pregnancy), however, then an *oral glucose tolerance test,* or OGTT, can be done. In the nonpregnant person, the OGTT consists of taking a blood sample for fasting blood sugar level, having the person drink a measured amount of sugar (75 grams) as a very sweet drink, and testing blood sugar again, at least at 120 minutes later, sometimes with in-between samples drawn also. (The OGTT is done slightly differently in pregnancy.) According to World Health Organization criteria, diabetes is diagnosed if the value two hours after the oral glucose is over 200 mg/dl.

During pregnancy, diabetes is diagnosed by slightly different criteria (see

Table 1.   Blood Sugar Criteria for Diagnosing Diabetes Mellitus and Impaired Glucose Tolerance in Nonpregnant and Pregnant Adults

Diabetes mellitus in nonpregnant adults is defined as either:
> Random plasma glucose greater than or equal to 200 mg/dl with symptoms of hyperglycemia (thirst, excessive urination, weight loss)

or
> Fasting plasma glucose greater than or equal to 126 mg/dl at least twice[a]

or
> In a 75-gram oral glucose tolerance test, 2-hour plasma glucose greater than or equal to 200 mg/dl

Gestational diabetes mellitus is defined as:
In a 100-gram oral glucose tolerance test, 2 plasma glucose values greater than or equal to the following:

Fasting	105 mg/dl
1 hour	190 mg/dl
2 hours	165 mg/dl
3 hours	145 mg/dl

Impaired glucose tolerance in nonpregnant adults is defined as:
> Fasting plasma glucose less than 140 mg/dl

and
> In a 75-gram oral glucose tolerance test, 2-hour plasma glucose between 140 and 200 mg/dl

and
> At least 1 plasma glucose between 0 and 2 hours greater than or equal to 200 mg/dl

[a]This criterion for the diagnosis of diabetes was changed by the American Diabetes Association in June of 1997 so that a fasting plasma glucose of 126 mg/dl or greater, rather than the earlier level of 140 mg/dl or greater, will make the diagnosis.

Table 1 and Chapter 31), but it is especially important to know whether you do or do not have diabetes during pregnancy.

Often, there is confusion over whether *urine* testing can be used to diagnose diabetes, without testing the blood. While high blood sugar levels (over about 180 mg/dl) do ordinarily cause sugar to "spill over" into the urine, the presence of sugar in the urine is *not* by itself sufficient to diagnose diabetes. A blood sugar level must be obtained.

Using the specific blood sugar criteria, then, it is possible to say definitely whether you do or do not have diabetes. There are some levels of blood sugar, though, that are not quite high enough to be called diabetes but are not entirely normal, either. When the blood sugar level two hours after the oral glucose is between 140 and 200 mg/dl, for example, the condition is called impaired glucose tolerance (IGT). This is *not* diabetes, but it does indicate that there is an increased risk of getting diabetes at a later time.

We avoid using such terms as *borderline diabetes, a touch of diabetes, chemical diabetes,* or other phrases that beat around the bush. If a person actually does have diabetes, these terms tend to minimize it, to suggest that it really isn't very important. And if the person does *not* have diabetes—for instance, if the right diagnosis is really IGT—then the person should not be saddled with the label *diabetes,* since it may have a negative impact on health or life insurance availability, employment, and so on. Again, it's important to get the straight answer: do you or do you not have diabetes?

Another often asked question is whether a person who has diabetes at one time will *always* have diabetes. It's not so easy to answer this question. If normal blood sugar levels have resulted from an ongoing treatment, such as diet or pills, then the person still has diabetes, very well controlled by treatment. But in some people, weight loss will effectively "cure" the diabetes, at least for the time being. In others, completion of a pregnancy will "cure" it. But anyone who has a previous history of diabetes, even if they don't have it currently, is definitely at greater-than-normal risk of developing diabetes in the future.

Hearing the Diagnosis of Diabetes

The whole range of emotions may pour out when a person hears for the first time that he or she has diabetes. Fear, anger, and feelings of impotence or being out of control are common responses. Many people cry, others feel the emotional impact hours or even days later. Some people, though, seem almost unnaturally matter-of-fact, accepting the changes they will have to make without apparent concern. Emotional swings occur, even from hour to hour. What causes this spectrum of responses, and is there a "normal" or "abnormal" response?

We don't think that there is any one normal response. An emotional outburst is certainly the most common, as is overwhelming concern for how this new diagnosis will affect life and life expectancy. People do better if they feel support and sympathy both from their health care professionals and from their families. Reassurance is definitely helpful: there *are* effective treatments, you *can* control this very well, and in all likelihood you *will* lead a long and healthy life. There is no need to learn everything about diabetes or self-care in the first few days, although people often want to make a frantic run to the library, bookstore, or World Wide Web to learn all there is to know about diabetes immediately. There is time. Self-care can be learned gradually.

How you respond depends, first, on your own personality. If you are an unusually calm, easygoing person with lots of confidence in yourself, you are more likely to accept diabetes in a matter-of-fact way. People who are naturally nervous, or "hyper," will probably have to cope with a series of diabetes-related anxieties. If you tend to be depressed, this news may make things worse.

Some people feel so overwhelmed by the diagnosis of diabetes that they do become clinically depressed. It's important to recognize when a response goes beyond the bounds of normal, tipping over into frank depression. We talk about how to detect and deal with psychological problems in Chapter 18.

The state of your life generally is another strong influence on your emotional response to the diagnosis. If you have a steady job that you like, one that earns you a reasonable income, it obviously helps. If you are otherwise healthy, with no other serious medical conditions and few family problems, you will undoubtedly find that things go easier, since you'll have time to learn about your diabetes, and you'll have the support of family and friends.

We find that the most intensely negative emotional responses to the diagnosis usually pass within a few months, as people move through the period of crisis and adjust to daily life with diabetes, learning that they can in fact cope with it. But if you feel that you are suffering too much during this early adjustment period, get professional help. Not only will it make you feel better, but it may start you on the road to better self-care.

At least as worrisome to us as a highly emotional response is a response that in effect denies the diagnosis altogether. It's one thing to be stoic and another to pretend you don't have diabetes. We feel such sadness when we see people who have willfully avoided the diagnosis until they develop significant long-term complications.

Diabetes is an important illness that will affect your life. If not well cared for, it could shorten your life. There is no use denying these realities, or denying the diagnosis. But diabetes is also a disease that can be very well managed, and people often live to their full life expectancy with diabetes. It is something you can live with, something you can control.

As a start, you should begin to learn what blood sugar values really mean.

Blood Sugar Variations in Diabetes

Andy, who was diagnosed with diabetes not long ago, came to see us because he was worried by the fact that his blood sugar readings were never the same, even

when he tested at the same time of day. "One morning it's 90 and the next it's 105,"
he explained. "One evening after supper it's 110 and another it's 125. What am I
doing wrong?"

Sonia, who had had diabetes for more than 15 years, was also worried about blood
sugar variations. "I've been taking insulin for an awfully long time," she told us,
"but my blood sugars still don't always make sense. Okay, when I eat too much, it
goes high. But some days, it can be 300, and then I take some extra insulin, and in
almost no time at all it's 30. What's going on?"

Seeing your blood sugar levels bounce up and down in unpredictable
patterns can be one of the most frustrating things about having diabetes, especially when you are testing regularly and trying to do your best with your
diet and exercise patterns. It is one of the strains we put on ourselves by regular blood sugar testing, wanting to see how the glucose is doing. But if you
check your sugar regularly, you *will* see it bounce. The first thing to understand is that no one's blood sugar is constant. The human body isn't made
that way. And if the blood sugar readings are within normal limits—as is true
for Andy—then there's absolutely no need for anxiety.

What is a normal blood sugar concentration? This is a deceptively simple question, especially since many laboratory result sheets print out the
"normal values" for fasting blood glucose, usually about 70–115 mg/dl. Actually, the "normal" value is something like the "normal" speed of a car: it may
be 55 miles per hour on a freeway, but 10 miles per hour in rush hour traffic. Likewise, the blood sugar level varies depending on the exact situation.

When you haven't eaten for some time, say 8–12 hours, the normal
(without diabetes) "fasting" blood sugar is what the lab printout says: about
70–115 mg/dl. (The low side of this range is variable, and what's acceptable
here depends on the individual's situation: if the person is taking insulin, a
fasting blood sugar in the 60–70 mg/dl range may be too close to hypoglycemia; if the person is not taking insulin and is not bothered by symptoms
of being low, a fasting blood sugar in the 60s may be perfectly acceptable.)

After eating any meal that contains carbohydrate or protein, blood sugar normally rises, often to about 120–130 mg/dl, but generally not more than
140 mg/dl in the person without diabetes. Over two to four hours, blood sugar returns to baseline. Day in and day out, from hour to hour, the normal
blood sugar levels vary (Figure 1). If you chart blood sugar levels in a person
without diabetes, you won't get a flat line but rather a series of hills and val-

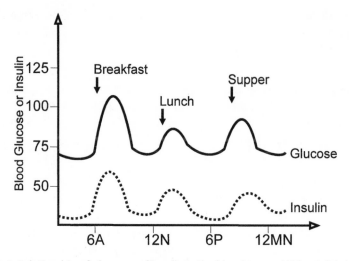

Figure 1. Relationship of glucose and insulin in the bloodstream. Without diabetes, the pancreas functions like a thermostat for the blood sugar. There are minor variations in levels, but overall blood sugar is kept within a tight range. When the blood sugar starts to go up with ingestion of a meal, the beta cells of the pancreas put out insulin, bringing the level of sugar down in the bloodstream. When the meal is complete, the beta cells put out just a little bit of insulin to take care of the sugar that the liver makes. The blood sugar is kept in the normal range: 70 to 115 mg/dl and less than about 140 mg/dl after a meal.

leys. And these are the variations that occur *without* diabetes; the swings are always much wider with diabetes.

To understand *how* and *why* blood sugar varies so much even in a person without diabetes, you have to understand something about insulin. Insulin is the wonderful hormone that comes out of the beta cells of the pancreas. Its purpose is to help the cells of the body *burn sugar* for energy. As the blood sugar rises after a meal, from the carbohydrate being absorbed, this triggers a release of insulin from the pancreatic beta cells. The insulin then opens the doors of the cells to glucose, allowing the sugar to leave the bloodstream and enter the cells, where it is used as fuel. (Figure 2 diagrams this process.) As the sugar enter the cells, the blood sugar level comes back to normal, and glucose is fuel for all the cell functions.

When there is relatively low blood sugar level, as happens before a meal, the beta cells are put at rest and insulin is not secreted. The cells turn to other sources of fuel they have kept in reserve, such as stored fat or carbohydrate.

In the person without diabetes, this is a finely tuned system: blood sugar is relatively low and beta cells are at rest overnight and before a meal, with

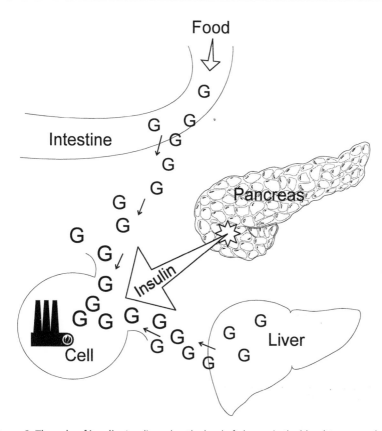

Figure 2. The role of insulin. Insulin makes the level of glucose in the bloodstream go down by allowing glucose to enter the cells of the body, serving as fuel for the cell. Insulin binds to a spot on the cell surface called a *receptor*. When this happens, glucose is able to pass through the cell membrane into the cell, where it is then used for energy. Some people liken this to a lock and key. Insulin is the key that opens up the lock (receptor) so that glucose can pass through the door into the cell. Using this analogy, in Type I diabetes, someone stole the keys (no insulin is made by the pancreas). In Type II, the door won't open fully even with the right key (insulin resistance).

the cells burning alternative fuels; as soon as the person eats, blood sugar levels rise, the beta cells wake up and make insulin, this insulin circulates and opens the cells up to glucose, and the cells use the available glucose as fuel, bringing the blood sugar level back to baseline.

The basic problem in diabetes is that not enough insulin is made by the pancreas. Sometimes the beta cells don't make any insulin at all, and the person has to take injections of insulin; sometimes the body is resistant to the insulin made, and the pancreas, try as it might, can't put out enough insulin.

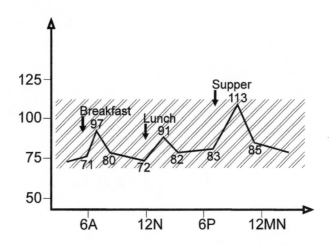

Figure 3a. No diabetes. The blood sugar level fluctuates, rising some after meals, but stays in the normal range, 70 to 140mg/dl, throughout the day. The average blood sugar in this case is 86 mg/dl.

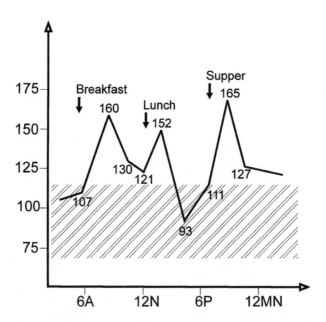

Figure 3b. Stable, well-controlled diabetes is characterized by mild variations in blood sugar levels, which remain in the normal range most of the time. The average blood sugar in this case is 129mg/dl.

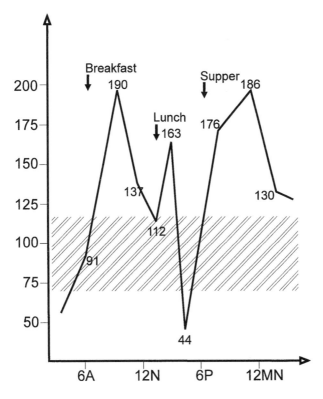

Figure 3c. Unstable, well-controlled diabetes is characterized by more abrupt changes in the blood sugar level throughout the day. At one minute it may be in the 200s and within the hour it may drop to 60. But the average is good in this case, at 136mg/dl.

In either case, if there is not enough insulin made, the blood sugar has a strong tendency to rise, since it is not exiting the bloodstream to enter the cells as fuel.

How much, and how quickly, do blood sugars rise and fall in a person with diabetes? This is an unanswerable question. There is just too much variability from person to person, from day to day. But let's discuss some generalizations, which are diagrammed in Figure 3. To begin with (Figure 3a), if you don't have diabetes, blood sugar level will start the day below about 115 mg/dl and will not rise above about 140 mg/dl. How high the level goes after each meal, and how soon it returns to baseline, depends largely on what the meal contains.

Figure 3b shows the pattern that might be seen in someone with "stable" diabetes well controlled. This could be a person with diabetes that is mild

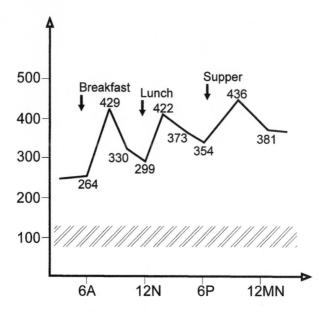

Figure 3d. Stable uncontrolled diabetes is characterized by persistently high blood sugars. They don't fluctuate much, but just stay high—in this case, 365mg/dl.

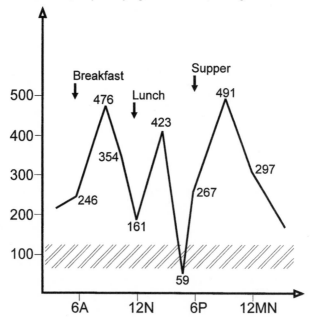

Figure 3e. Unstable uncontrolled diabetes is characterized by blood sugars that fluctuate wildly, and are, on average, high. In this case the average blood sugar is 275mg/dl.

(the person makes almost, but not quite, enough insulin). You can see that the blood sugar tends to start higher than normal and rises somewhat higher after meals, returning to normal more slowly. It is less finely tuned than normal, and on average it is higher.

When you look at the pattern labeled "unstable" diabetes (Figure 3c), you see the kind of fluctuations that made Sonia throw up her hands in despair. Even though on average it is well controlled, there are times in the day when the blood sugar is actually over 300. Sonia also feels the effects of a definite low just before supper. This is frustrating, to say the least. And the pattern she had today may not be much like the pattern she had yesterday or will have tomorrow. But there are reasons for the rises and falls, and if these reasons are understood, the peaks and valleys may be smoothed out. Much of this book will be devoted to helping people smooth out their blood sugar control. On a positive note, while Sonia's blood sugar was bouncing from low to high and back again, the average throughout the 24-hour period was actually not bad at all. This person has good average blood glucose levels, unstable as the sugars are hour to hour. She may have difficulty dealing with the highs and lows, but she is doing a good job of reducing her risk of long-term complications.

Finally, Figure 3, d–e, illustrates "uncontrolled" diabetes. In uncontrolled diabetes the blood sugar level starts high, goes higher, and stays high. The average for this person is 305 mg/dl. She is undoubtedly feeling the symptoms of uncontrolled diabetes: she is thirsty, urinating all the time, has blurred vision, and is generally without energy. What's more, if these levels continue year in and year out, she is very likely to develop serious complications from diabetes. The difference between Figure 3d and Figure 3e is that in Figure 3d the blood sugar is high but stable, not varying much, while in Figure 3e it is high and unstable, crashing up and down. This degree of uncontrolled diabetes is not rare: in fact, many people used to live for decades with average blood sugars over 200–300 mg/dl. On the whole, these are the people who suffered the worst complications of diabetes.

Few tools were available in the old days to help people control their blood sugar. Fortunately, it doesn't have to be that way any longer. Diabetes is definitely controllable. In this book we'll help you learn how to do it and give you lots of good reasons for following our—and your own doctor's—advice.

Chapter 2

Types of Diabetes

- *"I used to be controlled with diet, and then pills. But now I take insulin, because my sugar went way up. Why do they still say I have non–insulin-dependent diabetes when I definitely need insulin?"*

- *"People talk about types of diabetes. I'm not sure what type I am. When I talk to doctors, I don't get a straight answer, and I don't see why it matters, anyway."*

It is usually easy to diagnose diabetes, but deciding what *type* of diabetes you have can be confusing to doctors and patients alike. As we will discuss, even the names used for the two most common types of diabetes are misleading. Some people just don't fit neatly into the diagnostic "boxes." Whatever the reasons, patients, and often their health care professionals, are confused.

In this chapter, we will look at the different kinds of diabetes. We will discuss the rationale behind the formal names, as well as the practical implications of the different types. At the Johns Hopkins Medical School, we show second-year medical students a simple diagram that includes some very complicated theories and debates about diabetes (Figure 4). The diagram considers diabetes one disease, defined by high blood glucose (hyperglycemia), with many different primary causes, all leading to an inadequate amount of insulin from the pancreas. The hyperglycemia causes acute (immediate) complications and also long-term complications (these complications are the subject of Part IV).

Figure 4 is an oversimplification, because in reality there are different types of diabetes, and they behave differently in important ways. But diabetes of any type, whatever the cause, may produce any and all of the symptoms or complications. Thirst, fatigue, weight loss, and frequent urination, for example, occur whenever the blood sugar is elevated above about 200 mg/dl, regardless of what kind of diabetes the person has. Complications in-

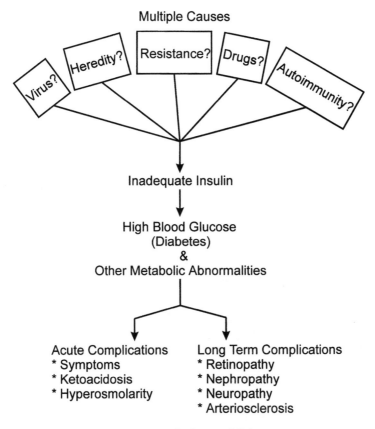

Figure 4. Overall schema of diabetes.

volving the eyes, kidneys, and nerves have also been found in all kinds of diabetes.

As you will see, the basic distinction made between Type I and Type II diabetes is that people with Type I diabetes do get ketoacidosis. But even this does not always hold. Many people with Type I diabetes, adequately treated, have never had ketoacidosis, and some people with Type II diabetes do develop ketoacidosis, especially if they are under severe stress.

The Classification System

In thinking about the kinds of diabetes, you should distinguish four general types:

—*Type I diabetes* is due to the complete or almost complete destruction of the pancreatic beta cells (the cells that make insulin) by immune mechanisms.

—*Type II diabetes* is due to the body not responding so well to the insulin made by the pancreas.

—*Other types of diabetes* include those kinds of diabetes with relatively well-known causes.

—*Gestational diabetes mellitus (GDM)* is the form of diabetes that first appears in pregnancy.

It is worth emphasizing that such other diagnoses as impaired glucose tolerance (IGT), borderline results, and previous history of diabetes mellitus do not mean that the person has diabetes. As mentioned in Chapter 1, these terms refer to conditions that put a person at *increased risk* of developing diabetes, though that person does not yet have diabetes.

What difference does it make what kind of diabetes you have? A major difference is how each kind of diabetes is treated:

—*Type I diabetes* will need insulin right away.

—*Type II diabetes* may not need insulin or pills until weight control is given a good try.

—*Other types of diabetes* may be helped by treating their underlying cause.

—*Gestational diabetes* must be treated aggressively with diet and then insulin in order to give the developing fetus every chance.

An accurate diagnosis does matter. There are differences in the approach to treatment, which we'll discuss in more detail later. First, let's look more closely at the different types of diabetes.

Type I Diabetes

- *"We were flabbergasted! There was no diabetes on either side of his family, he was a perfectly healthy kid, when all of a sudden he began to lose weight, was thirsty all the time, and spent half the night urinating. Once he started to take insulin, though, he settled right down, and it has been very easy to keep his sugars normal for three months now."*

Type I, or insulin-dependent, diabetes was previously called *juvenile onset diabetes*. It is the kind of diabetes that comes on in younger people, with onset most often in childhood but extending up to about 30 years old or even older. It occurs in people who are usually of normal weight or thin, and everyone with this type of diabetes must be treated with insulin. If you have diabetes and you fit these characteristics, the chances are that you have Type I diabetes. Most people can determine for themselves whether they have Type I diabetes by looking at the typical features of Type I diabetes listed in Table 2.

The beta cells in the pancreas are the only cells of the body that produce insulin, and in Type I diabetes they are destroyed. The beta cells are located in the islets of Langerhans, first discovered in 1869 by Paul Langerhans. Cells in the islets of Langerhans make several other hormones as well, and they are located among the acinar cells of the pancreas, which make digestive enzymes.

In 1901 a Johns Hopkins pathologist, Eugene Opie, was the first to discover the key point that beta cells produce an internal secretion needed to avoid diabetes. He noted that if the pancreatic beta cells were gone, the person had diabetes. Twenty years after that, Drs. Banting, Macleod, Best, and Collip, working in Toronto, successfully extracted the substance that those beta cells contain—insulin—and gave it to people with Type I diabetes. A marvelous account of this epic discovery, summarized in Chapter 12, can be found in the book *The Discovery of Insulin* by Michael Bliss (University of Chicago Press, 1982). The book was dramatized on television by the Public Broadcasting System in 1993.

In a person with Type I diabetes, the beta cells of the pancreas are destroyed by autoimmune processes, so virtually no insulin is produced. (The autoimmune process is discussed more fully later in this chapter.) When no insulin is produced in the pancreas, a person must be given insulin by injection. This is why Type I diabetes is called "insulin dependent": there is an absolute requirement, or dependence, on insulin treatment. In the absence of insulin treatment, or when far too little insulin is given, the result is diabetic ketoacidosis (Chapter 23).

The formal definition of Type I diabetes, then, is that form of diabetes which, in the absence of insulin treatment, causes ketoacidosis and ultimately death. Today, Type I diabetes is entirely treatable, and ketoacidosis is preventable by taking the right amount of insulin.

Since there is no insulin coming from the pancreas, a person with Type I diabetes will have *labile* blood sugars, meaning that the blood glucose will

Table 2.   Typical Features of Type I Diabetes

	Typical Features of Type I Diabetes	Comments
Age of onset	Under 40 years old, most common in childhood	Not always: some older people develop Type I.
Body weight	Thin to normal weight	
Presentation	Relatively quick onset, with symptoms developing and worsening over weeks to months	Thirst, frequent urination, and weight loss may progress to ketoacidosis.
Family History	Usually no known history of Type I diabetes in family	Unusually, there may be Type I diabetes in the family.
Risk factors	No major risk factors for Type I diabetes. Some protective factors such as African American ethnicity.	Risk is increased if strong family history of Type I diabetes, and mildly increased with a single family member having Type I diabetes. Eating sugar does not cause Type I diabetes
Insulin treatment	Always needed to control the diabetes and prevent keto-acidosis. Usually needs more than 1 shot a day.	Diabetes does not respond to pills for more than a year or so.
Blood sugar control	Up and down, hard to keep in ideal range	Blood sugar is very sensitive to small changes in diet, exercise, and insulin dose. Frustrating!
Honeymoon period	Usually starting within a few months of onset, a time when the diabetes is more stable, easier to control	Usually lasts 3–12 months
Laboratory tests	Blood sugar high, usually over 200 mg/dl if thirsty. Glyco-hemoglobin ususally high. Islet cell antibodies and/or GAD antibodies and/or insulin autoantibodies present about 80%–90% of people at time of diagnosis.	The antibody tests may be done at the onset of diabetes if there is doubt as to whether it is Type I or Type II. A positive result confirms Type I.

(continued)

Table 2.   *(continued)*

	Typical Features of Type I Diabetes	Comments
Cause	A combination of heredity and exposure to some factor during life triggers an auto-immune destruction of the insulin-producing beta cells in the pancreas.	Details of both the hereditary factor and the environmental factor are not well understood.

tend to shoot up and crash down. (See Figures 3C and 3E.) *Brittle diabetes* is another term used to describe the same thing—the blood sugar bouncing up and down. Sometimes people are diagnosed as having brittle diabetes, as though it were a specific, different kind of diabetes. We think, rather, that la-bility, or "brittleness," is a spectrum. Even people on the far end of this spec-trum, with very unstable blood sugars, can be reasonably well controlled by careful attention to the details of self-management. So we prefer not to con-sider brittle diabetes as a different form of diabetes.

To understand what causes lability, consider the following metaphor. A thermostat turns the furnace on or off depending on just what the room's tem-perature is, whether too warm or too cold. But if you're using a woodstove to heat the room, you don't have the benefit of a thermostat, and you have to guess how much wood to put in the stove each morning. Unless you guess very well every time, the room may well be too hot or too cold. The healthy pancreas op-erates under thermostatic control, sensing just when the blood sugar goes up and putting out just the right amount of insulin to bring it back to normal. In-sulin injections are more like stoking the stove with wood—you have to make your best guess about how much you will need as the day progresses.

The normally functioning pancreatic beta cell does its job with great pre-cision, secreting just the right amount of insulin to keep the blood sugar in the normal range, no matter the diet, the exercise, or the stress level. Insulin by injection rarely achieves this precision, even with the best intentions. (In-sulin pumps, discussed later, also lack the feedback control of a normal pan-creas, because "glucose sensors" are not yet available. When glucose sensors are developed, pumps will work by automatically adjusting the insulin flow to the body's need.) Lacking the natural feedback control of a normal pan-creas, the person with Type I diabetes is always struggling to estimate how much insulin to take and how much to eat, and to factor in exercise and stress as well. Treatment is difficult and imprecise. As the person with Type I diabetes knows, the great and wonderful discovery of insulin was not in fact a cure for diabetes.

What Causes Type I Diabetes?

This common question is very hard to answer. We do know certain things:

> —Insulin-dependent diabetes mellitus occurs in people with a genetic susceptibility, even when (as is usually the case) there is no known family history of Type I diabetes.
> —It requires exposure to something in the "environment," so it is not entirely hereditary.
> —Most important, it is an autoimmune disease.

Each of these facts requires further discussion, and each can be hard to comprehend fully, mainly because a lot more research will be necessary before we really understand the causes of Type I diabetes.

Consider, first, the hereditary factor. The best way to find out if heredity is involved in a disease is to see if the disease tends to run in families. The final proof is to see the disease occurring more often in identical twins than in nonidentical twins. If the condition were 100 percent genetic, then if one identical twin had Type I diabetes, the other, having exactly the same genes, would have it, too. Studies show that, indeed, the "concordance rate" in identical twins is high: in about 35% of identical twin pairs, where one twin has diabetes, the other twin does, too. But it is not 100%, so Type I diabetes is not entirely genetic.

It is unusual for several people in the same family to have Type I diabetes, but most people who have a child with Type I diabetes in the family want to know what the chance is that another child will get it. Table 3 provides the best available figures. Blood tests for autoimmunity, including islet cell antibodies (see below), can be run on first-degree relatives of people with Type I diabetes, to see if any of the relatives show evidence of damage occurring to their islet cells and therefore are likely to develop Type I diabetes.

A national study is under way to determine whether it's possible to prevent progressive damage of the islet cells once it has started (Chapter 33). People wanting to have the islet cell antibody test done (for instance, in brothers and sisters of a child with diabetes) must understand that there is at present no known way to prevent the development of Type I diabetes if these tests

Table 3. Risk of Developing Type I Diabetes If a Relative Has Type I Diabetes

	Risk of Type I Diabetes	Comments
Entire U.S. population	<0.2%	Lower in African Americans, higher in Scandinavians
Type I diabetes in second or third degree relative	<1%	Grandparent, cousin
Type I diabetes in mother	2% to 3%	Risk is higher if mother developed diabetes before the age of 11
Type 1 diabetes in father	6%	Risk is higher if father developed diabetes before the age of 11
Type I diabetes in one sibling	3% to 15%	Most studies find 3% to 10%
Type I diabetes in identical twin	35% to 50%	Risk in non-identical twin equals that of having one non-twin sibling with Type I

NOTE: These figures represent a range of figures drawn from various studies, with factors such as age and ethnic heritage factored out. The exact numbers vary from study to study.

are positive. This may be information that will worry you without giving you any way to affect the outcome On the other hand, if the tests are negative, you may be able to relax a little.

Another way of looking at the identical twin data—a perspective that concentrates on the good news—is that even with exactly the same genes, less than half of the unaffected twins ever get Type I diabetes. This suggests that something in the environment plays a role. It isn't all in the genes. Precious little is known about just what this factor really is, what a susceptible person is exposed to that sets off the reaction that causes beta cell damage and eventually diabetes. It may be a virus, although exposure to any particular virus has not been regularly found in people with Type I diabetes. It could be a toxin of some sort in the diet or in the air. There is no evidence that emotion or stress causes Type I diabetes, or that it is caused by excess sugar intake. The fact is, we just don't know what triggers Type I diabetes in the susceptible person.

Somewhat more is known now about what happens once the genetic predisposition and the environmental factor are established. The path to Type I diabetes is an *autoimmune* destruction of the pancreatic beta cells. This means that the body's immune system, which is responsible for recognizing and destroying outside invaders such as viruses or bacteria, begins to think that its own pancreatic beta cells are "foreign" and sets off a response that ends up destroying them. This destructive process is detected by a laboratory test known as the *islet cell antibody test*. The antibody measured, and several more like it, may in fact be either the cause or the result of the autoimmune process going on in the pancreas—we don't know which. But either way, a positive test is evidence of the autoimmune process and developing Type I diabetes.

The positive islet cell antibody test, which is evidence that beta cells are being destroyed in this way, shows up several years before Type I diabetes does. This means that the problem is developing for quite some time, not just over the few weeks the person has symptoms of diabetes. While the stress of a recent virus or cold may bring out Type I diabetes for the first time, it is not the *cause* of Type I diabetes. If the person had been tested before the virus or cold, the test results would have been positive for islet cell antibodies.

Another typical feature of Type I diabetes is the "honeymoon period." Just after coming down with Type I diabetes, the pancreas seems to recoup, and the person may be very stable or even not require insulin at all for a period of a few months to a year. Both the early phase of Type I diabetes, when the islet cell antibody tests are positive but diabetes has not actually developed, and the "honeymoon" period provide "windows of opportunity" in which, if we could safely interrupt the autoimmune process, we might save enough beta cells for the pancreas to deliver adequate amounts of insulin. In other words, if the procress that is destroying beta cells can be headed off, we might prevent the appearance of Type I diabetes altogether. Research is focusing on these time frames, as Type I diabetes is destroying beta cells.

Type II Diabetes

- *"My feet were becoming more and more numb, and I was having real problems with sexual activity—I just couldn't hold an erection. I attributed it to age, but then my doctor told me, 'It's your diabetes.' Well, to be perfectly honest, I didn't even know I had diabetes. He may have said something about a little sugar, but it had never sunk in. This was the first time I really heard that I had diabetes."*

Type II or non–insulin-dependent diabetes, previously called *adult onset diabetes* or *maturity onset diabetes,* is very different from Type I diabetes, even though it is capable of causing all the symptoms and all the complications found in any other form of diabetes. The typical features are presented in Table 4.

To begin with, Type II diabetes is much more common than Type I: over 90% of all diabetes is Type II, while less than 10% is Type I diabetes. Type II diabetes usually comes on in people over 40 years old, is much more common in overweight people, and is influenced more by heredity than Type I diabetes. Certain groups, such as African Americans, Hispanics, and, particularly, Native Americans have especially high rates of Type II. The best predictor of the frequency of Type II in a given population, however, is obesity.

The typical person with Type II, then, is older, overweight, with a strong family history of diabetes. Unlike Type I diabetes, which usually shows up abruptly (even though, as discussed, it has been developing for several years), the high blood sugar in Type II diabetes may develop very slowly, over many years. It is usually virtually impossible to discover exactly when the diabetes began. This is why we made such a point in Chapter 1 of the fact that exact criteria do exist to determine whether or not a person has Type II diabetes. We believe that a person should not be followed for years with a vague diagnosis—a "touch of sugar" or "just a little diabetes." With its gradual onset, Type II diabetes can be easily ignored or minimized. But to do so is dangerous, since serious long-term complications can occur before people are even aware that they have diabetes.

For many, many years the name *non–insulin-dependent diabetes* has been synonymous with Type II diabetes, but it is a confusing name for the simple reason that as many as 30% of people with Type II, "non–insulin-dependent" diabetes, actually *do* take insulin. Does taking insulin transform the person who previously had Type II diabetes into a person with Type I diabetes? Absolutely not. (We wish we could get this fine point across to most students and practitioners of medicine!) We have already mentioned some features that make Type II diabetes a fundamentally different disease from Type I diabetes, and we will mention more below. Just remember that many people with non–insulin-dependent diabetes do in fact take insulin.

The formal definition of Type II diabetes is that form of diabetes which does not require insulin treatment to avoid ketoacidosis. Except under unusual stress, the person with Type II diabetes should not get ketoacidosis even when a needed insulin treatment is withdrawn. The reason for this is really quite simple and basic to Type II diabetes: the pancreas of the person with Type II diabetes

Table 4.   Typical Features of Type II Diabetes

	Typical Features of Type II Diabetes	Comments
Age of onset	Over 40 years old, most common in older adults	Not always: some younger people develop Type II, particularly a hereditary form called MODY (maturity onset diabetes of the young)
Body weight	Overweight	Occasionally occurs in normal-weight people
Presentation	Usually slow onset, with symptoms developing over months to many years	Thirst, frequent urination, and weight loss may not be noticed. This can be a "silent disease."
Family History	Usually Type II diabetes in the family	
Risk factors	Clear, well-defined risk factors that put people at increased risk of Type II diabetes	Risk is increased if you have a history of diabetes during pregnancy, are overweight, have a strong family history of Type II diabetes, or are of Native American, African American, Hispanic, or Japanese American descent.
Insulin treatment	Often needed to control the blood sugar	Treatment usually starts with diet and exercise, progressing if needed to pills and later to insulin.
Blood sugar control	Usually easier to control, without the ups and downs found in Type I diabetes	Blood sugar may get very high and lows are also seen. But there are fewer peaks and valleys than in Type I diabetes.
Honeymoon period	Not seen in Type II diabetes	
Laboratory tests	Blood sugar may be very high, but is typically only mildly to moderately elevated. Glyco-	The antibody test may be done at the onset of diabetes if there is doubt

(*continued*)

Table 4. *(continued)*

	Typical Features of Type II Diabetes	Comments
	hemoglobin mildly or moderately elevated. Islet cell antibodies, GAD antibodies, and insulin autoantibodies.	as to whether it is Type I or Type II. A positive result confirms Type I.
Cause	A poorly understood combination of heredity, insulin resistance, and deficiency of the insulin-producing beta cells of the pancreas.	Not due to autoimmunity

does make some insulin, just not enough. With even a small amount of insulin, the uncontrolled breakdown of fat that causes ketoacidosis (see Chapter 23) is restrained. And, most important, the edge is taken off the rises and falls of blood sugar.

Relative stability, then, is a feature of Type II diabetes. Whatever amount of insulin is secreted by the pancreas comes out at just the right time, when the blood sugar rises, and stops at the right time, when the blood sugar falls. This normal pancreatic insulin secretion is a big advantage, providing some underlying stability to blood sugar levels, even if they are persistently too high (as in Figure 3D).

Finally, although any of the long-term complications can occur in Type II diabetes, the frequency of specific complications is quite different from that in Type I diabetes (these are discussed in more detail in Part IV). Such complications as circulatory problems, stroke, heart attacks, and hypertension are more common in Type II diabetes than in Type I. Presumably, the reason for this is simply the age factor: people in their 60s, 70s, and 80s are much more prone to hardening of the arteries than people in their teens, 20s, and 30s. (As noted, Type II diabetes usually begins in people older than 40.) The importance of this is that special attention has to be paid to preventing hardening of the arteries in people with Type II diabetes.

What Causes Type II Diabetes?

As with Type I diabetes, our understanding of what causes Type II diabetes is far from complete. We know certain facts, some already mentioned:

—Type II diabetes runs in families and certain ethnic groups.
—It occurs far more often in people who are overweight.
—The pancreas does make some insulin, although not enough.
—The cells of the body are resistant (respond less well) to insulin.

Discussion of these basic facts about Type II diabetes provides some insight.

The genetic influence in Type II diabetes is much stronger than in Type I diabetes. Returning to the identical twin model used above, we find that at least 90% of identical twins will both have Type II diabetes if one has it. The family history of people with Type II diabetes is routinely positive for Type II diabetes in other members of the family. Table 5 gives some numbers indicating the risk of other family members developing Type II diabetes when one person already has it. This strongly hereditary nature of Type II diabetes is partly but not wholly explained by inheritance of obesity. It is best illustrated in the greatly increased risk that specific ethnic groups have, regardless of body weight.

The importance of obesity as a cause of Type II diabetes, though, cannot be overemphasized. Although we don't know why, it is clear that the muscle cells of obese people (where most of the sugar breakdown occurs) are far less responsive to insulin than are the muscle cells of thinner people. This condition, called *insulin resistance,* means that a unit of insulin has less effect in lowering blood sugar. Consider the case of Anne.

> *When Anne was 35, she was of normal weight, nondiabetic, and her pancreas could put out 30 units of insulin a day, enough to do the job. With her last pregnancy, she had mild diabetes, but it went away entirely after the delivery. At 50, though, she became overweight and became resistant to her own insulin. Now the same 30 units of insulin that her pancreas could put out was not enough. To overcome her own resistance to insulin, she would have to make closer to 50 units of insulin, and her pancreas was not up to the challenge, so Anne developed diabetes. The obesity had caused insulin resistance, and had increased the demands on the pancreas, asking it to produce more insulin than it could.*

Put yet another way, if a person is obese, his or her pancreas has to put out heroic amounts of insulin to keep blood sugars normal. (The obese person without diabetes has a strong pancreas indeed.) So if the pancreas is in any way limited, if it is not able to make this large amount of insulin, then diabetes occurs when the person becomes obese. The good news is that if some

Table 5.   Risk of Developing Type II Diabetes If a Relative Has Type II Diabetes

	Risk of Type II Diabetes	Comments
Entire U.S. population	<6%	3% diagnosed, 3% undi-agnosed; higher in Native Americans, African Americans, Hispanics
Type II diabetes in father *or* mother	4% to 7%	Higher if mother has diabetes than if father has diabetes
Type II diabetes in father *and* mother	12%	
Type II diabetes in one sibling	13%	
Type II diabetes in identical twin	up to 90%	Risk in non-identical twin equals that of having one non-twin sibling with Type II

NOTE: These figures represent a range of figures drawn from various studies, with factors such as age, body weight, gender, and ethnic heritage factored out. The exact numbers vary from study to study.

of that weight is lost, the insulin output of the pancreas may very well be sufficient, and the person may no longer have diabetes.

There are many other causes of insulin resistance, some mentioned above, under the discussion of other types of diabetes. Perhaps the most common (other than obesity) is pregnancy. The insulin resistance caused by placental hormones gives rise to gestational diabetes when the woman's pancreas is unable to produce enough insulin to overcome this resistance (see below).

In addition to insulin resistance at the cellular level, some limitation of insulin secretion also occurs in Type II diabetes. The debate continues as to which comes first, the pancreatic problem or the resistance problem.

When People Don't Fit Neatly into Type I or Type II

- *"I'm 35 years old and recently got diabetes. I am mildly overweight, and am responding so far to diet and exercise, although my blood sugar is beginning to creep up. I have one grandparent who may have had diabetes. Do I have Type II diabetes or Type I diabetes, and how do you know?"*

It would be nice if every person with diabetes were easily and obviously classifiable, but this is not the case. Some people, like this one, seem to be in between. We cannot, of course, just stop treatment to see if the person develops diabetic ketoacidosis in order to make the "gold standard" diagnosis (ketoacidosis = Type I diabetes, no ketoacidosis = Type II diabetes.) But considering the case of the person quoted above can be valuable in sorting out the most important distinctions between Type I diabetes and Type II diabetes.

It is clear, for instance, that the age criterion is not very reliable. There are some definite exceptions to the general rule that diabetes occuring in the young is Type I and diabetes occuring in older people is Type II. There is a form of diabetes called maturity onset diabetes of the young (MODY), for example, that comes on during the teenage years but is not Type I diabetes. MODY is seen more often in African Americans and is now known to be due to a specific genetic defect which is unrelated to Type I diabetes. Likewise, we are increasingly aware that, when older people get diabetes, it is not always Type II. Even in the elderly, Type I diabetes, with autoimmune destruction of the pancreas, can occur. So age alone is not a reliable way to distinguish Type I diabetes from Type II diabetes, and the older terms "juvenile onset" and "adult onset" are better left in the archives.

We have emphasized that taking insulin does not mean you have Type I diabetes. Even obesity, so characteristic of Type II diabetes, is not a sure diagnostic sign of Type II diabetes. There is nothing to say that a person with Type I diabetes can't become overweight, and some people with Type II diabetes have normal body weight.

One of the most reliable indicators of Type II diabetes, as we have pointed out, is relatively stable blood sugars. This gets at the fundamental difference between Type II diabetes and Type I diabetes, which is at the level of the pancreas: people with Type I diabetes are not making any insulin, while those with Type II diabetes are. The pancreatic insulin, secreted at just the right time, produces more stability in blood sugars of people with Type II diabetes. If it is necessary to determine whether someone is making insulin, pancreatic insulin can be measured in the blood directly, either by testing the insulin level if the person is not taking insulin by injection or by testing a substance called C-peptide in the blood if the person is taking insulin. In practice, we don't use these tests very often, since the "honeymoon period" of Type I diabetes can confuse the issue, and the test results usually do not affect our initial management of diabetes.

Early in the course of diabetes, the best way to distinguish Type I from Type II diabetes is probably to look for islet cell antibodies in the blood as the indication of Type I diabetes. But at least 20% of people with Type I diabetes do not have positive islet cell antibodies at the time of diagnosis, so a negative test is not as helpful as a positive test in making this distinction.

So there are some people in whom, at the start, we can't make a definite diagnosis of Type I or Type II diabetes. But if we wait several years, beyond any "honeymoon period," it usually becomes clearer: the blood glucose is either quite stable (Type II diabetes) or quite labile (Type I diabetes), and the person either will respond well to diet and pills (Type II diabetes) or, within a year or so, will clearly need insulin (Type I diabetes).

Gestational Diabetes Mellitus

- *"Diabetes came on toward the end of my pregnancy. The doctors seemed very concerned, but after I delivered a healthy little girl, it just went away altogether."*

Diabetes during pregnancy is so important that it is discussed in a chapter of its own (Chapter 31). Here we will just say, first, that gestational diabetes mellitus (GDM) refers to new diabetes discovered first during pregnancy (as opposed to established diabetes in a woman who then becomes pregnant). It is so important to diagnose and treat GDM properly because if the disease is left untreated, the pregnancy is at greatly increased risk of ending unsuccessfully.

Gestational diabetes signals that a person has a relatively weak pancreas, with a high chance of developing permanent diabetes later. The woman with a perfectly normal pancreas overcomes the stress of pregnancy and does not develop diabetes. The woman with a borderline pancreas, on the other hand, develops diabetes during pregnancy.

Other Types of Diabetes

- *"I had diabetes in my family but never had it myself until I started using the diuretics called thiazides for high blood pressure. Was there any relationship?"*

The answer is yes. Thiazides are a classic cause of increased blood sugar, and therefore thiazide-induced diabetes is a classic form of "other diabetes" with known cause. In fact, all the "other types" of diabetes are those in which the cause is known. If the entire pancreas is surgically removed because of a serious abdominal injury, that person will have diabetes, since there is no other organ that can make insulin. Severe chronic pancreatitis (in which the pancreas is persistently inflamed, causing chronic pain), unusual tumors, or a disease of overabsorption of iron called hemochromatosis can also damage the pancreas to the point that it cannot make insulin.

More examples of other types of diabetes include diabetes brought about by drugs such as steroids (for example, prednisone taken for poison ivy or severe arthritis), or the above-mentioned thiazide diuretics, such as hydrochlorthiazide, mentioned above. In these cases it is more a question of the drug bringing out diabetes, since the person probably would not have developed it from taking thiazides or steroids if he or she did not have an underlying predisposition to diabetes.

Finally, there are some very uncommon diseases, such as Cushing's syndrome and acromegaly, that cause diabetes by counteracting insulin's effect. There are also some rare causes, such as hereditary conditions in which all the cells of the body lack receptors to insulin. This is like having the door key (insulin) but not having the lock (the receptor).

There are several different "types" of diabetes, some with a relatively well-defined cause, called other types, and then the two major types, with less well understood cause, called Type I (insulin-dependent diabetes mellitus) and Type II (non–insulin-dependent diabetes mellitus). Type I diabetes involves autoimmune destruction of the pancreatic beta cells, making the person dependent on insulin for life; people with Type II diabetes have some ability to make their own insulin but are resistant to it and do not make enough. Most of the differences in symptoms, in treatment, and in implications between Type II and Type I diabetes derive from these underlying differences. As we improve our understanding of the basic problems through medical research, we will be in a position to treat people better and, ultimately, to prevent and cure these two forms of diabetes.

Part II

Controlling Diabetes

It's all a balancing act. You don't want the blood sugar to go too high and you can't let it get too low. You don't want to eat too much or too little. Every medication you take must be in the right dose, not underdosed or overdosed.

To be successful in this balancing act requires a pretty good understanding of what you're doing. We'd be the first to agree that knowledge isn't everything, but you wouldn't get behind the wheel of a car without knowing the brake from the accelerator. Likewise, you can't take good care of your diabetes if you don't have a clue how you feel when your blood sugar is high or low, you don't know what the pills or insulin do, or you wouldn't know a carbohydrate if it jumped off the plate at you.

In fact, there are some fine points to managing your diabetes, things you may not have thought much about. Part II goes through all the important information you might need to take care of your diabetes. Some of it may be too basic for you, some may not be relevant to you. But the information is there, simply stated. If you pick up only a few pointers that make a difference for you, then it's all worthwhile. So use what you can, and come back for more later.

Being successful in the balancing act of self-care, in the long run, allows you to live a full and healthy life with diabetes. It does not mean perfection, especially if that perfection comes at the cost of being obsessed with your diabetes. Remember that you control your diabetes, it does not control you.

Chapter 3

Goals of Treatment and How to Reach Them

- *"What should my blood sugar be?"*
- *"I thought normal was 70 to 115, but my doctor says 150 is okay."*
- *"I just want to be healthy so I can see my grandchildren grow up."*
- *"I'm going to jog at the mall. Fifty minutes, seven mornings a week. I swear I am!"*

A goal is where you would like to be—a destination, an objective. Reaching the goal implies planning and action: you have to set it, and then you have to act to get there. If the goal is unrealistic (like the person who swears he'll jog in the mall every day), there are problems at the start. If it's not your goal but someone else's imposed on you, there is also trouble.

We talk a lot about goals in our diabetes management program at Johns Hopkins, and all kinds of specific ideas come up: some people want to avoid potato chips, some want to give up smoking, others seek to improve their cholesterol levels, and still others just want to stay healthy. Goals may range from the very specific to the very general.

We find it helpful to think of four broad categories of goals:

—Goals that deal generally with your quality of life
—Goals that deal with particular aspects of your health
—Specific blood sugar goals
—Goals that relate to your own self-care in action

Quality of Life

We're willing to bet that you'd prefer to live a long and healthy life. You want to have a good quality of life. That is about as general a goal as you can imagine, but it also may be the worthiest goal of all. And it *is* entirely possible with diabetes. But there are sure to be some differences between your life with diabetes and the life you would lead without it. There are adjustments and sacrifices you make because of your diabetes. We want to put these adjustments in perspective.

As you think about life with diabetes, you may want to reconsider what you think of as the good life. You may be used to thinking that the best thing in life is relaxing in front of the television, drinking beer and eating fast food. You may have defined quality of life in terms of how little physical exertion you could get away with or how quickly you could roll out of bed and into the car to get to work. You may have lived, to put it bluntly, the most unhealthy of lifestyles.

Let's talk about adjusting those notions of the good life. You might find that you have fun getting out and exercising; you might enjoy arriving home in time to have a well-cooked dinner with your family or getting up in time to have a leisurely breakfast while you read the newspaper. Diet drinks may not be so bad after all, and you can probably be just as happy without the 14-hour days spent at work eating pizza for lunch and supper. You may learn to value some of the little joys of life: throwing a ball with your kids, gardening, bowling, or square dancing. We know a lawyer who writes people's wills. She says she has yet to find the person who, at the end of their life, says their only wish is that they had not spent so much time with their family.

We are talking about redefining the quality of life. We admit to looking through rose-colored glasses, downplaying the things you can't do or eat that you used to love. There's no denying that some things ought to be avoided, some of life's patterns ought to be adjusted. But none of this has to impair your quality of life. You have the choice. You define quality. You set the goals.

Setting Health Goals

Basic to your quality of life is not only what you can do but also how you feel. By "health goals," we mean the goals you set for your own physical well-being. "I want my energy back. I don't want to be tired and running to the bathroom all the time." "I want to be healthy as I get older, able to climb the stairs, able to play with the grandchildren." These are health goals.

We believe that avoiding the acute symptoms of diabetes, feeling generally well, is achievable for virtually everyone. Actually, freedom from thirst, frequent urination, vaginal infections, and so on is the minimum health goal you should set. If you suffer from these symptoms of high blood sugar, reevaluate your treatment. For a first health goal, tell yourself, "I want to be free of the symptoms of diabetes. On a day-to-day basis, I want to feel well."

Another health goal we are sure you share is avoidance of the long-term complications of diabetes: kidney disease, visual impairment, nerve damage, blood vessel disease, and so on (described in Part IV). This is a more complicated goal, requiring better blood sugar control than just enough to avoid symptoms. Keeping blood sugars always between 150 and 200 mg/dl, for instance, will keep you free of symptoms but may not be good enough to avoid long-term complications. As well as blood sugar control, healthy habits, such as not smoking, exercising regularly, and controlling blood pressure and cholesterol levels, are an important part of controlling long-term complications.

Finally, if you already have some long-term complications from diabetes, the health goal should be to keep them from progressing and becoming disabling. Specific ways to manage complications are described later in this book; the good news is that most long-term complications can be effectively treated.

Blood Glucose Goals

Given the availability of self-monitoring of blood glucose and the new world of "blood glucose awareness," one of the most common questions we are asked is: "What should my blood sugar be?" It is certainly a fair question, one that you should raise with your own health care professional. But the answer isn't so easy. It needs individualization and quite a bit of discussion.

As mentioned previously, "normal" blood glucose levels are about 70–115 mg/dl before eating and up to about 140 mg/dl after eating. The normal blood glucose levels refer to what a person without diabetes has, day in and day out. Tight control means blood sugars that are kept in a relatively narrow range that is close to normal. Loose control or poor control means the opposite—sugars that usually run high. Lability or brittleness means that the sugars bounce up and down a lot, whatever the average is. As far as we know, it is the *average* that determines the long-term complications, not whether you have periods of highs and lows. An 8- to 12-week average is most easily tested, as we will describe, by the hemoglobin A1c (glycohemoglobin) test, although frequent self-monitoring of blood glucose will also provide a good indication of average.

Blood sugar control can be labeled as excellent, good, fair, or poor, depending on how close the sugar levels are to normal. But the terms don't mean much unless they are tailored to the individual circumstances. One size does not fit all. What is good or excellent for one person in one situation may not be so good for another person or even for the same person in a different situation.

This individualization of blood glucose goals is frustrating for many people. Not only do the targets change from one person to another, but they can change from time to time for the same person. Let's look at some examples.

> *Sam is 38 and has had Type I diabetes since he was 12. He has always had very good control, with intensive management especially since adulthood. Blood sugars were rarely above 200 and quite often less than 100. But lately he has had a series of severe insulin reactions. His wife and children are alarmed, and so are his co-workers. Sam's doctor suggests that he "back off" a bit, trying to keep his sugars always above 100, even if he is over 200 some of the time. At the moment the insulin reactions are more of a threat than somewhat higher sugars. But Sam is resistant—he has always prized lower glucose, and he does not want "bad control."*

Circumstances change, and what was good for Sam in previous years has to be modified now. It could be that he will regain the awareness of his hypoglycemia and be able to go back to even tighter control later. But for now, loosening up is necessary.

> *Naomi's daughter is 12 years old and has Type I diabetes. Mother and daughter struggle to keep most of the sugars under 200, but they aren't always successful by any means. But in her doctor's waiting room she talks to an older man, Chester, who proudly announces that it's no problem for him to keep his sugars always under 140 and usually under 120—he just takes his pills and doesn't drink so many soft drinks. To Naomi, the very thought of averaging 120 is ridiculous—she knows that her daughter would be sent home from school with insulin reactions on a daily basis. Naomi is upset and depressed by the conversation.*

Naomi's response is natural, and Chester's insensitivity does not make it any easier. But she has to understand that Chester has stable Type II diabetes. His blood sugar targets have nothing whatever to do with what Naomi's daughter can achieve. Probably the most important individual consideration in setting blood glucose goals is what kind of diabetes a person has.

As we have said, people with Type I diabetes inevitably have widely fluctuating blood sugars. The goals they set must recognize this fact. Even with the most intensive treatment and the best of self-care, the blood sugars of a person with Type I diabetes will vary more than those of most people with

Type II diabetes. Often, less tight target blood sugars are a more reasonable goal.

How intense a person is about controlling blood sugars is also a highly individual trait. The terms *intensive control* and *intensive therapy* came into popular use during the Diabetes Control and Complications Trial (DCCT), the trial that specifically compared an intensive treatment approach with a less intensive, "standard care" approach. We believe there is no one "intensive" regimen; instead, individualization is the key.

Peter has heard about the DCCT and is worried. He takes two insulin injections a day, with very good results. His hemoglobin A1c is regularly within 1% of normal, and his sugars run in a very good range. But he wants to know whether he should be on an "intensive" treatment program, taking three or four shots a day.

We would tell Peter, "You're doing great. Don't change a thing." There is no reason to "intensify" a treatment program if what you are doing is working for you. The bottom line is the blood glucose control.

Stephanie is taking two injections a day and doing okay but complaining of middle-of-the-night lows, highs in the morning, and a lot of fluctuation before dinner. She would like to become pregnant. What do we think?

Stephanie has definite patterns of when she's high, when she's low, and when she fluctuates too much. Furthermore, planning a pregnancy is a time when most women with diabetes are motivated to work the hardest. We would intensify the regimen, increasing the number of shots per day, and work on all aspects of self-care.

There are many other factors that should be taken into consideration as you set blood glucose goals. The list could go on indefinitely. But it might help to list some of the characteristics that cause us to lean one way or the other—toward tighter, more intensive targets or toward looser, more relaxed blood glucose goals:

Tighter control may be indicated if you:

—Have symptoms of high blood sugar
—Have noticed a worsening of your blood sugar control
—See patterns of highs and lows
—Are thinking about pregnancy
—Are more "into" your diabetic control, for whatever reason

—Don't mind the glucose monitoring or injections as much as you used to and are ready to step to another level of control

On the other hand, less tight blood sugar targets may be indicated if you:

—Have lost your awareness of hypoglycemia and are increasingly prone to severe insulin reactions

—Have other serious medical problems, such as coronary heart disease, a psychiatric disorder, or substance abuse, so that the risks of hypoglycemia are increased

—Are elderly, with relatively recent onset diabetes, and are not so concerned about long-term complications that may occur 20 years down the road

—Have something coming up, such as an important meeting, exam, presentation, or long drive, when the most important thing is not to go too low

—Are recovering from surgery, not eating much, and it's more important not to go too low

How to Tell Whether Your Treatment Is Working

Once you have set goals for yourself, the central issue becomes how to know when your treatment is working and when it is not. This isn't as easy as it might seem at first glance, but here are some guidelines: First, are your "numbers" in a good range? Second, are you helping yourself avoid or manage complications? And third, do you have the sense that diabetes is not running your life?

Since there are no absolute standards for good blood sugar control, and no one with diabetes can achieve perfectly normal blood sugars, we recommend individual targets, such as "I want to be in this range a certain percentage of the time." For example, you may decide that your target is having 50% of readings under 140 mg/dl and 90% under 200 mg/dl.

Next, your treatment is working if you are doing your best to avoid disabling complications and to manage any complications you may already have. You are taking good care of your feet, having an annual eye examination, and so on.

Finally, if the treatment plan is working, you will feel that your diabetes is kept in perspective, at least most of the time. You will generally feel that diabetes is in its place in your life and that your life has a place for diabetes, as well as much more.

What to Do When Your Treatment Isn't Working

Let's say that you *have* set realistic standards for evaluating your treatment and that, by these standards, you're not sure your treatment is working. Major problems in any of the areas we looked at above—reasonable numbers on blood sugar testing, avoidance of complications, and a reasonable frame of mind about diabetes—deserve your attention. But what should you do? There are three common sources of treatment failures: stress and its consequences, self-care problems, and failure to get the most out of health care providers. Interactions with health care professionals are discussed in Chapter 19. Here we'll look at first stress and then self-care.

Stress and Diabetes

Stress will undermine your treatment. Physical stress, such as surgery, illness (a cold or the flu), or, for women, the normal hormonal variations of the menstrual cycle, can send blood sugars out of control. Blood sugars destabilized by stress can be hard to straighten out. Fortunately, these physical stresses tend to pass, so their effect on blood sugar control is temporary. But emotional stress can also destabilize blood sugar levels.

> *Mike uses an insulin pump. He was having problems with blood sugar control and was often under tremendous stress at work. His supervisor, he said, was "the boss from hell," a screamer, not just insensitive but positively boorish, a bully, inconsistent, and stupid as well. The only good news was that the boss was on the road about half the time, so people in the office could get things done. It finally dawned on Mike that when the boss was in the office his blood sugars shot up. He had to double the amount of insulin his pump delivered. When the boss left the country, down the sugar levels would come, stabilizing on less insulin every time.*

Emotional stress can hit in two ways: by pushing blood sugar up, through stimulation of adrenaline, and by keeping you from practicing self-care. Mike is a classic example of the former. An example of the latter is the person who feels she has to eat every time she's under stress. One thing you can do is take control by working to restabilize your blood sugars. This involves recommitting to good self-care.

Self-Care Goal Setting

"Cheating" and Diabetes Self-Care

Typical self-care problems include difficulty taking medication and monitoring blood glucose, and difficulty in sticking with a healthy diet and exercising. Notice that we didn't say *cheating*. We find that even thinking in terms of cheating is really not a useful way to look at a problem. Who is being cheated? Some people carry huge burdens of guilt when they deviate even slightly from ideal regimens, while others may proudly announce, "Of course I cheat," as if it were a badge of independence or machismo. Sometimes people begin their office appointment with us by saying that they "cheated bigtime" the night before. We assume they are making a statement of defiance or obstinate denial, and we often talk with them about what's going on.

In self-care, you set the goals, do what you can, get the help that you need, and that's it. Please don't think of it as a character issue. You may have a good nature but not stick to your regimen so well. Or maybe you're very careful about your diabetes but otherwise a scoundrel. There is no necessary link between good self-care and overall character.

Self-Care Behaviors

Behavior is where the rubber meets the road. All the lofty talk, all the sound intentions are for naught if you don't put into practice some good self-care behaviors. So think about how you'll actually behave, as you set goals for good health and good blood sugar control. It makes no sense to target bedtime blood sugars between 100 and 150 mg/dl if you don't measure your blood sugar at bedtime. It makes no sense to say you want to avoid damaging your feet in a way that could lead to amputations, but you can't take the time to inspect your feet and your shoes each day.

Sometimes people get confused about their motivation: they think they should change behavior to make the *doctor* happy. Let us remind you that this isn't the point; the point is to keep *yourself* feeling and functioning well. Doctors can tell you how, they can tell you why, and they can motivate you. But you have to do it.

Setting behavior goals requires very personal decisions. You have to be realistic and not make a promise you know you can't keep, but you also have to push yourself. You have to trust that just because you seldom raise yourself from the couch nearest the television to go get some exercise doesn't mean you *can't* get up and out. So think hard about what you can do to help your own health, and think specifically about behaviors. Even write yourself a contract or create a diary ready to be filled in.

Let's close the chapter with a few more anecdotes of people with various goal-setting issues:

Seymour was given thirteen different instructions by his doctor at his last office visit. Unfortunately, they weren't written down, and he forgot most of them before he left the examining room. But he recalls that he was told to check his sugar four times a day, and he never could seem to do it more than once a day. So Seymour has been avoiding going back to his doctor, afraid of the lecture he'll get. In fact, it's five years now since the last visit, and his monitoring strips gave out two years ago. He doesn't want to hurt his doctor's feelings by choosing another doctor, but he's feeling pretty thirsty these days and thinks things aren't going so well.

We hesitate to place blame, but this is a broken relationship. Seymour is carrying around enormous guilt, feeling bad about himself, and heading straight for some major problems. The question isn't who's at fault, whose feelings will or won't be hurt; the issue is how Seymour can get himself under good care before it's too late. His immediate goal should be to pull himself together and get in to see a good health care professional, either the doctor he saw before or someone else.

Sam knows that his blood sugars aren't meeting the targets he agreed to with his nurse educator. So he writes down other results in his diary—just makes them up. His nurse educator seems perfectly happy. Sam has successfully fooled her.

We hope that people like Sam realize who is being hurt and who is not. We hope that Sam understands that he's missing the point and turns to reasonable goal setting for himself, not his nurse.

The variety of personalities never ceases to amaze us. And if we were to ignore the variety, we would be trying to put a lot of square pegs into round holes. Let's compare two people we know:

Lauren does very well with her blood sugar control. She approaches her diabetes like everything else in her life—in a careful, measured, and methodical way. Roxanne, in contrast, is an artist, in profession and in personality. She's very successful with her photography but struggling with her blood sugars. Mainly, the problem is that when she's in the creative mood she just doesn't think about lunch (or dinner or snacks), and she thinks about nothing but eating when she's not feeling creative.

Goal setting for these two women has to be very different. For Lauren, we might suggest a little fine tuning here and there, taking some calories from lunch and putting them into the 3 P.M. snack or adjusting the bedtime insulin according to blood sugar. For Roxanne, it is more reasonable to target just one good sandwich between noon and 1 P.M. and to do some sugar testing so we can see when she's highest and lowest.

We have long since given up trying to remake personalities. If they were uptight, regimented, and disciplined before they got diabetes, they'll probably be the same afterward; if they were loose and free-flowing before, we're unlikely to make them into compulsive recordkeepers. Instead, we want goal setting to be realistic and practical. Our own goal is to take people from wherever they are up to the next level of self-care (and then, hopefully, to the next, and the next.)

You most likely have no problem buying into the big goals: a long and healthy life of good quality. You must realize by now that good self-care is the best way to realize these goals. You now know that specific blood glucose targets should be tailored to your own individual situation: the type of diabetes you have, your age, your ability to recognize hypoglycemia, your medical condition, and your own personality.

Once you've thought about goal setting, with the help of a good health care professional, you reach for these targets with specific, short-term behavior goals. Your short-term goals may be to monitor more often, to eat more regularly, or to get more exercise. To make the changes, a step-by-step approach is best, and realism is essential. You won't be able to do it all at once, you will need help, and you won't be perfect. But, step by step, success by success, you *will* get there. Believe it.

Chapter 4

Blood Glucose Monitoring

- *"What's going on with my diabetes right now? Am I low or high?"*
- *"How's my control overall?"*
- *"What happens to my blood sugar when I exercise?"*
- *"When during the day is my blood sugar highest, and how does it respond to pasta?"*
- *"I feel really sick. Is this an emergency?"*

A person's blood sugar varies from hour to hour, sometimes almost from minute to minute. Since you're reading this book, we know that you're a person who wants to know what's going on in your own body. To find out what's happening with your blood sugar—whether it's high, low, or just right—you need to know about monitoring.

The symptoms of high blood sugar and low blood sugar are usually obvious. You feel thirsty, dry, and tired when the sugar is high; you feel shaky or sweaty or have other telling symptoms when it's low. But even if you are a pro at recognizing these symptoms, waiting for them is definitely not the best way to monitor your sugars day in and day out. One problem is that the symptoms don't come on until the sugar is very high (over 200–250 mg/dl) or very low (under about 60 mg/dl). (Some people who are used to much higher sugars feel low even when the glucose level is in the vicinity of 90 mg/dl.)

Another problem is that there is a wide range—too wide a range—of blood glucose levels that don't produce any symptoms at all. On the high side, you may "get used to" blood sugars in the 200s or even 300s. You can feel perfectly well as your body is slowly suffering irreversible complications. And on the low side, the problem is that if you are regularly near low at a particular time of day, then every now and then, maybe one day in ten, you will go very low at that time. Three serious insulin reactions a month is way too many. So don't count on your symptoms to tell you when you're out of control. Poor control can be a "silent disease." Check your blood sugar.

Monitoring provides accurate, dependable answers to two questions: "What is my blood sugar right now?" and "How am I doing, on average, over time?" There are several different tests for monitoring blood glucose. We discuss them in this chapter, beginning with self-monitoring, which provides much more reliable and useful information than simply watching symptoms.

Self-Monitoring of Blood Glucose

Mary, 45 years old, came into the office with a medical mystery. She monitors her blood glucose three times a day, and everything seems fine. Her usual evening routine consists of exercising on a stationary bike, eating a small snack and taking her bedtime insulin, and then going to bed. Lately, however, she has been having nightmares, and she sleeps restlessly, with drenching sweats. She doesn't understand these nightmares. Naturally, she wonders about menopause. Mary asked us, "Are the nightmares related to my blood sugar and, if so, am I high or low?" Together, we decided that Mary should find out. She sets her alarm for 2 A.M. three nights in a row and finds that her blood sugar readings are 65, 53, and 60 mg/dl. So there's the answer: she's low! No amount of estrogen replacement therapy or air conditioning is going to help that. Mary reduces her evening insulin dose and does fine.

Mary's case is a simple example, but a telling one. With blood glucose monitoring, you can find out if you are high or low, you can find out what makes your sugar go high or low, and you can find out how you're doing day in and day out. It's hard to overestimate the importance of this tool.

At present it's not possible to self-test blood sugar without sticking a finger to get a drop of blood; nor is it possible to keep continuous track of blood sugar. Like everyone, we hope that a noninvasive glucose monitor will come into general use in the near future. Such a monitor would allow a person with diabetes to check blood sugar continuously without a finger stick. (For more about this, see Chapter 33.) Really, though, self-monitoring of blood glucose is not that hard to do and not *that* painful. It is such a powerful tool for good self-care that people with diabetes have taken to it in droves. It allows them to know just where they stand and to take better control of their diabetes.

How the Meter Systems Work

All the systems available today use an enzyme (either glucose oxidase or hexokinase) to react with the glucose in the drop of blood you put on the strip. In most systems, a color develops once the blood is applied to the strip. The more glucose, the darker the color. The colored strip is then measured by the meter, which translates it into a blood sugar reading. Some of the systems have strips that don't develop a color; instead, they measure the electrical current generated by the enzyme.

Developing this bit of chemistry and making it practical was no small technological feat. By now, though, several companies produce dependable systems, so there are a number of competing products to choose among.

How to Do Self-Monitoring of Blood Glucose

There's no avoiding the facts: self-monitoring requires a drop of blood, a drop of blood requires a finger stick, and a finger stick can hurt. We aren't unsympathetic to these facts of life with diabetes. If you've been resisting self-monitoring because of the finger stick, though, we need to tell you that thinking about it usually hurts more than doing it. Just about everyone gets used to the finger sticks. For a long time many doctors discouraged self-monitoring because they were afraid that their patients couldn't stand the prick. In fact, most people who self-monitor get so accustomed to it that they really don't notice any pain at all (Figure 5).

Once you've decided to just do it, you'll have some questions: to wash your hands or not? to use an alcohol pad or not? It can't hurt to have a clean finger, assuming that you remember to dry your finger completely before you take the drop of blood (otherwise you'll be diluting the blood with water or alcohol). To tell the truth, it's not really necessary to have a clean finger, since infections due to self-monitoring are virtually unknown. We suggest that if your hands are unusually dirty or if you have any history of infected fingers, you should wash up. Otherwise, there's no need.

Don't stick your finger with a hand-held needle or one of those little bayonets. Use a lancing device. The spring-loaded, pen-shaped devices are calibrated to control the depth of penetration. There are many different models. Find one you like, and learn how to get a good drop of blood with minimal discomfort.

To avoid pain, speed is the key. Nerve endings don't become as irritated with a quick action as they do with one that is prolonged, so a quick stick doesn't hurt as much as slowly inserting the lancing device and slowly taking it out. Another trick is to experiment until you find the location on the fingertip that works best for you. Most people prefer the side of the fingertip, not in the middle of the ball of the finger. There are said to be fewer nerve

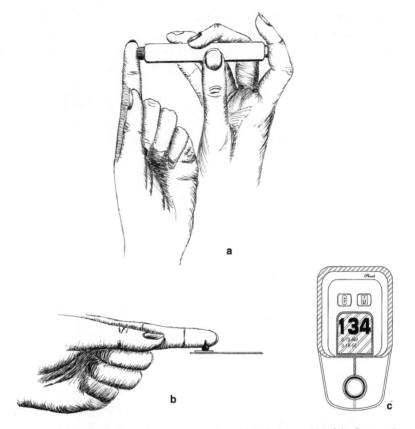

Figure 5. Technique of blood glucose monitoring. (a) Prick the outside of the finger using a lancing device to decrease the pain. (b) Milk the finger if necessary to get a large drop of blood to appear on the fingertip. Apply the blood to the glucose reagent strip. (c) Blood sugar result

endings on the sides than in the middle (fewer nerve endings means less pain), and there are plenty of little blood vessels on the side. Also, sore fingertips make it uncomfortable to type or use your fingers for other things.

You may have to stick a little deeper than you think, and you may have to squeeze the finger gently to extract some blood. You need to get a drop of blood large enough to cover the test strip pad in one big drop. Be sure the drop is thick enough not to dry out on the pad during the test.

Sometimes it seems like the blood just doesn't want to flow. Remember that there *is* definitely blood in those fingers—all you have to do is find it! Here are some tips:

—Wash your hands with warm water to stimulate circulation to the fingertips.

—With your arms at your sides, shake your hand back and forth below the level of the heart. This will force more blood into the fingertips.

—Stick a little deeper. Some people literally have thick skin.

—Use centrifugal force: swing your arm in a circle a few times

—In extreme cases, use a rubber band like a tourniquet at the base of the finger. Take it off immediately after you get the blood.

—Rotate your fingers (not literally, of course). We know one person who has his Monday, Tuesday, Wednesday (and so on) finger, his morning, noon, and night side of the finger, and his other hand as backup! You really *don't* have to hit the same spot twice in a short period of time.

After you get the drop of blood, you are home free. In less than a minute, in most cases, the meter does the work and gives you a reading of your blood glucose.

Can You Trust Your Meter Reading?

If the meter is used properly and with reasonable expectations, you can trust the reading. The specifications for the meters—how accurate they should be when used properly—are plus or minus about 10% of the actual blood sugar. This means that if the most accurate of laboratories found a blood sugar of 100 mg/dl, your meter should read between 90 and 110 mg/dl. At the extremes of glucose—say, over 400 mg/dl or under 50 mg/dl—the meters are much less accurate; in those cases the reading will not tell you *exactly* what your blood sugar number is and should be counted on simply to tell you that you're too high or too low.

That said, we need also to admit that several things can go wrong in the technique, so a healthy level of skepticism is needed. Consider Jerry's experience:

> *Jerry's blood sugars were always unstable but in a reasonable range. All of a sudden, he began to get crazy readings. When he was pretty sure he was low, the meter read 180 mg/dl; when he felt definitely high, it read 60 mg/dl. He knew something was wacky. First, Jerry bought new strips. This didn't seem to make any difference. So he got an old meter out of the closet, cleaned it up, and compared the results. The old meter was much closer to what he thought was his reading. He sent the defective meter to the manufacturer through his pharmacy. He never heard*

*what the problem was, but he received a gleaming new meter in the mail shortly
and has not had a problem since.*

Jerry apparently knew that it is more common for strips to go bad than
for meters to break down, and that's why the first thing he did in trou-
bleshooting was replace his strips. But the main thing Jerry had going for him
was that he kept his wits about him: he knew that his readings didn't reflect
how he was feeling. Anyone who is self-monitoring needs to be on the watch
for odd things like this. After all, if the speedometer in your car suddenly
started showing 100 mph when you could see and feel that you were only
going about 25 mph, you wouldn't believe the speedometer and slam on the
brakes. In the same way, you have to realize that sometimes the blood glucose monitoring systems break down.

For accurate results, you'll need to observe the following rules:

1. *Read the directions*—even if you are the kind of person who doesn't read
   directions—and follow the directions!
2. *Keep the meter clean.* Meter manufacturers usually provide written
   instructions for cleaning which specify what kind of cleaner to use and
   which parts of the meter are most sensitive. Alcohol can cause an
   irreversible fogging of the window, so be careful.
3. *Calibrate the meter* with each new batch of strips. Also called *coding* or
   programming, calibrating is a procedure in which the machine is
   adjusted for each batch of strips. Just as paint color can vary slightly
   from one can to the next, different packages of test strips may vary.
   Calibration factors in the difference in the batches of strips, so for
   accurate results, it's an essential step.
4. *Use the check strips or control solutions supplied by the manufacturer.* If the
   result does not come up in the range specified, either the strips are bad
   or the machine is broken or needs to be cleaned.

Finally, here's a caution that must be followed not for accurate results but
for your safety. Whatever you do, *don't share meters with anyone else.* Every
now and then, someone will come into our office and say, "Oh, all those highs
weren't mine—they were Uncle Joe's. I let him use the meter." It gives us chills
to hear that. Uncle Joe could have an infectious disease like hepatitis, he
could have the virus that causes AIDS, or he could have any other infection
that can be passed through blood from one person to another. These viruses
can survive on the surface of a meter and can enter your own bloodstream as

you place your pricked finger down on the meter during testing. Even if you don't see a blood stain, microscopic amounts of blood do end up on every meter, so there is no way you can be sure that your meter doesn't carry disease unless you keep it to yourself.

What Should I Do with the Blood Glucose Reading?

Many meters will automatically store the test result in your meter's computer memory for later discussions with your health care professional, or you can keep a written diary of blood sugar results (Figure 6, a and b). Usually, even if you have a meter with memory, it's a good idea to write down the results and look them over for yourself (Figure 6c). With a written log, you can see the patterns and *adjust your treatment regimen based on the reading you get.*

Did we say adjust your own treatment regimen? We sure did. As you will see in Chapters 11 and 12, we are strong believers in teaching people how to adjust their self-care, within safe limits, to fit the circumstances. It is especially important to learn to translate blood sugar readings into an action. After all, you're not doing all this finger sticking to make the doctor happy, you're doing it to keep yourself well. So when you find that the reading is especially low, or especially high, at a particular time of day, *do something about it!* Modify your diet or modify your insulin. If you're not sure what to do, ask your health care professional.

Many research studies have shown that blood sugar testing is most valuable if it leads to rational, thoughtful changes in self-care.

A word about the office blood glucose determination. A blood glucose determination drawn at the doctor's office may have some use, but it is certainly not an adequate way to follow a person's diabetes day in and day out. The blood is usually taken from an arm vein in the fasting state. It indicates what the blood sugar level is at that particular moment, but you know that when you eat your next meal, it will go up. The tendency is for the patient to think, "Gee, my blood sugar was 260 six months ago when I was in the doctor's office and now it's 255. I must be doing better." As you know, your blood sugar didn't stay at 260 *or* 255 very long. It may have been crashing up and down on an hourly basis for three months, but a one-time blood glucose test done at the doctor's office will never give you that information.

In general, the fasting blood sugar is a more reliable measurement of the all-day average for Type II diabetes than for Type I, because blood glucose varies so much more in Type I. But you have a right to be skeptical if your health care provider thinks that an occasional office blood glucose measure-

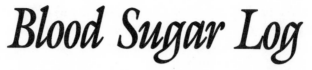

Sunday's Date:

	Breakfast	**Lunch**	**Supper**	**Bedtime**
SUNDAY	▨		▨	
MONDAY	▨		▨	
TUESDAY	▨		▨	
WEDNESDAY	▨		▨	
THURSDAY	▨		▨	
FRIDAY	▨		▨	
SATURDAY	▨		▨	

Sunday's Date:

	Breakfast	**Lunch**	**Supper**	**Bedtime**
SUNDAY	▨		▨	
MONDAY	▨		▨	
TUESDAY	▨		▨	
WEDNESDAY	▨		▨	
THURSDAY	▨		▨	
FRIDAY	▨		▨	
SATURDAY	▨		▨	

a

Figure 6 (a and b). Blood sugar logs.

ment is a perfectly good way to monitor your diabetes control. You ought to get involved with self-monitoring of blood glucose and ask your health care professional to test your glycated hemoglobin.

Glycated Hemoglobin and Fructosamine Measurements (Hemoglobin A1c, Glycohemoglobin)

Glycated hemoglobin, hemoglobin A1c, and glycohemoglobin are used to measure the overall control of diabetes in the preceding 8–12 weeks. Although there are some differences in laboratory technique among the three, for all intents and purposes they are the same test.

Here's how glycated hemoglobin monitoring works. The hemoglobin in your red blood cells is what makes them red. Each red cell "lives" about four

BLOOD SUGAR RECORD

DAY	BREAK BS/ MED	MEAL, ACTIVITY, OTHER	LUNCH BS/ MED	MEAL, ACTIVITY, OTHER	DIN BS/ MED	MEAL, ACTIVITY, OTHER	BED BS/ MED	3 AM BS/ MED
SUN								
MON								
TUE								
WED								
THUR								
FRI								
SAT								

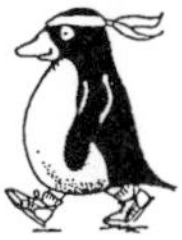

.b

Figure 6 (*continued*)

months from the time it comes out of the bone marrow, where it is made. During that time, the hemoglobin in the cell becomes more and more *glycated*, meaning that glucose molecules stick to it. The higher the glucose level in the blood over the months, the more glucose is stuck to the hemoglobin, and the higher the glycated hemoglobin.

Thus, glycated hemoglobin paints the big picture. It indicates the person's average glucose control over recent weeks to months. As you know well by now, the blood glucose measurement itself only gives you information

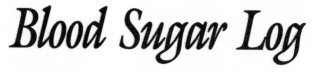

Sunday's Date:

	Breakfast	**Lunch**	**Supper**	**Bedtime**
SUNDAY	126 N✗✗ RS	Exer. 52	207 R6	147 N6
MONDAY	161 N✗✗ R6	102	182 R6	121 N6
TUESDAY	107 N✗✗ RS	87 wK	72 RY	133 N6
WEDNESDAY	138 N✗c R6	78	140 RS	182 N6
THURSDAY	209 N✗✗ R7	128	68 RY	100 N6
FRIDAY	111 N✗✗ RS	92	80 RY	158 NL
SATURDAY	141 N✗✗ RS	70	168 R6	101 NL

Sunday's Date:

	Breakfast	**Lunch**	**Supper**	**Bedtime**
SUNDAY				
MONDAY				
TUESDAY				
WEDNESDAY				
THURSDAY				
FRIDAY				
SATURDAY				

Figure 6(c). Example of completed blood sugar log.

about blood glucose at that moment, and the reading will be different in a matter of hours. Glycated hemoglobin, in contrast, changes only over a matter of weeks.

To understand the meaning of the glycated hemoglobin result, you have to know the "normal value" of the laboratory doing the test. In many labs the "upper limit of normal" is about 6.4%. This means that people without diabetes, people with normal blood sugars, would have a glycated hemoglobin of up to 6.4%. If your glycated hemoglobin is in that range, then you know that most of the time your blood sugars are in an excellent, nondiabetic range. A result of 7.5% would be very good but not normal, and 9% would not be very good. Some labs, however, have normal values up to about 8%. In that case, 7.5 would be excellent, and 9% would be pretty good, too. For this rea-

Histogram

Name: Samuel Zaccari   Report Date: 1/3/97 - 2/3/97

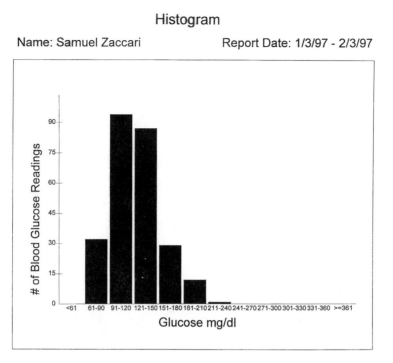

Target Range: 65 - 200

Figure 6(d). Histogram. Computer-generated printout of blood sugar readings recorded in the monitor memory. This graph shows the relative quantity of readings in segmented ranges. This example illustrates excellent blood sugar control.

son, you have to know the upper limit of normal *for your laboratory* to make sense of your result.

How is this test used? In the old days, it was used to "catch cheaters" who would come into the doctor's office after a few days of working hard and controlling their diet but who before that had been way out of control. We don't think of the test that way anymore. Instead, we use the glycated hemoglobin to see how control is going on average. No one checks blood sugar continuously, so this adds information to the results of self-monitoring. If we find a discrepancy—say the once-a-day blood sugar tests look good, but the glycated hemoglobin is quite high—we'll want to find out why. We usually get a glycated hemoglobin two to four times a year, but if the result is high we may want to test more often.

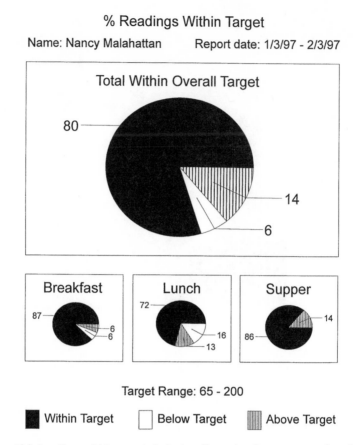

% Readings Within Target

Name: Nancy Malahattan   Report date: 1/3/97 - 2/3/97

Total Within Overall Target

80

14

6

Breakfast   Lunch   Supper

87   72   14
6   16   86
6   13

Target Range: 65 - 200

■ Within Target   □ Below Target   ▓ Above Target

Figure 6(e). Readings within target. A pie chart illustrating the percentage of readings below target, within target, and above target. This example illustrates very good blood sugar control. Only a small percentage of blood sugar readings are above or below the target that was set.

If glycated hemoglobin provides the big picture, it doesn't give the *whole* picture. It does not, for example, tell you whether the overall control is fairly stable at a particular level or whether you have many highs averaged with many lows. Self-monitoring of blood glucose is the only way to get these answers.

Fructosamine is a blood measurement that provides information similar to that obtained by the glycated hemoglobin, except that the "view" provided by fructosamine is shorter—in the range of two weeks instead of several months. This test measures the glucose that is bound to proteins other than

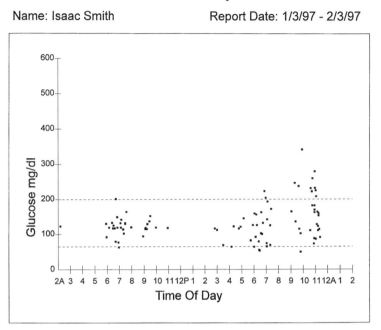

Standard Day

Name: Isaac Smith   Report Date: 1/3/97 - 2/3/97

Target Range: 65 - 200

Figure 6(f). Standard day. This computer-generated graph plots every reading by value and time of day. It is helpful in spotting trends and visualizing degree of fluctuation in control. This example illustrates very good blood sugar control with a trend of slightly higher readings in the evening.

hemoglobin, and these other proteins don't have as long a life span as hemoglobin.

Fructosamine assays have not been used very widely, though they can provide useful information, especially if a person's blood glucose control has changed quickly in recent weeks or if it's desirable to get a short-term average—for example, during a pregnancy. We usually rely on the glycated hemoglobin instead of fructosamine, but we don't object to having both tests done.

Urine Glucose Testing

The ancient Egyptians, we are told, diagnosed diabetes by putting urine near an anthill. If the ants were attracted, the patient was told that he had diabetes.

If that seems a bit crude, it is at least more aesthetically pleasing than the seventeenth-century doctor's approach, which was to taste the urine. Sugar spills into the urine when the blood glucose reaches a certain level, usually about 180 mg/dl, and testing urine for sweetness, as these examples show, is a time-honored procedure.

Athalia was brought up testing urine glucose, and naturally she prefers it to measuring blood glucose: there's no finger stick involved. Her diabetes has become more unstable lately, though. She finds, for example, that she feels low before lunch, but when she checks her urine, it is 2+ for sugar. She complains to her doctor that her urine no longer reflects her blood sugar, and she worries that her kidneys are bad.

In fact, Athalia's kidneys are fine, as her doctor points out. What's happening is that her blood sugar is going up after breakfast (spilling glucose into the urine) and then crashing down before lunch (causing her to feel low). So when she tests the urine before lunch, it is really showing her the after-breakfast rise. Athalia will be much better off when she begins checking with blood glucose monitoring.

The test for urinary sugar (called *glucosuria* or *glycosuria*) is done by dipping a reagent stick into a fresh sample of urine. The pad on the end of the stick contains glucose oxidase, the same enzyme used to test blood glucose. Glucose oxidase turns a deeper color depending on how much sugar is in the urine.

For many years, urine testing was the only way to monitor blood glucose. Further, many children with diabetes were brought up thinking they should always spill at least some sugar in their urine, to avoid insulin reactions. Simple and straightforward as that advice was, it meant that these children were always running blood sugars over about 180–200 mg/dl. We can do much better than that, of course, with direct blood glucose testing.

We consider urine glucose testing to be history. It's time to put this time-honored test to rest. As a measure of diabetic control, it has several limitations:

—Since the urine is formed slowly, when you empty your bladder you are testing urine from several hours earlier. As you know, your blood sugar can be very different now than it was then. The urine reading for sugar could be low at just the time the blood sugar is going high.

—Urine testing is imprecise. The *renal threshold* (the blood sugar level at which glucose is spilled into the urine) changes markedly from person to person and from time to time.

—You can't tell if you are normal, low, or near to low. Testing urine glucose only tells you if you're high.

—Finally, the concentration of your urine makes all the difference in urine testing: if you drink two glasses of water and dilute your urine, the glucose level in the urine will seem to be lower, when in fact your blood sugar hasn't changed.

Adding up these limitations, we conclude that urine testing for sugar can provide only a rough measure of glucose control. There are much better ways of monitoring blood glucose levels.

Urine Testing for Ketones

Ketones in the urine can signal danger. They can be a sign that your diabetes may be badly out of control and approaching the medical emergency called *ketoacidosis* (explained more fully in Chapter 23). On the other hand, urine ketones may *not* be an indication of trouble. Ketones reflect fat breakdown for use as fuel. When you haven't ingested any carbohydrate and you don't have much insulin circulating, the body turns to fat as a source of fuel and produces ketones as the fat is broken down. In a normal fast—for instance, when you skip breakfast and haven't eaten in 12–16 hours—you may spill some ketones in your urine, but this doesn't mean that you are in danger of going into diabetic ketoacidosis.

Testing urine for ketones, then, is a way to tell how far out of control your diabetes is and whether a true emergency exists. If there is a moderate or large amount of ketones in your urine *and* your blood sugar is high (or urine sugar is positive, if you don't test the blood), then you need medical help quickly. Don't be fooled into complacency by blood sugars that are only moderately increased, since some people develop ketoacidosis with sugars only in the 200s.

When should you check your urine ketones? Keep updated test strips on hand at home all the time. There is no reason to test ketones on a daily basis, though, because the test will be meaningful only when you are really approaching trouble, and you should know when that is happening: your symptoms or your blood sugar levels will warn you. Test ketones if you're sick or if you think your diabetes is way out of control. If you are positive for ketones in your urine at that time, then be sure to take at least your usual amount of insulin and *seek help*.

Rational Use of Testing

In this chapter we've described self-monitoring of symptoms, self-monitoring of blood glucose, office blood glucose testing, glycated hemoglobin testing (hemoglobin A1c or glycosylated hemoglobin), urine glucose testing, and urine ketone testing. The whole point of testing, of course, is to learn about your diabetic control and to use that knowledge to avoid trouble. So let's summarize when and where each should be done:

Symptom recognition.   You should definitely know the symptoms of highs and lows, so you can tell when you're in trouble even before you test. But knowing the symptoms is not a substitute for actual blood sugar testing. It's too easy to fool yourself into thinking everything is okay when it's not.

Self-monitoring of blood glucose.   This is the mainstay of modern diabetic testing. We recommend that it be done on a regular basis by everyone with diabetes. How often is "regular"? It depends on your kind of diabetes, and especially on how unstable your diabetes is. If you have very stable Type II diabetes, the sugars may be in a normal range virtually all the time, and all you need is to be sure they don't drift out of range. It may be perfectly adequate to test once a day in the morning and let your health care professional know if you see a drift high or low. If you have unstable Type I diabetes, however, or if your treatment is changing, you will probably want to test much more often, maybe three to four times daily or even more. This is because, between the morning and later in the day, the blood glucose may vary widely.

We ask people to monitor upon rising in the morning, before meals, and at bedtime. Some people alternate the times by checking before breakfast and dinner one day, before lunch and bedtime the next; others do "profiles," checking four times a day twice a week. Usually we are not very interested in the levels taken within an hour or two after a meal. At these times, the sugar levels are changing rapidly, and your reading will depend on exactly what you ate and when you check. Fifteen minutes earlier or later can make a big difference. We prefer to know what the glucose levels are *going into a meal* rather than just after a meal.

In general, then, we recommend self-monitoring as often as you are willing to do it, short of becoming obsessive about testing and disrupting your life and your psyche with it. Try to develop a pattern of testing; don't do it just "every now and then." Make it a part of your routine, like brushing your teeth. Try to think of the results objectively, as free as possible of emotion-laden terms. Perpetually judging yourself only causes aggravation: "Oh, I'm awful today" or "Gee, I must have been really bad, but I don't even know what I did." The objective approach will be easier to maintain if you think in terms of *action:* "Well, if I'm high, I'd better take a little longer walk tonight" or "That 65 isn't making me feel bad now, but it's getting pretty close. Tomorrow, I'll eat a bigger lunch."

Doctor's office blood glucose testing. We attach little importance to testing the blood sugar in the office. Office testing may be useful in checking your meter to make sure that it's not way out of range. And if you have very stable diabetes, it may be a way to get a quick look at control. But, to return to our earlier example, it's like looking at the speedometer on your car only once a month or so. It won't tell you a whole lot about how fast you drive.

Glycated hemoglobin (hemoglobin A1c or glycosylated hemoglobin). We find it very useful to perform this test of long-term control about every three to six months. It is a true validation of whatever other testing you do, showing your overall blood glucose. If your doctor hasn't been testing the glycated hemoglobin, you may want to find out why, and then ask that it be done. It is a part of regular diabetes care.

Fructosamine. Because it provides information that is very similar to the information from glycated hemoglobin, but with coverage for a shorter period, this test is optional. It can be done as often as every month or so. We don't use it much for our patients.

Urine glucose testing. This is the poor and distant relative of blood glucose testing. Check the urine if you want to, but we don't recommend that you rely on the results.

Urine ketone testing. Check urine ketones when you are sick, when your blood sugar is running unusually high, or when you think for any other reason that you may be in trouble. Urine ketone testing is the way to find out whether you are on the road to ketoacidosis—a road you definitely do not want to travel.

Remember that feeling good day to day, being free of symptoms, is only the first goal of diabetes treatment. The second goal is to stay free of long-term complications. This requires keeping your blood glucose levels in a pretty good range most of the time. Just what range you can target, what goals you should strive for, were discussed in Chapter 3. But you'll never know if you don't look. Testing is like looking at the speedometer of the car, so you can hit the brakes or the accelerator as needed.

Fortunately, the options for monitoring are much better than they were some years ago. Blood glucose monitoring may be the most important advance in diabetes care in 50 years. In the near future monitoring is likely to become even easier and may not require the finger stick. But take advantage of what is available today, so you can use what comes along tomorrow. The ability to monitor blood glucose is a boon to people with diabetes.

Chapter 5

Hypoglycemia

- *"When I go low I don't have any control over anything—what I'm doing or saying or whatever's going on around me."*
- *"When I think my husband is low, I'll suggest that he test his blood. If he jumps down my throat, I know he's having a reaction."*
- *"Hypoglycemia used to come on slowly; I'd have lots of warning so I could deal with it. Now I get blindsided: one minute I'm fine and the next I'm completely out of it."*

You may know it as an *insulin reaction*, a *hypo*, a *reaction*, or simply a *low*. But by whatever name, hypoglycemia means trouble. It is by far the most common complication of insulin treatment, estimated to occur an average of once a week in people taking insulin. For many people, mild hypoglycemia is much more common even than that. Most hypoglycemia is fairly mild, but it can be serious enough to cause coma or seizure. More common in people with Type I diabetes, hypoglycemia can also occur in people with Type II diabetes who take insulin or pills.

Hypoglycemia is always unpleasant. It can interfere with your thinking, making normal activities—such as driving a car, riding a bicycle, or operating machinery—dangerous or impossible. Fear of hypoglycemia can cause a person to maintain high blood sugar levels all the time, increasing the risk for long-term complications. Finally, hypoglycemia that causes antagonistic behavior or results in a medical emergency is not just a momentary problem. It can affect family relationships, friendships, or even employment.

In this chapter we will describe the symptoms of different levels of hypoglycemia. We will identify common causes of hypoglycemia and discuss more fully the potential consequences of low blood sugars. Then we will review the steps for avoiding, recognizing, and treating hypoglycemia, including suggestions for family members and friends who must deal with a loved one's hypoglycemia.

But first, a definition. Technically, on laboratory reports, hypoglycemia often is defined as a blood sugar level below 60 mg/dl. We resist the notion of defining hypoglycemia solely by a specific blood glucose level, however, because the clinical effects of low blood sugar occur at very different levels from person to person. Instead, we define hypoglycemia as a blood sugar low enough to make you *feel* or *act* hypoglycemic.

Symptoms of Hypoglycemia

The common symptoms of hypoglycemia are quite typical, even though each person may have his or her own "personal" symptom. It is very important for everyone at risk of hypoglycemia (generally, everyone taking insulin or pills for diabetes) to know the symptoms of hypoglycemia, what they mean, and what to do about them.

Hypoglycemia causes symptoms that come and go rapidly, usually within a matter of several minutes. These symptoms fall into three categories: physical, mental, and emotional.

Physical Symptoms

The most common physical symptoms of hypoglycemia include:

—Trembling (sometimes a visible fine tremor, sometimes described as an "inner trembling")
—Lightheadedness or dizziness
—Pounding or rapid heartbeat
—Poor coordination

Less common physical symptoms of hypoglycemia include:

—Visual disturbances
—Sudden hunger
—Sudden, severe fatigue

In addition, there are what we call each person's "personal symptoms." One person will tell us he feels a tingle in his little finger, another a tickle at the back of the throat, yet another a feeling of "distance from the world." One man reported that his reliable sign of hypoglycemia was a sudden twitch in

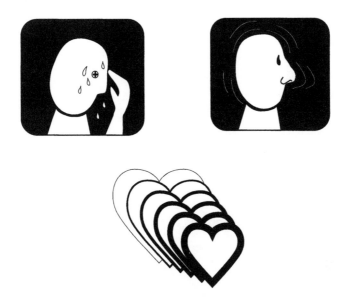

Figure 7. Hypoglycemia: adrenergic signs. For most people, when the blood sugar falls into the low range (hypoglycemia), the body will produce adrenaline—the "fight or flight" hormone. This hormone produces characteristic *adrenergic signs:* sweating, shaking, and nervousness and rapid heartbeat. The symptoms are uncomfortable, and are a clear sign that something is wrong. Action (taking a sugar) should be taken.

his left eye. He might be the only person who ever had this symptom, but it helped him know when he was hypoglycemic, and that was all that mattered.

Mental Symptoms

If your blood sugar level goes very low, you will develop the mental symptoms of hypoglycemia. These are much more serious than the physical symptoms, since at a minimum they impair your ability to think clearly, and sometimes they cause a level of confusion that keeps you from recognizing your own hypoglycemia. In the worst case, they cause coma or seizures. The mental, or "cerebral," symptoms of hypoglycemia include:

—Difficulty concentrating
—Headache
—Dizziness
—Confusion
—Slurred or slow speech

—Extreme fatigue
—Lack of coordination
—The feeling of being out of your body

Emotional Symptoms

Some people, and many spouses of people with diabetes, report that low blood sugars affect the mood. It can cause a person to feel irritable or start to "act funny." Family members often tell us that mood changes are the first sign the person is hypoglycemic. Emotional lability (sudden crying, inappropriate giggling, anger) is very commonly associated with hypoglycemia.

The Pitfalls of Using Symptoms as a Guide to Blood Sugar Levels

Unfortunately, counting on symptoms to identify hypoglycemia can be tricky and unreliable at times. First of all, people differ in their symptoms of low blood sugar. Second, many of the symptoms are so nonspecific that they are caused by any number of other situations as well as by hypoglycemia.

> *Joan, a 19-year-old college freshman with Type I diabetes, was about to go into a big exam at 10 o'clock one morning. She had taken insulin that morning but was so anxious about the test that she couldn't really remember what she had eaten for breakfast. As exam time approached, Joan's heart felt as though it were beating out of her chest. She had sweaty palms. Almost as a kneejerk reaction, she reached for the glucose tablets in her purse. But then, Joan thought, "Hey, I'd better just check, to be sure." Two minutes and one finger stick later, Joan had the answer: her blood sugar was 140 mg/dl—not low, not high, just right. The blood sugar check reassured her that her rapid heartbeat and sweaty palms were probably no more than the nervousness that all her classmates were feeling heading into this test. Even more important, it also kept Joan from taking a lot of sugar to treat a nonexistent hypoglycemic reaction. Her mind relieved, Joan did well on her exam.*

The most serious problem with counting on warning symptoms is that they may not occur until it's too late—until you are too confused to treat yourself. We discuss this situation, called *hypoglycemia unawareness,* in more detail later.

What Causes These Symptoms?

In order to keep you functioning well, your body has strong defenses against hypoglycemia. When your blood sugar goes too low, certain hormones,

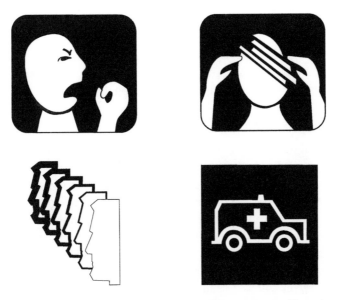

Figure 8. Hypoglycemia: neuroglycopenic signs. Other symptoms of hypoglycemia are caused by the lack of sugar to the brain. When the brain doesn't get enough sugar, the following symptoms may develop: crankiness, confusion, trouble speaking or thinking clearly, and even loss of consciousness. These are called the *neuroglycopenic signs*.

called *counterregulatory hormones,* are released that stimulate your liver to make glucose, bringing the blood glucose back to normal. In other words, the counterregulatory hormones hold the blood sugar *up,* acting in opposition to insulin (which, of course, lowers blood sugar).

Glucagon, cortisol, and *growth hormone* are all counterregulatory hormones, released in response to hypoglycemia. Another is *epinephrine,* also called *adrenaline.* Adrenaline, you'll recall, is the same hormone your body releases when you are in any stressful situation ("fight or flight"). This all makes sense, when you think about it: if you are about to enter a fight, you want lots of available fuel (glucose) in the blood, and adrenaline will raise the blood sugar. But it also means that the symptoms of hypoglycemia and the normal "adrenaline rush" in response to stress are identical, because they are caused by the same hormone—adrenaline. Joan's dilemma, discussed above, was actually that she *did* have adrenaline pouring out—she just couldn't tell, without checking her sugar, whether the adrenaline rush was due to hypoglycemia or simple stress.

The mental, or cerebral, symptoms of hypoglycemia are due to the fact that the brain needs a certain amount of glucose to function normally. When blood sugar falls too far, the incredibly complicated functions we call consciousness begin to break down. It is actually quite remarkable that almost the moment the blood sugar is brought back to normal, the brain recovers (assuming there was no severe, prolonged hypoglycemic coma).

Severity of Hypoglycemia

Insulin reactions vary in severity from a minor nuisance to a major disaster. Many people we know "feel a little low" at some point most days and simply treat the feeling with a little food. For others, insulin reactions are not a medical danger but can be a significant embarrassment—having to excuse yourself abruptly so you can go get some sugar in the middle of an important meeting, for instance. Then there are the true medical emergencies, when a person is confused or even in coma, dependent on another person for treatment.

We are often asked whether hypoglycemia can be fatal. The answer is yes, but very, very rarely. Usually, the danger is due not to the hypoglycemia itself but to what happens as a result of the hypoglycemia. These dangers include motor vehicle accidents (the number-one danger), seizures, and breathing into the lungs any fluid mistakenly given to a comatose person (called *aspiration*).

Because the range of severity of hypoglycemia varies so enormously, it is now broadly classified into three categories:

Mild hypoglycemia.   When you are mildly hypoglycemic, the symptoms are mainly physical: sweating, trembling, and so on. You can recognize them. You may notice that you aren't thinking as clearly as you usually do or that you aren't behaving quite normally, though others might not notice these subtle changes. Even mild hypoglycemia can be distressing, but most people don't find these episodes terribly upsetting.

Moderate hypoglycemia.   When you are moderately hypoglycemic you may become confused or act inappropriately, but you can still treat the low blood sugar yourself.

Severe hypoglycemia.   When you are severely hypoglycemic you are no longer able to self-treat. You are too confused to know what's going on. You may even fall into a coma or suffer a seizure.

Common Causes of Hypoglycemia and How to Prevent It

Hypoglycemia is usually caused by one or a combination of several factors: tight control, too much insulin, too little food, or too much exercise. Other, less common causes include alcohol consumption or slowed absorption of food from the stomach.

Tight Blood Sugar Control

There's no doubt about it: intensive regimens designed to keep your blood sugars as close to normal as possible do increase your risk of hypoglycemia. That's because there is a much smaller margin of safety if you are aiming for near normal blood sugar levels than if you are at higher levels. You are driving down a narrow road with plenty of curves. You have to be especially careful. The Diabetes Control and Complications Trial (DCCT) found three times as much hypoglycemia in participants who practiced "intensive" treatment.

This increased risk of hypoglycemia does not in any way mean that you should give up on good blood sugar control. It just means that you should be aware of the risk and should stay alert. Be aware of the near lows. If you always tend to run 60–75 mg/dl during the day or at night, once in a while it'll be 50 mg/dl, and you will be in trouble. Don't try to cut it too close.

There are also times when it makes sense to ease up a little on your blood sugar control. Let the situation guide you. If you have been having lots of lows, back off on your insulin dose for a few days. There will also be certain times when a low blood sugar would be so unwelcome that you might choose to run a little high: a key meeting, a long drive, an athletic event, or a camping trip.

> *We thought it was time for David to go on an "intensive" regimen, by which we meant taking Regular and NPH insulin before breakfast, Regular insulin at lunch and dinner, and NPH insulin at bedtime. David agreed, since he did not particularly mind the shots. But for the first month he found himself always on the verge of hypoglycemia at lunchtime—if he didn't eat by noon, he felt low—and again at about 4 P.M. He checked his sugar for a few days at about 11 A.M. and 4 P.M. on days when he was not actually having symptoms and found it to be between 60 and 70 mg/dl. David called us, and the insulin doses were changed. Specifically, the morning and lunchtime insulin were cut significantly. It was clear that even though the sugars he tested were not frankly low, the complete picture—an intensified regimen, quite frequent symptoms late in the morning and in mid-afternoon, and borderline sugar levels at that time—put him at risk of severe hypoglycemia if we did not change things.*

Too Much Insulin

In one sense, if you take insulin, then by definition you took too much if you become hypoglycemic. The fact that you skipped a meal, exercised more than usual, or did something else that resulted in a low might be the immediate reason why the insulin was too much. But there are certain things you should consider very carefully with regard to your insulin dose and hypoglycemia.

The most common insulin-related cause of daytime hypoglycemia is taking too much fast-acting insulin (Regular or other fast-acting preparations). Hypoglycemia overnight is usually due to too much presupper or bedtime insulin. (These issues are discussed in Chapter 12.) But bear in mind that we don't like to think of an insulin dose as one constant amount, day after day and year after year, especially when the blood sugar control is at all unstable. Frequent hypoglycemia, or a pattern of hypoglycemia at one time of day, should prompt you to talk with your health care provider about changing your insulin dose.

Hypoglycemia may also be the result of erratic or altered absorption of insulin. Sometimes you can control this—for example, by picking a nice fleshy spot to inject rather than a hard, tough area of the skin. But unpredictability of insulin absorption is not entirely controllable. Especially if you actively exercise a part of your body in which you have just injected insulin, the more rapid absorption may trigger hypoglycemia.

If you have switched from an old bottle of insulin, which had lost some of its potency, to a new bottle, taking the same dose may lead to a low blood sugar. Using more purified insulin or switching from mixed species to single-species or human insulin may also lead to lower blood sugars.

If you vary your dose of insulin according to your blood sugar (*sliding scale*), think clearly about whether your lows follow overtreatment of highs or too much insulin when you are in a good range.

> *George was told to take 6 units of Regular insulin before breakfast if his blood sugar is under 100 mg/dl, 9 units if 100–200 mg/dl, and 12 units if he is over 200 mg/dl. He finds that the 12 units work, bringing him down to a reasonable range by noon, but that if he takes 6 units when he's under 100 mg/dl, he is sure to be symptomatically low by 11 A.M. Solution? Cut down the low end of his scale, taking only 3 units if under 100 mg/dl.*

> *Tammy, on the other hand, when given the same sliding scale for her insulin doses, finds she goes low when she takes 12 units, even if she is over 200 mg/dl.*

Solution? Cut down the upper end of her scale, so that she never takes more than 10 units.

Too Little Food

Skipping meals, delaying meals, or eating meals with insufficient amounts of carbohydrate can result in hypoglycemia. Most people with Type I diabetes learn that they may go low even if a meal is late. People are at special risk for hypoglycemia if they wake up, take their insulin, and then go back to sleep without eating. The level of risk depends to a large extent on how unstable your sugars are in general. But most people who take insulin learn to be aware of the timing of their meals.

Too Much Activity

Unplanned physical activity and prolonged or high-intensity activity can also make you hypoglycemic. As we discuss more fully in Chapter 10, the hypo-glycemic effect of exercise can be immediate or delayed. It may last for as long as 24 hours. So if you are planning to exercise, test your blood first. If there is a reasonable chance you will go low during your activity, eat something before you start. Always have a source of fast-acting carbohydrate available when you exercise, in case you start to become hypoglycemic.

Alcohol

One of the less common causes of low blood sugar is drinking alcoholic beverages (even as little as 2–3 ounces). Alcohol suppresses glucose release from the liver and in this way increases the risk of hypoglycemia. If you are planning to drink alcohol, have something to eat first. That way you won't be depending on the glucose reserves in your liver to protect you from hypoglycemia. Remember also that some symptoms of hypoglycemia, such as confusion and slurred speech, can easily be mistaken for drunken behavior. People have ended up in jail for inebriation when in fact they were hypoglycemic. So please be careful not to drink in excess: it's too much of a risk for a person with diabetes.

Oral Hypoglycemic Agents

We have so far talked almost exclusively about hypoglycemia due to insulin. But what if you don't take insulin? What if you only take pills for diabetes? They can be a problem, too. The longest acting pill, chlorpropamide, is the most notorious for causing hypoglycemia. The fact is, though, that hypoglycemia is much less common from the pills than from insulin.

Other Medications

Drugs such as the beta blocker propranolol may mask some of the counter-regulatory warning signs of low blood sugar and predispose a person to severe hypoglycemia. If you are taking a medication that masks symptoms of hypoglycemia, you may need to test your blood sugar more often or pay closer attention to other signs to keep you out of trouble.

Menstrual Cycle

Insulin requirements can fluctuate with the phases of a woman's menstrual cycle. For a few days before a period begins, insulin needs may increase; they may then drop dramatically when the flow starts. These fluctuations are probably the result of hormonal shifts: just before the menstrual flow begins, a woman's body secretes increased amounts of progesterone (another counterregulatory hormone). Once the period begins, progesterone levels go down again.

If you notice that your blood sugars tend to fluctuate with the phases of your menstrual cycle, you should keep very close track of the pattern. That way, you can raise and lower your insulin levels at the earliest possible moment and avoid high blood sugars just before your period and low blood sugars once your flow starts.

Gastroparesis

A form of diabetic nerve damage called *gastroparesis* delays the emptying of the contents of a meal from the stomach into the intestines. If you have this complication, your food will be absorbed more slowly, and any insulin you have injected may get into your system faster than the food. This increases your risk of hypoglycemia.

Gastroparesis is not common, but it can cause havoc with blood sugar control. If you have this complication, try to work out an insulin regimen with your health care professional that takes into account the slower rate at which you absorb the food you eat.

Hypoglycemia Unawareness

The key to managing your own hypoglycemia without undue problem is to be aware of your own symptoms and pay close attention to them. But what if you don't have symptoms anymore? What if you are completely unaware that you are getting low until you become confused, disoriented, and unable to care for yourself? This is called *hypoglycemia unawareness*.

Hypoglycemia unawareness usually develops after many years (generally more than 15–20) of diabetes. In mild forms, people will just notice that the insulin reactions "sneak up" on them with less warning than before. There may be recognizable symptoms, such as dizziness, lack of coordination, tiredness, visual disturbance, and difficulty concentrating. But if you *start* with confusion, you may not be able to treat your own hypoglycemia. It may progress to the point where there really are no symptoms at all before total confusion sets in.

The condition of hypoglycemia unawareness is considered to be due to nerve damage (neuropathy), which blunts the usual nerve-stimulated release of adrenalin. With defective glucose counterregulation, you may no longer have such symptoms of hypoglycemia as sweatiness, pounding heart, trembling, and nervousness, which are triggered by the release of adrenalin. You may have only the mental (cerebral) signs, due to your brain not getting enough glucose.

The treatment for hypoglycemia unawareness involves rigorously avoiding low blood sugars for a period of days or weeks. This seems to rejuvenate some of the ability to detect hypoglycemia.

Blood Glucose Awareness Training

A recently developed technique called blood glucose awareness training (BGAT) holds promise for people who are not good at recognizing when they are going low. In essence, BGAT teaches people to increase their ability to avoid, detect, and rapidly treat hypoglycemia, using internal and external cues, such as the ones we have discussed. The internal cues for BGAT include physical symptoms, performance cues, and moods and feelings. Typical of the external cues are the combinatin of insulin dose, time of day, and last blood sugar reading or the combination of food intake, time, exercise, and last blood sugar reading.

The results of BGAT research are impressive. People who completed the training program improved their ability to detect low and high blood sugar levels and had fewer low blood sugars, fewer episodes of nighttime hypoglycemia, fewer automobile accidents, fewer traffic violations, and no deterioration in long-term blood sugar control.

Treating Hypoglycemia

Since anyone taking insulin or even hypoglycemic pills is at risk of hypoglycemia, you should by all means know how to treat it. In theory, treatment is simple: at the earliest sign, you should quickly take in some food. In reality, many people get themselves in trouble by either undertreating or overtreating.

All too often, people ignore the early warning signs of hypoglycemia or tell themselves they can hold out another 10 minutes (or 30 or 60 minutes). This mistake can lead to a severe reaction or at least a more severe reaction. The answer, of course, is to *treat early symptoms immediately.* Don't be caught anywhere without fast access to quickly absorbed carbohydrate. Always be prepared for hypoglycemia. Have glucose tablets or other reaction antidotes in your pocket or purse, in your car, at your office, and by your bed at night.

Overtreating is also a common problem. In the midst of an insulin reaction, there is an almost irresistible urge to eat everything in sight. The result can easily be to careen from too low right up to too high. You may then take more insulin to bring the sugar back down, and off you go on a roller-coaster ride of too low–too high–too low.

There are a few things you can do to avoid overtreatment of lows. First, remember that it will take a few minutes (often 15–20 minutes) for anything you eat or drink to be absorbed through the stomach and raise your blood sugar. So eating continuously until the sugar comes up does not help. You might be able to curb the tendency to overtreat if you prepare your "hypoglycemia first aid package" in advance. Set out exactly the right carbohydrate in the right proportion to treat your insulin reactions (usually 10–15 grams of carbohydrate; see below). You may use commercially prepared glucose tablets and gels, which are less appetizing than many foods, so you are less likely to overuse them. Or you may pack just enough food to do the job. You might also consider the approach one of our patients uses. As she waits for the food she has eaten to bring her blood sugars back up, she repeats to herself, "You took the right amount. Just wait until it works. You'll feel fine in a few minutes." She tells us that this simple, reassuring message really works to keep her from overtreating.

Specific Suggestions to Treat Hypoglycemia

Mild and even some moderate hypoglycemia can be treated with 10–15 grams of fast-acting carbohydrate. Some examples are:

—2 or 3 glucose tablets (5 grams each)
—$\frac{1}{3}$–$\frac{1}{2}$ of a 30-gram tube of glucose gel
—4–6 ounces of orange juice
—4–6 ounces of regular soda
—$\frac{1}{4}$–$\frac{1}{3}$ cup of raisins
—5 Lifesavers candies

Repeat this treatment in 15–30 minutes if your low hypoglycemic symptoms persist or if your blood sugar level is not above 60 mg/dl. Neither chocolate nor ice cream is a good choice for treating hypoglycemia because the fat they contain can reduce the rate at which your body absorbs the sugar you need.

Moderate hypoglycemia requires the same treatment as mild, though it may take more than one treatment and it may take longer for the person to fully recover.

If you are severely hypoglycemic, by definition you cannot treat yourself. That's why it's essential that your family, friends, and co-workers know what to do. It is always frightening to see someone severely hypoglycemic, especially for people who have not seen it happen before. So even if you are not especially prone to insulin reactions, it would be a good idea to rehearse with your family what to do if one should occur. It's like a fire drill: it's better to practice and be prepared, even if the fire never happens.

It is very important that *no one put anything in your mouth unless you are sitting up and able to swallow.* The consequences of trying to pour something sweet into the mouth of a semiconscious person can be tragic. Most people can be coaxed into eating or drinking something sweet, even if they are severely hypoglycemic. If not, *don't force anything into the mouth.* Call 911 or inject glucagon.

Glucagon is to be given only when the hypoglycemic person is unresponsive, so it is always given by another person, who must be trained and prepared to do the injection. Be sure glucagon is available and that a family member knows when and how to give it to you. The injection is not difficult, since it can go into any muscle. Glucagon is not glucose; it is one of the hormones, mentioned earlier, that cause the liver to release glucose into the bloodstream.

Glucagon is safe to use and is available by prescription. When stored in the refrigerator, it is good for several years. Since you probably won't need it very often, be sure to check the expiration date now and then, and periodically review the instructions for administering glucagon with the person or people who might be doing the injection. Here are some guidelines for using glucagon:

—Make sure the person administering the glucagon knows to call for emergency assistance if you don't respond to treatment within 15–30 minutes.

—Your stomach may be upset after you have received glucagon; you may even vomit.

—As soon as you are alert and able to swallow, you should be offered something light, such as soda or crackers. Eating will restore the glucose supply in your liver.

—As soon as you are able to hold down food, you should eat something more substantial, such as a sandwich or some milk.

—If nausea persists, follow your plan for sick days and contact your health care provider.

Finally, in preparing to manage severe hypoglycemia, make sure everyone in your family, even children as young as four years old, knows how to call 911 if you become unconscious or are otherwise unable to care for yourself. We know of cases in which preschoolers have saved their parents from serious hypoglycemic peril by calling for emergency assistance.

When you are away from home, always wear a medical alert identification bracelet or necklace or carry an identification card to advise anyone coming to your aid that you have diabetes and take insulin.

Nighttime Hypoglycemia

More than half of all episodes of severe hypoglycemia occur during the night. This is the most dangerous time to go low, because you're asleep and not aware enough to treat the condition immediately. In addition, the insulin requirements of most people are lowest (often 20–30% lower than at other times) in the middle of the night. Finally, NPH or Lente insulin taken at dinner often peaks at this time. To avoid nighttime hypoglycemia, test your blood before you go to bed, and eat a snack if the reading is less than 120 mg/dl, especially if you were unusually active during the day. It's also a good idea to check your predawn blood sugar levels from time to time.

For Family and Friends

You are probably already aware that low blood sugar causes changes in behavior. Often, it starts with just a little change in the person's voice or speech pattern or a look in the eye that only you are aware of. Your family member may become negative, stubborn, irritable, or even verbally or physically abusive. Severe hypoglycemia may make the person disoriented, causing him or her to bump into things, aimlessly pick things up and put them down, or just sit and stare into space.

When you see this happening, try to keep two things in mind: first, you are probably right that it is hypoglycemia; second, like it or not, you are the person on the spot with a clear head, responsible for doing the right thing. The hypoglycemic person is really out of control.

It is often difficult to convince a person who is mentally confused or emotionally charged to treat his or her low blood sugar. He or she may refuse to cooperate or may even fight you, stoutly maintaining that there's no problem, telling you to mind your own business. But you have to trust your own instincts. At the very worst, treating with something sweet won't hurt. So have a plan and the means for treatment.

Dealing with the person whose emotions are spilling out can be especially trying. None of us likes to be called names, be accused of things we didn't do, or have to deal with a person emotionally out of control. The natural tendency is to fight back, to argue, to be defensive. But just keep telling yourself, "He's not himself. This is a person under the influence of hypoglycemia. He doesn't mean it." You must find a way to deal with your own feelings when this responsibility is thrust upon you. Resist the natural temptation to lash out or to walk away from the whole mess. Remember that you are the one with a normally functioning brain, so you need to use it.

Last but not least, you need to know how to administer glucagon. It's frightening to think of being responsible for giving your loved one a shot, not knowing if you will succeed in bringing him or her back to consciousness. But prompt use of glucagon can provide your loved one the fastest possible treatment. It can also allow you to avoid the trauma and expense of dealing with emergency medical personnel and hospital staff.

Hypoglycemia is inconvenient at best and frightening or even life-threatening at worst. We hope that what you've learned from this chapter will help you better avoid low blood sugars and treat them more quickly and effectively when they do occur.

Chapter 6

Introduction to Nutrition Therapy
Planning and Understanding the Diet

- *"None of my favorite foods are on the list of what I should eat. What are they thinking?"*
- *"I don't understand this concept of exchanges. Just tell me what to eat."*
- *"Now that I'm eating healthy, I feel so much better."*

Eating is a central part of life. It makes us feel comfortable, safe, and warm. No wonder, then, that when your diet becomes medicalized—when what you can eat is dictated by a medical condition—you're likely to put up some resistance. You're not the first person to think: "End my midnight snack and you end life as I've known it!"

We can't deny that to maintain your good health with diabetes, you'll need to make some changes in your way of eating. But these changes don't have to spell the end of the good life—on the contrary. Nutrition therapy means treating disease or illness at least in part through diet. The goals of nutrition therapy these days include planning a diet just for you, one that will keep you healthy *and* have you eating you the foods you like, or most of them. Your food preferences, traditions, and preferred seasonings, your ethnicity and your social patterns of eating: these are factors that a skillful nutritionist will build into your diet plan. If you add your own understanding about foods to the guidance provided by the nutritionist, you can manage your diet and your diabetes, and still enjoy your food to the fullest.

The 1994 American Diabetes Association position statement titled "Nutrition Recommendations and Principles for People with Diabetes Mellitus" stated the goals for nutrition therapy as follows:

1. Maintenance of as near normal blood glucose levels as possible by balancing food intake with insulin (your own or by injection) or oral diabetes medication and activity.
2. Achievement of optimum levels of fat in the blood (cholesterol and triglycerides) to decrease the risk of cardiovascular disease.
3. Provision of adequate calories to maintain or attain reasonable body weight for adults, to achieve normal growth and development rates of children and adolescents, to meet increased needs during pregnancy and lactation, or to recover from illness. Reasonable body weight is the level of weight that individuals and health care providers see as achievable and maintainable for both the short and long term. This is in contrast to desirable body weight, which is an ideal based on height and frame size.
4. Prevention and treatment of the acute complications of insulin-treated diabetes, such as hypoglycemia, short-term illnesses, and exercise-related problems, and of the long-term complications of diabetes.
5. Improvement of overall health through optimal nutrition.

In this and the following three chapters, we'll explain how the food you eat and when you eat it can help you feel better and achieve good control. We start here with background information, by looking at food categories: carbohydrate, fat, protein, and the "micronutrients," such as vitamins and minerals. Then, we'll talk about how to put this information together into a good, healthy diet.

What Do You Eat, and What Do You Need?

Calories, protein, fiber, chromium, monounsaturated fats, macronutrients, sugar, carbohydrates: there are so many words used to describe food, it's enough to give you indigestion! In truth, though, the terms that are used to describe what's in food aren't that hard to understand. A calorie, for example, is the energy value of food—how much energy you get when you "burn" that amount of food. The problem is that you don't always burn the calories right away, and if you consume more than you burn, the excess is stored in your body as fat. That's why calories count: too many calories and you gain weight, too few calories and you lose weight. Calories are generally found in three kinds of food: carbohydrate, fat, and protein.

Carbohydrates

Carbohydrates include such foods as pasta, potatoes, grains and cereal, and the sugar in fruit, candy, milk, and cookies. The building blocks of all carbohydrates are sugar molecules, such as glucose and fructose. When only one or two sugar molecules are held together, as in sucrose (table sugar), the result is called a *simple sugar. Complex carbohydrates,* on the other hand, are very long, branching chains of sugar molecules. They do not taste sweet, and they have to be digested in the stomach and intestine before being absorbed.

How many calories do carbohydrates have? It depends, of course, on how much carbohydrate you're talking about. But the rule is: 1 gram of carbohydrate (simple or complex) has 4 calories.

Simple sugars.   The one or two sugar molecules stuck together as simple sugars also go by the name of *concentrated sweets.* Sucrose is the most common. Its effect on the blood sugar is simple: the sucrose is easy to digest into its two sugar molecules (glucose and fructose), which are easily absorbed, and the blood glucose level goes up.

Given their sweet taste, it is not surprising that simple sugars show up all over—as table sugar and in candy bars, honey, molasses, and hard candy, for example. You also often hear about "hidden sugars," which usually means that sugar has been slipped into something like a spaghetti sauce or salad dressing to make it taste better.

When simple sugars are in the form of "fruit sugar" (mainly fructose) or sorbitol, they are digested more slowly.

Complex carbohydrates.   These are the carbohydrates that don't taste sweet: starches, pasta, cereals, breads, and so on. Because they are composed of long strings of glucose molecules, for the body to absorb them it has to digest them down to their sugar building blocks, which then pass through the wall of the intestine into the blood.

Are carbohydrates good or bad?   Many people think that carbohydrates are fattening. Even the innocent baked potato has gotten a bad rap! With only 4 calories per gram (as compared to 9 calories per gram of fat), carbohydrates are a pretty good deal in the energy equation. It's the fat that's often loaded on top of the carbohydrate (butter and sour cream on the baked potato, cream or meat sauce on the pasta) that can do you in.

Carbohydrates do make the blood sugar rise after a meal, but this is normal, and the right amount of insulin brings it back down. It is just plain wrong, then, to think of carbohydrates as a forbidden food. The cells of the body, with the help of insulin, easily burn glucose for energy. Current recommendations are for 50%–60% of our dietary calories to be in the form of carbohydrate, although there is controversy about this. Some specialists think that there should be less carbohydrate in the diet, in the range of 35%, with more monounsaturated fat. Their logic is that eating less carbohydrate may reduce blood triglyceride levels. At present, however, this is a minority view. We'll go with the 50%–60% carbohydrate diet, unless individual circumstances, such as high triglyceride levels, dictate otherwise.

Since insulin, either from the pancreas or by injection, is needed for the body to utilize carbohydrate, people who depend entirely on insulin by injection often do better when they learn to measure the amount of their carbohydrate intake precisely. This approach, called carbohydrate counting, is discussed in Chapter 8, since it applies most often to people with Type I diabetes.

What about sugar (I'm talking sweets)?　In 1994 the American Diabetes Association went out on a limb. It issued a report that emphasized all sorts of important and well-proven dietary recommendations, stressing individualization of the diet to the person. But a small comment slipped in, allowing people some concentrated sweets. Predictably, the press picked up this little tidbit, and many people with diabetes were led to believe that after all these years, it was now okay to eat sweets. At the risk of being spoilsports, we beg to differ. Here's the story.

Several careful studies on hospitalized subjects showed that, gram for gram, there isn't much difference between the blood sugar rise from complex carbohydrates and the blood sugar rise from simple sugars. In other words, 20 grams of carbohydrate from pasta might raise the blood sugar about the same amount as 20 grams of table sugar. But (and here's the kicker) people tend not to eat the same number of grams of concentrated sugar as they do of complex carbohydrate. When you get into candies and pies, you usually eat a lot more grams of carbohydrate than you would with pasta or potatoes. For example, one fast-food milkshake and three medium-sized baked potatoes each contain about 60 grams of carbohydrate, and one nondiet soda and about two cups of cooked spaghetti each contain about 40 grams of carbohydrate.

Get the picture? You are a lot more likely to order a small shake or a soft drink than three baked potatoes or two cups of spaghetti. And your blood sugar will show the difference, unless you take just the right amount of insulin to cover the large carbohydrate load. "So," you say, "I'll take the right amount of insulin to cover the sweet." And we say, "Okay, do that—if you can figure it out." If you check your blood sugar and it is in an acceptable range, terrific. But do you know exactly how much sugar is in this candy bar or that one, this piece of pie or that one, this doughnut or that one? Almost certainly not. It isn't easy to tell.

There are other problems with concentrated sweets: they are usually highly caloric, so will tend to put weight on you; they don't provide any of the important nutrients (that's why they're referred to as "empty calories"); and, of course, they are bad for the teeth. The upshot is that we don't have a problem with your eating an occasional cookie or scoop of ice cream, if it means a lot to you and you can make a reasonable adjustment in your insulin dose if you take insulin. Or you could use the sweets as exchanges allowed in a meal plan, trading them off for other foods. You could, for instance, have $\frac{1}{2}$ cup of sweetened cereal instead of $\frac{3}{4}$ cup of unsweetened cereal. But we strongly recommend that you fight off the notion that you have a "sweet tooth" that depends on a constant flow of sugars, because your blood glucose control will suffer. We would much prefer that you learn to love diet drinks, fruits, and other nonsugary foods. It'll pay off in the long run.

Fat

Fat on your waistline, fat in your french fries, fat in your blood: it's hard to find much good to say about fat. Yet fatness is sometimes considered a sign of prosperity; it's by far the most efficient way for the body to store calories; and, at least for primitive human beings, it was a lifesaver. In times of plenty, when there is lots to eat and lots of insulin to burn the carbohydrate ingested, the body stores away the extra calories as fat. When the famine comes, insulin levels in the body drop, and all that fat becomes the main energy source.

The natural purpose of fat, then, is to store calories efficiently. But in an overfed society, storing fat is not much of a benefit. In fact, too much body fat carries definite risks, chiefly an increased risk of Type II diabetes. Too much fat in the blood, of course, is also a risk for heart disease and hardening of the arteries. So we are back where we started: there's not much good to be said for lots of fat.

What is fat?   Technically, fat is the class of chemicals that don't mix with water. Dietary fat is found in particularly tender beef and other meats, dairy foods, oils, butter and margarine, fried foods, bacon, nuts, and seeds. There are two important kinds of fat in the diet, the blood, and body fat: triglyceride and cholesterol. Triglycerides make up the majority of the fat we eat, as well as the fat in our bodies; these are the fats in a steak or in bacon, in oils and in dairy products. You probably eat between 40 and 100 grams of fat a day. Cholesterol, found especially in egg yolks and organ meats, comes in much smaller amounts; you eat perhaps half a gram of cholesterol a day.

Cholesterol in the blood has a lot to do with hardening of the arteries. But just like sugar (which comes both from the carbohydrates you eat and from the liver), blood cholesterol does not all come from the diet: the liver also makes cholesterol. To complicate the issue, there's the "good cholesterol" (HDL cholesterol), high blood levels of which *protect against* hardening of the arteries, and there's the "bad cholesterol" (LDL cholesterol), high levels of which *cause* hardening of the arteries.

Triglyceride also comes in various forms, generally called *saturated, monounsaturated,* and *polyunsaturated.* You probably already know that saturated fat (found in butter, lard, and fatty meats) is the bad stuff and that unsaturated fat (found in olive oil, margarine, and vegetable oils, for example) is good for you. It has been known since the 1950s that eating a lot of saturated fat increases the blood cholesterol level, while eating unsaturated fat lowers cholesterol, although it's still not known why this is so. It *is* known that having a low proportion of saturated fat in your diet will help keep your blood cholesterol low.

Monounsaturated fat does not raise cholesterol levels. Found primarily in olive oil and canola oil, it is a preferred form of fat. Polyunsaturated fat, found in safflower oil and other soft fats and oils, lowers cholesterol but has in recent years gone out of favor because it may lower HDL cholesterol, too. Dietary fat guidelines are summarized in Table 6. Remember that there are nine calories in a gram of fat, more than twice as many as in a gram of carbohydrate or protein.

Table 6. Recommended Intake of Fat

Type of Fat	Recommended Intake
Total fat	Less than 30% of total calories
Polyunsaturated	Up to 10%; preferably 6%–8% of total calories
Saturated	Less than 10% of total calories
Monosaturated	10%–15% of total calories
Cholesterol	Less than 300 mg per day

Does fat affect the blood sugar?   The answer is no. Eating a pure fat meal does not increase or decrease blood sugar. But dietary fat has an indirect effect on blood glucose. Because it takes some time to be digested, it will delay the glucose rise from the carbohydrate components of the meal. This means that if a portion of bread would cause the blood sugar to rise to a peak, say, 45 minutes after eating, the peak would be delayed to about 60 minutes if the bread were eaten with significant amounts of fat. We don't think of this as a very important effect. We think that dietary fat can strongly affect your total calorie intake, your waistline, and your blood cholesterol level; its effect on blood sugar is small.

The preferred oils are canola and olive, because of their high monounsaturated fat content. When selecting margarines, check to see that the first ingredient is liquid canola, corn, safflower, soybean, or sunflower oil and that saturated fat is less than 1–2 grams per tablespoon. Reduced calorie or "light" salad dressings definitely require close inspection. They differ greatly in caloric value and often have increased amounts of sodium. Sugar, corn syrup, or other forms of sugar or starch may be added. Each product must be individually evaluated.

Protein

The days are long gone when protein was considered a muscle-building, power-giving, pregame performance enhancer. To be sure, some protein in the diet is necessary, and protein deficiency is a serious problem in undernourished people living in developing countries. But, as with fat, in the overfed populations of prosperous nations, there is more than enough protein in the average diet to meet nutritional needs.

Protein contains 4 calories per gram and is a large component of such foods as seafood, chicken, turkey, beef, milk, pork, egg whites, peanut butter, and legumes. Egg whites, for instance, are almost entirely protein. In contrast, a medium-fat hamburger may contain about 88 calories as protein but 130 calories as fat.

The human digestive system breaks protein down into its building blocks, called amino acids. These are absorbed, providing nitrogen to the body. The amino acids are also, to some extent, converted to glucose. Therefore, protein will raise the glucose level—but not much and not quickly.

For adults with diabetes, 10%–20% of the total daily caloric intake should be in the form of protein (roughly 36–90 grams, depending on the number of calories consumed). There is some evidence that excessive protein intake accelerates the progression of kidney disease in diabetes, so when someone has nephropathy, dietary protein is usually restricted to between 7% and 10% of total calories, or 0.8 gram per kilogram body weight. Protein requirements are increased during childhood and adolescence, during pregnancy, and in physical conditioning with exercise. Higher protein intake is also recommended in cases when tissue breakdown is likely to occur, such as after surgery, in the elderly, and during weight-loss diets.

Micronutrients

These are the things you eat that don't add significant calories but are nevertheless important parts of a normal diet. Examples of micronutrients are vitamins and minerals, including iron, sodium, calcium, chromium, magnesium, and the so-called antioxidants.

Vitamins.   Vitamins have been known to be essential parts of the diet at least since the late eighteenth century, when British sailors in the 1770s learned to avoid scurvy by taking a good supply of sauerkraut, and later on, citrus fruit, on long voyages as a source of vitamin C. But vitamins are needed in only very small amounts to avoid the specific diseases caused by vitamin deficiency. And these trace amounts of all the vitamins are found in the foods that make up a normal, balanced diet. Believe us, you will not suffer from vitamin deficiency diseases if you eat a normal American diet.

Where, then, did all the vitamin hype come from? In some cases, it is just that—hype without scientific evidence. In a few cases, there is some evidence that amounts higher than the minimum requirement may be beneficial. For example, vitamin C is a powerful antioxidant, and some studies have suggested that the symptoms of colds may be reduced by taking extra Vitamin C. In pregnancy, with its special nutritional demands, a single daily multivitamin pill is usually recommended.

Do high-dose vitamins (so-called megavitamins) provide any health benefits? Our answer is to be cautiously noncommittal. We just don't know of any good evidence showing that high-dose vitamins do any good, and we do know that very high doses can sometimes do harm. So, provided the high doses are not extreme, we won't discourage people from taking vitamin tablets daily, but we can't say that there is much benefit.

Iron.   The body needs iron, particularly for the formation of hemoglobin in red blood cells. Through blood loss, some people, especially women with heavy menstrual periods, can easily become iron deficient and anemic. It's relatively simple to determine with laboratory tests whether your iron level is normal, so if any doubt exists, a few tests should tell you if you need iron supplements. Again, in pregnancy, iron pills are essential.

Sodium.   Sodium is one of the micronutrients that Americans seem to have no trouble getting enough of—even too much of—in the form of salt. The minimum sodium needed for the body is only 220 mg per day, while the typical intake is 4,000–8,000 mg per day and the recommendation is that sodium be restricted to less than 3,000 mg per day. (One teaspoon of salt contains about 2,300 mg of sodium.) The recommendation is made because sodium can cause the body to retain water, and in people who tend to have high blood pressure, it will worsen that tendency.

While many people just urinate out any excess sodium they take in, it is not unusual for fluid retention or high blood pressure to be worsened by salt intake. So be sure to cut down your salt intake if you have hypertension; otherwise, consider getting in the habit of not ingesting too much salt. In rare cases, some people actually need a high sodium intake, if they have low blood pressure associated with dizziness.

Calcium.   Calcium is an essential nutrient and is usually present in adequate amounts in a normal diet. It is found in foods like dairy products and leafy vegetables. A person who is on a "tea and toast" diet may not take in enough calcium, and anyone who is prone to osteoporosis (thinning of the bones) should be sure to get enough calcium. A supplement is a good idea if there's doubt about the adequacy of your intake.

Chromium.   Not a week goes by where we don't have at least one question about chromium and glucose control. The question stems from the observation that in animals who were purposely fed diets deficient in chromium, blood sugar control suffered and then improved with replacement. However, chromium supplementation in persons with diabetes has not resulted in improved control. This suggests that most people with diabetes do not have a chromium deficiency, and we believe there is no benefit from routinely taking a chromium supplement.

Magnesium.   Magnesium deficiency can be part of an unusual but vicious cycle. Poor control of diabetes can lead to magnesium deficiency, and magnesium deficiency can lead to insulin insensitivity. In people with a documented deficiency, magnesium supplements may improve control.

Antioxidants.   You may have heard that antioxidants are considered to protect against a variety of diseases. For example, the common antioxidants vitamins C, E, and A (beta carotene) have been thought to protect against heart disease. Should you be taking them as supplements? The short answer is that the jury is still out. Studies on animals show that these antioxidants inhibit the oxidation of LDL cholesterol and can slow the progression of atherosclerotic disease. In humans, this has not been proven. Two large randomized trials recently failed to show any benefit of beta carotene and even suggested that among smokers it may be dangerous. Evidence is lacking to recommend antioxidants to everyone. But consider that vitamin E is found in vegetable oils and cereal grains; vitamin C is found in many fresh fruits and vegetables; and beta carotene is found in carrots, winter squash, broccoli, and many green leafy vegetables. To us, this sounds like another good argument for a healthy, well-balanced diet.

Fiber.   Fiber is the indigestible carbohydrate that comes primarily from plant cell walls. There are two kinds of fiber, water-insoluble and water-soluble. Water-insoluble fiber is found in whole wheat products, wheat bran, and fruit and vegetable skins. Its action is in the large bowel, where it draws water into the feces. This type of fiber is helpful for constipation, diverticulosis, and irritable bowel syndrome. It may also prevent colon cancer.

Water-soluble fiber is found in fruits, vegetables, oats, beans, and peas. There is evidence that large amounts of soluble fiber have a beneficial effect on fat levels in the bloodstream.

Sweeteners.   The sweeteners, of course, give a good taste to food. But you have to be careful, because there are two very different kinds of sweeteners: those that contain calories (nutritive) and those that do not (nonnutritive).

Table sugar, called sucrose (discussed above), is the classic caloric sweetener and, in our opinion, one to avoid. You may think that if you choose a "more natural" sweetener, such as unrefined sugar, honey, fruit juice, or molasses, you're doing yourself a favor. But it doesn't work that way. There is no evidence that these sweeteners offer any advantage over sucrose when it comes to calories and blood sugar control. They are not "freebies." Other sweeteners that are just about the same as table sugar are corn syrup, dextrose, and maltose. See Table 7 for a list of other sweeteners.

Fructose seems to cause less of a rise in blood glucose than sucrose, but there is some evidence that if taken in large quantities, it may raise LDL cholesterol levels. There is no reason to avoid fruits and vegetables in which fructose occurs naturally.

Consuming the sugars sorbitol, mannitol, and xylitol may result in lower and slower glucose and insulin rises than consuming glucose or sucrose. However, these sugars are high in calories and may cause cramping and diarrhea if taken in large amounts.

In marked contrast to the nutritive, caloric sweeteners, the nonnutritive

Table 7. Sweeteners

Acesulfame K	A noncaloric sweetener 200 times as sweet as sucrose. Acesulfame K can be used in baking and cooking.
Aspartame	A protein sweetener 180 times as sweet as sucrose. Now available for consumer use in the United States. Technically, aspartame is caloric; however, it is so sweet that the amount used per serving of food is likely to supply almost no calories.
Carob powder (carob flour)	Produced by grinding the pod of the carob tree. Tastes similar to chocolate. 75% is made up of sucrose, glucose, and fructose, which are all caloric.
Cyclamates	*Noncaloric* sweeteners approximately 30 times as sweet as sucrose. Cyclamates were banned from use in the United States in 1970 because of questions about their possible cancer- and tumor-causing properties. They are still used in some foreign countries, and the risk associated with moderate use is considered by many to be very small.
Dextrin	Chains of glucose molecules. Their effect on blood sugar has not been well evaluated, but may be similar to glucose. Caloric.
Dulcitol	A sugar alcohol. Caloric.
Fructose (fruit sugar, levulose)	One of the most common naturally occurring sugars, particularly found in fruit and honey. Half of table sugar is fructose. Fructose is not associated with a rapid and high rise in blood sugar in well-controlled diabetes. The sweetness of pure fructose varies, but under certain conditions it can be almost twice as sweet as sucrose. Caloric.
Glucose (corn sugar, dextrose, grape sugar)	A naturally occurring sugar that normally causes a fast and high rise in blood sugar. About half as sweet as table sugar. Carbohydrates (starches) break down to glucose during digestion, as do all sugars eventually. Glucose is the form of sugar that the body uses for energy and other purposes, and it builds up in the blood if diabetes is poorly controlled. *Dextrose* is the commercial name for glucose and will often be seen on food labels, including those of some sugar substitutes. Caloric.

Glucose syrups (corn syrup, corn syrup solids, sorghum syrup, starch syrup, sugar cane syrup)	Liquid sweeteners produced by the breakdown (hydrolyzation) of starch. They contain a mixture of glucose, maltose, and longer chains of glucose molecules and can be produced from a variety of starches (hence, the varied names). *Corn syrup solids* are the crystallized form of corn syrup. Caloric.
High fructose corn syrups	Produced from corn syrups. They contain differing amounts of fructose, ranging from 42% to 90%. The remaining part of the syrup is primarily glucose. The effect of the highly refined type (90% fructose) on blood sugar has not been well evaluated, but, theoretically, it should not cause high and fast rises of blood sugar in people whose diabetes is well controlled. The 90% type is the only one that might prove to be an acceptable sweetener for people with diabetes. Caloric.
Honey (comb honey, creamed honey)	A natural syrup that varies in sugar and flavor depending on many factors. It is primarily glucose (about 35%), fructose (about 40%), and water, and, by weight, is about 75% as sweet as sucrose. Additional glucose is sometimes added to some honeys. Caloric.
Lactose	Milk sugar. It comprises about 4.5% of cow milk. About 30% sweet as sucrose. Caloric.
Maltose	Two glucose units linked together. It is only 30%–50% as sweet as sucrose. Caloric.
Mannitol	A naturally occurring sugar alcohol that causes less of a rise in blood sugar than sucrose or glucose. It is about half as sweet as sucrose and is slowly absorbed into the blood. In large amounts, it can cause diarrhea. Caloric.
Maple syrup (maple sugar)	Made from the sap of the maple and other trees. It is mostly sucrose with some invert sugar (see sucrose) and trace amounts of other compounds. The crystallized syrup is *maple sugar*. Caloric.
Milk chocolate (bitter chocolate, bittersweet chocolate)	Produced by the addition of milk, sugar, and cocoa butter to bitter chocolate. *Milk chocolate* is approximately 43% sugar and *bittersweet chocolate* is about 40% sugar. The sugar is caloric.
Molasses (blackstrap, golden syrup, refiners' syrup, treacle, unsulfured)	The sugar drawn from sugar crystals as they are refined into pure sucrose. Different types are usually produced during sucrose refinement. All types, however, contain 50%–75% sugar (sucrose and invert sugar) and should be avoided by those with diabetes. The sugars are caloric.

(continued)

Table 7. *(continued)*

Saccharin	One currently used *noncaloric* sweetener in the United States. It is about 375 times as sweet as sucrose.
Sorbitol	A naturally occurring sugar alcohol found in many plants; commercially produced for glucose. It is about half as sweet as sucrose and more slowly absorbed than glucose. In individuals whose diabetes is well controlled, it causes only a small postmeal rise in blood sugar. In large amounts it may cause cramping and diarrhea. It is widely used in the manufacture of dietetic foods and dietetic hard candies. Caloric.
Sucrose (beet sugar, brown sugar, cane sugar, confectioner's sugar, invert sugar, powdered sugar, raw sugar, saccharose sugar, sugar, table sugar, turbinado)	A naturally occurring sugar that is composed of equal parts of glucose and fructose linked together. It is produced from sugar cane or sugar beets. *Invert sugar* is made of sucrose that has been broken down to equal parts of glucose and fructose (with some fructose left intact). *Brown sugars, raw sugar,* and *turbinado* do all contain some molasses.
Sweetened condensed whole milk (sweetened condensed skim milk, sweetened condensed whey)	Produced by reducing the water content of milk by about half and adding sugar. The finished product is about 44% sucrose, which is caloric. This means a 14-oz can of condensed whole milk contains the equivalent of 8 tablespoons of sugar and 2½ cups of milk.
Xylitol	A naturally occurring sugar alcohol produced by xylose (bark sugar). It is slowly absorbed and causes less of a rise in blood sugar than does sucrose or glucose. Depending on how it is used, it is as sweet or less sweet than sucrose. Studies show it to be less cavity-inducing than other sugars. Like sorbitol, large amounts may cause diarrhea. This amount varies. In children, it may be as little as 5–10 grams. (One piece of hard candy can have about 3 grams of sugar alcohol.) Caloric.

SOURCE: "Alias Sugar," advanced information series, American Diabetes Association.

sweeteners—saccharin, aspartame, and acesulfame K—have no calories and no effect on the blood sugar level. They are therefore considered "free": you may eat and drink as much as you want of them (within reason, of course). They are approved by the Food and Drug Administration and are considered safe for use.

Drinking diet drinks with aspartame (Nutrasweet) is no worse than drinking water, if the labels say the drinks have zero calories. So go for it! We would even suggest that you keep trying different brands until you find one you really like.

Summary of Food Components

Nutrition may seem a complicated science, but if you concentrate on it for a while, you very quickly learn to distinguish a carbohydrate from a fat, a non-nutritive sweetener from a sugar, and a micronutrient from a microchip. Still, it really helps to talk to a professional in nutrition, such as a registered dietitian. Your local chapter of the American Diabetes Association or the American Association of Diabetes Educators may be able to provide some recommendations about a qualified professional in your area, or you can call the American Dietetic Association.

Dietary Recommendations: General Guidelines

In the next three chapters, we discuss recommendations for people with special requirements, but first it's important to tie together the information presented above about what the different foodstuffs are with basic information about how much of them you should consume and why you should include them in your diet.

How Many Calories Do I Need?

This depends on your height and activity level. A larger person needs more calories to maintain body weight than a smaller person; a person who has a high level of physical activity needs more calories to maintain weight than a less active person of the same size; and a person who is trying to lose weight needs less than a person who is trying to maintain or gain weight. In other words, to maintain body weight unchanged, you need to take in the same number of calories that you expend; to lose weight, you need less intake than expenditure; and to gain weight, you need to take in more calories than you expend.

Here is one method of estimating the caloric requirements for weight maintenance for a nonpregnant, nonlactating adult: 10 calories per pound of body weight, plus 20% for sedentary lifestyle, or plus 33% for light physical activity, or plus 50% for moderate physical activity, or plus 75% for heavy activity.

This rough guide does not even take into consideration age and gender, so it must be considered only a rough estimate. Nevertheless, it can indicate roughly what your weight-maintenance caloric intake should be. For example, a 120-pound woman who engages in low levels of physical activity would require 10 × 120 = 1,200 calories + 33% (1,200 × .33 = 400) = 1,600 calories per day to maintain body weight. We emphasize that this is an example and a rough estimate. Pound for pound, women require slightly fewer calories than men to maintain body weight. Also, obese people require slightly fewer calories than lean people to maintain their weight.

Once you have an estimate of how many calories you need to consume every day to maintain your weight, you can calculate how many calories to cut back if you want to lose weight. Each 3,500 calories represent 1 pound of body weight. If you eat 3,500 calories less than you require—over whatever period of time you're comfortable with and is healthy for you—you lose 1 pound. For example, if during a one-week period your diet contains 500 calories a day fewer than your requirement, you will lose 1 pound.

Does Water Matter?

Water is necessary for life, and pure water must be one of the "safest" of all substances to ingest. How much do we recommend? You should be drinking enough fluid to keep from feeling thirsty. Most people drink about 2 quarts a day. If you find yourself unusually thirsty, of course, the first thing to consider is that your blood sugar may be high.

Alcohol

Alcohol is a touchy subject, wrapped in mystique, morality, and merriment. Let's deal with the facts, some of which you may find surprising:

—Alcohol is not necessary. People do very well without it.
—In moderation, alcohol is not intrinsically harmful. A large body of scientific evidence indicates, to the contrary, that one or two drinks a day may reduce the risk of heart attacks.
—Alcohol acts to *potentiate* insulin. With insulin, alcohol can cause

hypoglycemia. We know one very careful person with Type I diabetes who two years in a row had his only significant hypoglycemic reaction on New Year's Day, after imbibing the night before. Rather than reduce the insulin dose, we recommend eating something along with a drink of alcohol.

—In excess, alcohol can not only cause severe insulin reactions but also damage the liver, causing cirrhosis. People with any liver disease, therefore, are routinely counseled to avoid alcohol. Excessive alcohol intake is also the major cause of traffic fatalities and family breakdown, and drunkenness can easily be confused, as we note elsewhere, with an insulin reaction.

The calories consumed as alcoholic beverages can add considerably to your total daily caloric intake, even leaving aside the peanuts, cheese, or chips that people tend to munch on as they drink. The number of calories in an alcoholic drink depends on the proof of the alcohol. If you are interested in knowing approximately how many calories you are consuming, try this formula:

$$0.8 \times \text{proof of the drink} \times \text{number of ounces} = \text{calories}$$

For example, if you drink two 4-ounce glasses of 86 proof bourbon, that's 550 calories ($0.8 \times 86 \times 8 = 550$). One 6-ounce glass of 12.5% alcohol wine (which is equivalent to 25 proof) would contain 120 calories ($0.8 \times 25 \times 6 = 120$). Finally, one 12-ounce can of 6% alcohol beer (12 proof) contains 115 calories ($0.8 \times 12 \times 12 = 115$).

The bottom line? We stop short of recommending alcohol but are supportive if our patients want to build a drink or a beer or a glass of wine into their regular diet. A moderate amount of alcohol is defined as 1.5 ounces of distilled liquor, 4 ounces of wine, or 12 ounces of beer. Much has been said about red wine being higher in sugar than white wine, but we are not impressed with the data and support a glass or so of either red or white. We recommend strongly against excessive drinking, which we define as more than one or two drinks daily. Pregnant women, people with a history of alcohol abuse, and people with conditions such as gastritis or high triglycerides or a history of pancreatitis may also be well advised to avoid alcohol. Talk with your health care provider to see if he or she agrees.

Using Exchange Lists

Exchange lists were devised decades ago to help people with diabetes recognize portions of food that are more or less equivalent. Some people find them very helpful, and some find them totally useless. We like to encourage those who are motivated to learn exchanges to do so. Used skillfully, they can keep your diet stable at the same time that they provide variety. A nutritionist will work out a meal plan specifying food choices (exchanges) for meals and snacks based on your food preferences. By following the plan, you will get the recommended proportions of protein, fat, and carbohydrates balanced throughout the day and consistent from one day to the next.

Essentially, the exchange lists are groups of foods that are alike in composition. There are six groups: starch/bread, meat and substitutes, vegetables, fruit, milk, and fat (see Table 8). Your dietitian can supply you with a set of exchange lists with your meal plan, or you can obtain a set from the American Diabetes Association. Each food within a list, in the quantity listed, is equivalent nutritionally and calorically to all others on the list. You pick and choose. Say, for example, that your plan calls for 2 starch exchanges. You may pick 2 slices of bread or 1 slice of bread and $\frac{1}{2}$ cup of cooked cereal or 1 cup of cooked cereal. Two meat exchanges could be 2 ounces of lean roast beef or 1 ounce of roast beef and $\frac{1}{4}$ cup of cottage cheese or $\frac{1}{4}$ cup cottage cheese and $\frac{1}{4}$ cup tuna. Making varied choices within the lists from day to day helps to ensure an adequate intake of the micronutrients.

Rather than simply complementing a meal plan, exchanges can form the basis for a meal plan. (For another system, carbohydrate counting by the gram, see Chapter 8.) Looking at the exchange list, you'll notice that the fruit, starch, and milk lists are the high-carbohydrate foods and have about equal grams of carbohydrate. Therefore, you could decide periodically to have 4 starch exchanges instead of 2 starch exchanges, 1 fruit, and 1 milk exchange. (That's how you can get in a plate of spaghetti with your chicken cacciatore!) Because fat and protein do not affect the blood sugar greatly, some of the fat and meat exchanges can periodically be moved to another mealtime for a special occasion. The total amount of carbohydrate at a meal should not be altered.

Reading Labels

No discussion of food would be complete without some comments about food labels. The labeling laws that went into effect in 1994 made label reading much easier than it used to be. You'll find that if you bypass the colorful

Table 8.   Exchange List

Starch List
One starch exchange equals 15 grams carbohydrate, 3 grams protein, 0–1 grams fat, and 80 calories.

Bread

Bagel	½ (1 oz)
Bread, reduced calorie	2 slices (1½ oz)
Bread, white, whole-wheat, pumpernickel, rye	1 slice (1 oz)
Bread sticks, crisp, 4 in. long × ½ in.	2 (⅔ oz)
English muffin	½
Hot dog or hamburger bun	½ (1 oz)
Pita, 6 in. across	½
Raisin bread, unfrosted	1 slice (1 oz)
Roll, plain, small	1 (1 oz)
Tortilla, corn, 6 in. across	1
Tortilla, flour, 7–8 in. across	1
Waffle, 4½ in. square, reduced-fat	1

Cereals and Grains

Bran cereals	½ cup
Bulgur	½ cup
Cereals	½ cup
Cereals, unsweetened, ready-to-eat	¾ cup
Cornmeal (dry)	3 Tbsp
Couscous	⅓ cup
Flour (dry)	3 Tbsp
Granola, low-fat	¼ cup
Grape-Nuts®	¼ cup
Grits	½ cup
Kasha	½ cup
Millet	¼ cup
Muesli	¼ cup
Oats	½ cup
Pasta	½ cup
Puffed cereal	1½ cups
Rice milk	½ cup
Rice, white or brown	⅓ cup
Shredded Wheat®	½ cup
Sugar-frosted cereal	½ cup
Wheat germ	3 Tbsp

(continued)

Table 8.   *(continued)*

Starchy Vegetables

Baked beans	⅓ cup
Corn	½ cup
Corn on cob, medium	1 (5 oz)
Mixed vegetables with corn, peas, or pasta	1 cup
Peas, green	½ cup
Plantain	½ cup
Potato, baked or boiled	1 small (3 oz)
Potato, mashed	½ cup
Squash, winter (acorn, butternut)	1 cup
Yam, sweet potato, plain	½ cup

Crackers and Snacks

Animal crackers	8
Graham crackers, 2½ in. square	3
Matzoh	¾ oz
Melba toast	4 slices
Oyster crackers	24
Popcorn (popped, no fat added or low-fat microwave)	3 cups
Pretzels	¾ oz
Rice cakes, 4 in. across	2
Saltine-type crackers	6
Snack chips, fat-free (tortilla, potato)	15–20 (¾ oz)
Whole-wheat crackers, no fat added	2–5 (¾ oz)

Beans, Peas, and Lentils
(Count as 1 starch exchange, plus 1 very lean meat exchange)

Beans and peas (garbanzo, pinto, kidney, white, split, black-eyed)	½ cup
Lima beans	⅔ cup
Lentils	½ cup
Miso*	3 Tbsp

Starchy Foods Prepared with Fat
(Count as 1 starch exchange, plus 1 fat exchange)

Biscuit, 2½ in. across	1
Chow mein noodles	½ cup
Corn bread, 2 in. cube	1 (2 oz)
Crackers, round butter type	6
Croutons	1 cup
French-fried potatoes	16–25 (3 oz)

* = 400 mg or more sodium per exchange

Table 8. *(continued)*

Granola	¼ cup
Muffin, small	1 (1½ oz)
Pancake, 4 in. across	2
Popcorn, microwave	3 cups
Sandwich crackers, cheese or peanut butter filling	3
Stuffing, bread (prepared)	⅓ cup
Taco shell, 6 in. across	2
Waffle, 4½ in. square	1
Whole-wheat crackers, fat added	4–6 (1 oz)

Fruit List
One fruit exchange equals 15 grams carbohydrate and 60 calories.
The weight includes skin, core, seeds, and rind.

Fruit

Apple, unpeeled, small	1 (4 oz)
Applesauce, unsweetened	½ cup
Apples, dried	4 rings
Apricots, fresh	4 whole (5½ oz)
Apricots, dried	8 halves
Apricots, canned	½ cup
Banana, small	1 (4 oz)
Blackberries	¾ cup
Blueberries	¾ cup
Cantaloupe, small	⅓ melon (11 oz) or 1 cup cubes
Cherries, sweet, fresh	12 (3 oz)
Cherries, sweet, canned	½ cup
Dates	3
Figs, fresh	1½ large or 2 medium (3½ oz)
Figs, dried	1½
Fruit cocktail	½ cup
Grapefruit, large	½ (11 oz)
Grapefruit sections, canned	¾ cup
Grapes, small	17 (3 oz)
Honeydew melon	1 slice (10 oz) or 1 cup cubes
Kiwi	1 (3½ oz)
Mandarin oranges, canned	¾ cup
Mango, small	½ fruit (5½ oz) or ½ cup
Nectarine, small	1 (5 oz)
Orange, small	1 (6½ oz)
Papaya	½ fruit (8 oz) or 1 cup cubes
Peach, medium, fresh	1 (6 oz)

(continued)

Table 8.   *(continued)*

Peaches, canned	½ cup
Pear, large, fresh	½ (4 oz)
Pears, canned	½ cup
Pineapple, fresh	¾ cup
Pineapple, canned	½ cup
Plums, small	2 (5 oz)
Plums, canned	½ cup
Prunes, dried	3
Raisins	2 Tbsp
Raspberries	1 cup
Strawberries	1¼ cup whole berries
Tangerines, small	2 (8 oz)
Watermelon	1 slice (13½ oz) or 1¼ cup cubes

Fruit Juice

Apple juice/cider	½ cup
Cranberry juice cocktail	⅓ cup
Cranberry juice cocktail, reduced-calorie	1 cup
Fruit juice blends, 100% juice	⅓ cup
Grape juice	⅓ cup
Grapefruit juice	½ cup
Orange juice	½ cup
Pineapple juice	½ cup
Prune juice	⅓ cup

Milk List
One milk exchange equals 12 grams carbohydrate and 8 grams protein.

Skim and Very Low-fat Milk
(0–3 grams fat per serving)

Skim milk	1 cup
½% milk	1 cup
1% milk	1 cup
Nonfat or low-fat buttermilk	1 cup
Evaporated skim milk	½ cup
Nonfat dry milk	⅓ cup dry
Plain nonfat yogurt	¾ cup
Nonfat or low-fat fruit-flavored yogurt sweetened with aspartame or with a nonnutritive sweetener	1 cup

Table 8. *(continued)*

Low-fat Milk
(5 grams fat per serving)

2% milk	1 cup
Plain low-fat yogurt	¾ cup
Sweet acidophilus milk	1 cup

Whole Milk
(8 grams fat per serving)

Whole milk	1 cup
Evaporated whole milk	½ cup
Goat's milk	1 cup
Kefir	1 cup

Vegetable List
One vegetable exchange equals 5 grams carbohydrate, 2 grams protein, 0 grams fat, and 25 calories.

One-half cup of cooked vegetables or juice, or 1 cup of raw vegetables:

Artichoke
Artichoke hearts
Asparagus
Beans (green, wax, Italian)
Bean sprouts
Beets
Broccoli
Brussels sprouts
Cabbage
Carrots
Cauliflower
Celery
Cucumber
Eggplant
Green onions or scallions
Greens (collard, kale, mustard, turnip)
Kohlrabi
Leeks
Mixed vegetables (without corn, peas, or pasta)
Mushrooms
Okra
Onions
Pea pods
Peppers (all varieties)
Radishes

(continued)

Table 8.   *(continued)*

Salad greens (endive, escarole, lettuce, romaine, spinach)
Sauerkraut*
Spinach
Summer squash
Tomato
Tomatoes, canned
Tomato sauce*
Tomato/vegetable juice*
Turnips
Water chestnuts
Watercress
Zucchini

Meat and Meat Substitutes List

Very Lean Meat and Substitutes List
One exchange equals 0 grams carbohydrate, 7 grams protein,
0–1 grams fat, and 35 calories.

One very lean meat exchange is equal to any one of the following items:

Poultry: Chicken or turkey (white meat, no skin), Cornish hen (no skin)	1 oz
Fish: Fresh or frozen cod, flounder, haddock, halibut, trout, tuna (fresh or canned in water)	1 oz
Shellfish: Clams, crab, lobster, scallops, shrimp, imitation shellfish	1 oz
Game: Duck or pheasant (no skin), venison, buffalo, ostrich	1 oz
Cheese with 1 gram or less fat per ounce:	
Nonfat or low-fat cottage cheese	¼ cup
Fat-free cheese	1 oz
Other: Processed sandwich meats with 1 gram or less fat per ounce, such as deli thin, shaved meats, chipped beef,* turkey ham	1 oz
egg whites	2
egg substitutes, plain	¼ cup
hot dogs with 1 gram or less fat per ounce*	1 oz
kidney (high in cholesterol)	1 oz
sausage with 1 gram or less fat per ounce	1 oz

* = 400 mg or more sodium per exchange

Table 8. *(continued)*

Count as one very lean meat and one starch exchange:

Beans, peas, lentils (cooked) ½ cup

Lean Meat and Substitutes List
One exchange equals 0 grams carbohydrates, 7 grams protein, 3 grams fat, and 55 calories.

One lean meat exchange is equal to any one of the following items:

Beef: USDA Select or Choice grade of lean beef
    trimmed of fat, such as round, sirloin, and flank
    steak; tenderloin; roast (rib, chuck, rump); steak
    (T-bone, porterhouse, cubed), ground round   1 oz

Pork: Lean pork, such as fresh ham; canned, cured,
    or boiled ham; Canadian bacon*; tenderloin,
    center loin chop   1 oz

Lamb: Roast, chop, leg   1 oz

Veal: Lean chop, roast   1 oz

Poultry: Chicken, turkey (dark meat, no skin),
    chicken (white meat, with skin), domestic
    duck or goose (well drained of fat, no skin)   1 oz

Fish:
    herring (uncreamed or smoked)   1 oz
    oysters   6 medium
    salmon (fresh or canned), catfish   1 oz
    sardines (canned)   2 medium
    tuna (canned in oil, drained)   1 oz

Game: Goose (no skin), rabbit   1 oz

Cheese:
    4.5%-fat cottage cheese   ¼ cup
    grated parmesan   2 Tbsp
    cheeses with 3 grams or less fat per ounce   1 oz

Other:
    hot dogs with 3 grams or less fat per ounce*   1½ oz
    processed sandwich meat with 3 grams or less
        fat per ounce, such as turkey pastrami or kielbasa   1 oz
    liver, heart (high in cholesterol)   1 oz

(continued)

* = 400 mg or more sodium per exchange

Table 8. *(continued)*

Medium-fat Meat and Substitutes List
One exchange equals 0 grams carbohydrate, 7 grams protein, 5 grams fat, and 75 calories.

One medium-fat meat exchange is equal to any one of the following items:

Beef: Most beef products fall into this category (ground beef, meatloaf, corned beef, short ribs, Prime grades of meat trimmed of fat, such as prime rib)	1 oz
Pork: top loin, chop, Boston butt, cutlet	1 oz
Lamb: rib roast, ground	1 oz
Veal: cutlet (ground or cubed, unbreaded)	1 oz
Poultry: chicken (dark meat, with skin), ground turkey or ground chicken, fried chicken (with skin)	1 oz
Fish: any fried fish product	1 oz
Cheese: with 5 grams or less fat per ounce	
feta	1 oz
mozzarella	1 oz
ricotta	¼ cup (2 oz)
Other:	
egg (high in cholesterol, limit to 3 per week)	1
sausage with 5 grams or less fat per ounce	1 oz
soy milk	1 cup
tempeh	¼ cup
tofu	4 oz or ½ cup

High-fat Meat and Substitutes List
One exchange equals 0 grams carbohydrate, 7 grams protein, 8 grams fat, and 100 calories.

Remember that these items are high in saturated fat, cholesterol, and calories and may raise blood cholesterol levels if eaten on a regular basis.

One high-fat meat exchange is equal to any one of the following items:

Pork: spareribs, ground pork, pork sausage	1 oz
Cheese: all regular cheeses, such as American,* cheddar, Monterey jack, Swiss	1 oz

* = 400 mg or more sodium per exchange

Table 8.   (*continued*)

Other: Processed sandwich meats with 8 grams	
or less fat per ounce, such as bologna,	
pimento loaf, salami	1 oz
sausage, such as bratwurst, Italian, knockwurst,	
Polish, smoked	1 oz
hot dog (turkey or chicken)*	1 (10/lb)
bacon	3 slices (20 slices/lb)

Count as one high-fat meat plus one fat exchange:

Hot dog (beef, pork, or combination)*	1 (10/lb)
Peanut butter (contains unsaturated fat)	2 Tbsp

Fat List

Monounsaturated Fats List
One fat exchange equals 5 grams fat and 45 calories.

Avocado, medium	$\frac{1}{8}$ (1 oz)
Oil (canola, olive, peanut)	1 tsp
Olives: ripe (black)	8 large
green, stuffed*	10 large
Nuts	
almonds, cashews	6 nuts
mixed (50% peanuts)	6 nuts
peanuts	10 nuts
pecans	4 halves
Peanut butter, smooth or crunchy	2 tsp
Sesame seeds	1 Tbsp
Tahini paste	2 tsp

Polyunsaturated Fats List
One fat exchange equals 5 grams fat and 45 calories.

Margarine: stick, tub, or squeeze	1 tsp
lower-fat (30%–50% vegetable oil)	1 Tbsp
Mayonnaise: regular	1 tsp
reduced-fat	1 Tbsp
Nuts, walnuts, English	4 halves
Oil (corn, safflower, soybean)	1 tsp
Salad dressing: regular*	1 Tbsp
reduced-fat	2 Tbsp

(*continued*)

* = 400 mg or more sodium per exchange

Table 8.   *(continued)*

Miracle Whip Salad Dressing*: regular	2 tsp
reduced-fat	1 Tbsp
Seeds: pumpkin, sunflower	1 Tbsp

Saturated Fats List[†]
One fat exchange equals 5 grams of fat and 45 calories.

Bacon, cooked	1 slice (20 slices/lb)
Bacon, grease	1 tsp
Butter: stick	1 tsp
whipped	2 tsp
reduced-fat	1 Tbsp
Chitterlings, boiled	2 Tbsp (½ oz)
Coconut, sweetened, shredded	2 Tbsp
Cream, half and half	2 Tbsp
Cream cheese: regular	1 Tbsp (½ oz)
reduced-fat	2 Tbsp (1 oz)
Fatback or salt pork‡	
Shortening or lard	1 tsp
Sour cream: regular	2 Tbsp
reduced-fat	3 Tbsp

SOURCE: "Exchange Lists for Meal Planning," American Diabetes Association and American Dietetic Association, 1995.

 * = 400 mg or more sodium per exchange

 †Saturated fats can raise blood cholesterol levels.

 ‡Use a piece 1 in. × 1 in. × ¼ in. if you plan to eat the fatback cooked with vegetables. Use a piece 2 in. × 1 in. × ½ in. when eating only the vegetables with the fatback removed.

trappings boasting "No cholesterol!" or "No added sugar!" and go right to the Nutrition Facts section of the label, you'll learn a lot about the product. We'll take a look at each part of this label (Figure 9).

Serving size.   Start with the serving size: all the other information is applicable only for that amount. The serving size given may be small compared to what you consider to be a serving, so be aware that if you eat an entire package of something that contains four servings, you've just downed *four times* the amounts listed as "per serving."

Calories.   Calories are listed only for the serving size specified on the food container, not for an exchange or for other usual serving sizes.

Percent daily value.   This part of the label can be misinterpreted, because the single item does not represent all the foods eaten for the day. But it

Nutrition Facts

Serving Size 7 wafers (29g)
Servings Per Container About 8

Amount Per Serving

Calories 120   Calories from Fat 30

	% Daily Value*
Total Fat 3g	5%
Saturated Fat 0.5g	3%
Polyunsaturated Fat 0g	
Monounsaturated Fat 1 g	
Cholesterol 0g	0%
Sodium 170 mg	7%
Total Carbohydrate 22g	7%
Dietary Fiber 4g	15%
Sugars 0g	
Protein 3g	

Vitamin A 0%-Vitamin C 0%-Calcium 0%

Iron 8%-Phosphorus 10%

* Percent Daily Values are based on a 2,000 calorie diet. Your daily values may be higher or lower depending on your calorie needs:

	Calories:	2,000	2,500
Total Fat	Less than	65g	80g
Sat Fat	Less than	20g	25g
Cholesterol	Less than	300mg	300mg
Sodium	Less than	2,400mg	2,400mg
Total Carbohydrate		300g	375g
Dietary Fiber		25g	30g

Calories per gram: Fat 9 · Carbohydrate 4 · Protein 4

Figure 9. A nutrition facts label.

can be helpful if you are adding up how much fat, protein, or another nutrient you consume each day. Be aware that the calculation on the label assumes a total daily intake of 2,000 calories. Your actual intake may be more or less. For example, if your intake is 1,500 calories per day, then a food that provides 500 calories would be 33% of your daily intake, not 25% as labeled.

Total fat and cholesterol.   You need to keep fat consumption within the recommended guidelines. In interpreting the label, it may be helpful to go straight to the saturated fat grams, remembering that 5 grams of fat equals 1 teaspoon or pat of butter or margarine or 1 teaspoon oil, and that saturated fat is what raises blood cholesterol level.

Sodium.   Sodium is the part of table salt that some people have to cut down on if they have high blood pressure or ankle swelling. The sodium figure includes sodium from salt as well as other sodium-containing foods in the product.

Total carbohydrate.   Total carbohydrate is the carbohydrate from dietary fiber, sugars, and other (complex) carbohydrates. Dietary fiber has virtually no calories and therefore should not be factored in when counting carbohydrates or exchanges. Examples of sugars are sucrose, fructose, glucose, lactose, corn syrup, and honey. Other carbohydrates are the complex carbohydrates in the product. This amount may not be indicated on the label but can be calculated by subtracting the grams of dietary fiber and grams of sugars from the total carbohydrates.

Protein.   This section lists the total grams of protein.

Calories from fat, protein, and carbohydrate.   At the bottom of the label is the figure for the number of calories per gram of fat, protein, and carbohydrate. You can use this information to determine how many calories in the product come from each. Just multiply the total fat grams by 9, the total carbohydrate (minus the fiber) by 4, and the protein by 4.

Putting It All Together

Some people are visual learners. Once we see a picture, it all makes sense. For the visually inspired, the U.S. Department of Agriculture (USDA) has put together the Food Guide Pyramid to illustrate the relative proportions of different kinds of foods making up a healthy diet (see Figure 10). It is consistent with recommendations for persons with diabetes. As you can see, the base of the pyramid is made up of carbohydrate-containing foods: a large amount of bread, cereal, rice, and pasta; at the next level, there are slightly smaller amounts each of vegetables and fruits. Protein-containing foods, the milk and meat foods, appear on the next level, representing a moderate intake. Finally, at the tip—the smallest part of the pyramid—are the fats, oils, and sweets, obviously meant to be used sparingly.

Other people do better with words than pictures and might find the Dietary Guidelines for Americans from the USDA helpful in getting started on a healthy diet:

1. *Eat a variety of foods.* Eating a variety of foods is a way of ensuring that your intake of micronutrients is adequate.
2. *Maintain reasonable body weight.* Be careful of portion control. Daily

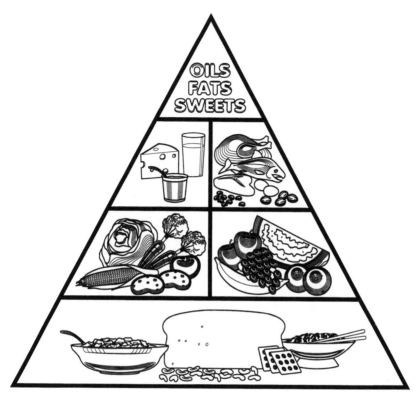

Figure 10. The food guide pyramid.

activities should be increased. Meals should be eaten at about the same time of day and not be skipped.

3. *Avoid too much fat, saturated fat, and cholesterol.*
    –Eat smaller servings of meat. Select fish and poultry more often. Choose lean cuts of red meats.
    –Prepare meats by roasting, broiling, or baking. Trim all fat off before cooking.
    –Avoid added sauces and gravies. Remove skin from poultry.
    –Avoid fried foods. Avoid adding fat during cooking process, including before broiling.
    –Eat fewer high-fat foods, such as cold cuts, bacon, sausage, hot dogs, spreads, nuts, salad dressings, ice cream, whole milk.
    –Drink skim or 1% milk and products made from these milks.

4. *Avoid too much sodium and salt.*
   –Reduce the amount of salt used in cooking.
   –Do not add salt at the table.
   –Eat fewer high-salt, high-sodium foods, such as canned soups and processed foods.
5. *Eat foods with starch and fiber.*
   –Choose dried beans, peas, and lentils more often.
   –Eat whole grain cereals, breads, crackers, brown rice, oat bran, or bulgur.
   –Eat more vegetables (raw and cooked) and fresh fruits (eat skins if possible).
   –Eat less sugar by avoiding regular soft drinks, table sugar, honey, syrup, jams, jellies, candy, sweet rolls, cakes with icing, regular gelatin desserts. Use artificial sweeteners, if needed, in place of caloric sweeteners.
6. *Drink only moderate amounts of alcohol.*

We have covered a lot of material in this chapter—facts, figures, and opinions. It will most likely take you a while to even begin to master nutrition. But remember that you're already very familiar with the foods themselves. We're just asking you to think a little more about the foods you eat every day, to learn what it is you're putting in your mouth. With the help of a good professional nutritionist, you will discover a multitude of healthful foods that taste good, too.

Chapter 7

Dietary Health for Type II Diabetes

- *"I asked my doctor to treat my diabetes, and my doctor said I need to lose 20 pounds. I know I need to lose weight, but that's not what I went to see the doctor for."*

- *"Being overweight isn't my fault. Everyone in my family is heavy. It's in our genes."*

- *"Are there good and bad ways to lose weight? Every time I open a newspaper or magazine I see more ads about weight loss."*

- *"I'll never be skinny, but my diet is better now, and I'm controlling my blood sugar and my cholesterol."*

Type II diabetes is a diet-dependent and exercise-dependent disease, and it is serious. In this chapter, we will encourage you to lose weight if you're overweight. This is not because we think everyone should have the physique of a movie star and not because we think it's the *easy* way to control blood sugar, but because we know from experience that a good diet is essential to the successful treatment of Type II diabetes.

As you know, there are additional treatment options in managing Type II diabetes, including several kinds of pills and insulin. It may be hard to understand, then, why we keep emphasizing diet and exercise. Many people would rather pop a pill than follow a diet. But with a good diet and some regular activity (plus pills or insulin, if necessary), Type II diabetes can almost always be effectively treated; without a reasonable diet and exercise, the pills and even insulin aren't successful.

So we will keep pounding home diet and weight control in this chapter, because it's the central problem for the vast majority of people with Type II diabetes. We will describe again the link between body weight and Type II diabetes (mentioned in Chapter 2), talk briefly about issues of genes and physiology as they apply to obesity, and describe the elements of a good diet for Type II diabetes and associated conditions, such as high blood cholesterol and high blood pressure.

Type II Diabetes and Obesity

Insulin Resistance and Obesity

The link between Type II diabetes and obesity is really quite simple: the fatter you are, on the whole, the more *resistance you have to your own insulin. Insulin resistance* means that a specific amount of insulin doesn't work as well as it should. If you give 10 units of insulin to a thin person, you might drop his or her blood sugar by 50 mg/dl; give the same 10 units to an obese person, and the blood sugar might drop by only 20 mg/dl. That's resistance to insulin.

You may like to think of insulin resistance with a story: John's riding a bike. If he's on a nice smooth bike path, the pedaling's easy, no resistance. If he rides off the road onto a beach, though, the wheels sink into sand, and there's lots of resistance. If John is strong, he can push through the sand and keep going. But if he's not so strong, the bike doesn't make it. What does this have to do with insulin resistance? A slim, physically fit body is like the smooth road, and a little insulin (like a little pedaling) does just fine. Add obesity, and you're in the sand, because obesity causes resistance to the insulin. If you have a strong pancreas that's putting out lots of insulin, it can overcome the resistance. But if your pancreas is weak, it can't make enough insulin, and you have diabetes.

Losing weight, if you are overweight to begin with, decreases the insulin resistance, like riding out of the sand and back onto the pavement. All of a sudden, your pancreas may be up to the job, and your blood sugars may be normal.

The Causes of Obesity

Isn't it well known that obesity is hereditary? Aren't some people just born to be overweight? If that's so, then you may well ask, as Ado Annie sings in *Oklahoma*, "How can I be what I ain't?" There is no doubt that heredity plays a role in obesity. Studies of twins prove it. We all know families in which both parent and child have a "weight problem." Scientists have even isolated an "obesity gene" (see Chapter 32). Furthermore, both people who are obese and people who are thin have a strong, innate homing mechanism: when they gain or lose weight on a rigid diet, they have a strong tendency to return to their original weight.

But as with so many human characteristics, genetics is only part of the story. Even if you have an inborn tendency to be overweight, you still have to ingest more calories than you burn if you are going to gain weight. And the amount of food people take in varies enormously in our culture, where food is available virtually everywhere all the time. So, yes, some people are genetically predisposed to obesity and some are not. But whatever genes you have, there is still a lot you can do to control your weight by controlling your behavior.

Type II Diabetes without Obesity

Excess body weight explains a lot of Type II diabetes, but not all. Many overweight people don't have diabetes, because their pancreas is very strong and puts out large amounts of insulin to overcome the resistance (like pedaling successfully in the sand). And some people with Type II diabetes are thin. Chances are their pancreas is not making much insulin. On the whole, thin people who develop Type II diabetes are more likely to end up needing insulin by injection, since their relatively limited insulin production by the pancreas makes them less likely to achieve control with diet and pills.

Type II Diabetes and Other Risk Factors

Type II diabetes tends to come on in older people who are at risk of other problems, such as heart disease, just because of their age. It should not be a surprise, then, that people with Type II diabetes do have more associated illnesses and risk factors. We emphasize throughout this book that blood glucose control is important in improving your chances of avoiding complications; but with Type II diabetes, even greater risks are added if the person smokes or has high cholesterol, high blood pressure, or a strong family history of heart trouble.

Especially in Type II diabetes, then, nutrition therapy must be *individualized.* This is true even if the person only has diabetes. Most often, the associated problems, such as hypertension or high cholesterol, need to be addressed in a specific diet prescription. But underneath it all will be the emphasis on healthy eating. This is the foundation of diet therapy for Type II diabetes.

Healthy Eating Habits

The key to healthy eating is to obey the adage "everything in moderation." This is a hard lesson to learn in our fast-moving, go-for-it society. It means checking that impulsive stop at the drive-through fast-food joint, where you can put down 1,000 calories in 10 minutes. It means restraining the impulse to grab potato chips off the supermarket shelf. It may mean targeting particular times of day or activities in the house that cause you to overeat, such as that 45 minutes when you first get home in the evening, or as you start cooking dinner. And it usually means thinking carefully about what you are putting in your mouth and what exercise you are doing to burn off calories.

You might consider using the USDA Food Pyramid (Chapter 6) to start guiding your healthy selections. There will, no doubt, be sacrifices. Yes, it may mean giving up the cream-filled doughnut picked up on the way to work. But consider eating fresh strawberries with skim milk and sweetener, and a warm low-fat bran muffin with a pat of margarine melting on top: is that such a hardship? Serve it on the fanciest plate in the house with a cloth napkin, and you're eating breakfast at a gourmet restaurant.

Don't skip meals. They don't have to be elaborate, but eating regularly is important to sustaining energy levels and especially to controlling appetite. Some people try to restrict calories by skipping breakfast and lunch. In our experience, these same people are so overcome with hunger and fatigue by evening that they eat everything not nailed down.

Selection of foods, preparation of foods, and portion control are three different things, and it is essential to know about each. At the start, when people are just getting into healthy eating, their selection may be way off. Consider Jack's case, for instance.

> *Jack's downfall was onion-flavored potato chips. Watching his favorite baseball team on television, he would go through a medium-large bag in the first five innings. He knew it was wrong, but it was a habit. The only way to break the habit, it turned out, was to ban onion-flavored potato chips from the house. Jack, his wife, and the kids all took the vow: no onion-flavored chips when you go to the supermarket. It worked! Jack still liked his ballgame in the evening, but he took to snacking instead on some celery and carrots.*

Sometimes, it is not so much the food itself, but how it's prepared. Take the inspirational case of Melissa, for example.

> *Melissa loved fried chicken—chicken for lunch, chicken for supper, chicken for a snack. She even sometimes ate leftover chicken for breakfast. The problem wasn't the chicken, it was the preparation. Fried chicken has an enormous amount of total and saturated fat, which is just what Melissa didn't need. Banning chicken from*

the house or eating small portions wasn't the answer, particularly since Melissa also bought the food in a fast-food setting where the portion sizes couldn't be modified. During Melissa's week at our Diabetes Center as she went through "fried chicken withdrawal" while substituting lower fat foods, Melissa's blood sugars started coming down. Months later, she was still "clean" and boasted that even the smell of fried chicken at a family gathering had made her feel sick. Melissa lost weight and, as a bonus, her insulin requirement went down.

Finally, there is the issue of portion size, especially when eating at home. We frequently hear the comment, "I'm eating good foods, but way too much." There are relatively few low-calorie, high-bulk foods like lettuce and other greens, where portion size isn't a problem. But most parts of the healthy diet—the pat of margarine, piece of meat, serving of spaghetti, or dollop of salad dressing—are healthy only if you control the quantity. You can definitely have good things in your diet, but you may also be taking in too much of a good thing! Many behavioral modification techniques (see below) are designed specifically to address this very point—how to help you eat in moderation.

This basic, healthy approach to diet says, "I can eat well, I can love eating, and I can still eat healthy." Eating in moderation is a diet prescription that will help with your health problems, whether diabetes, high blood pressure, or high cholesterol. And it is healthy not just for you but also for the whole family.

Most people with Type II diabetes need to do more than eat healthy, though. They also need to work on weight reduction followed by a fairly strict maintenance plan.

Slanting the Weight Curve by Trimming Calories and Increasing Activity

To slant the weight curve in your favor (downward), you have to create a calorie deficit. There's no way around it. But if you decrease your calories and increase your activity, your weight *will* start coming down. We introduced the arithmetic in Chapter 6, now let's play it out a bit. Remember that consuming 3,500 calories less than your weight-maintenance requirement will result in the loss of about 1 pound. If you consume 500 calories a day less than your requirement, you'll lose 1 pound in a week. But what happens if you add in a brisk daily exercise that burns off 200 calories? Then you only have to eat 300 calories less each day.

What will you see on the scale? Don't be upset if you don't see weight loss every day. Body weight can fluctuate several pounds from day to day, depending on things like your bowel habits, your menstrual cycle, and any tendency to retain fluid. Look at the longer range weight curve. If you are taking in, on average, less calories than you expend, your weight will trend downward over the weeks. Averaging just 1 pound a week sounds easy, but think about it. Four pounds a month, 25 pounds in six months, 50 pounds in a year. That would truly be a new you!

That's why our dietitian and the American Diabetes Association suggest a moderate caloric decrease, 250–500 calories less than what it takes to maintain body weight. They also recommend an increase in activity to burn up some calories. Your own dietitian will be your best resource to help you put together a plan of healthful eating with a moderate caloric restriction. It will include portion control and a reduction in the total amount of fat, especially saturated fat, as a way of decreasing caloric intake.

A great many "weight control plans" are out there, and great claims are often made for them. We aren't against them, and we certainly don't believe that the simpler, more gradual program we tend to favor is the only plan that works. Still, we want to give you our thoughts—pro and con—on some of the more popular approaches to weight loss.

Very Low-Calorie Diets

This approach usually refers to temporary diets in the range of 400 calories to 700 calories total per day. After the dieter reaches a certain target weight, the very low-calorie diet comes to an end. Clearly, such a diet cannot be maintained forever: that's not enough calories to maintain life in the long run. Under proper supervision, very low-calorie diets undoubtedly produce a sharp drop in body weight if the calorie restriction is adhered to. Blood sugar levels in people with Type II diabetes will drop dramatically as soon as they start such rigorous dieting. But since the very low-calorie diet has to be temporary, it is only as effective as what you do after it's over. If you go back to a very high-calorie diet, you will promptly gain the weight back, probably to about your previous weight or even more. So don't get involved in the very low-calorie diets unless you fully intend to pursue maintenance of a healthy follow-up diet and exercise program for the long run.

Commercial Very Low-Calorie Diet Programs

Commercial diet programs of the very low-calorie type are easy to find and often come packaged not only with their own brand name but with a series of support groups, nutritionists, and even health club memberships. Bear in mind that such a diet can be expensive. Very low-calorie foods don't have to come in a formula with a particular brand name. This said, if you can afford it and it makes sense to you, and if the program is medically sound, we have nothing against your enrolling in such programs. It may just mean changing the way you spend your available money—away from activities that have harmed your health and toward activities that improve it.

Fasting

Fasting is an extension of the very low-calorie diet. Fasting is even riskier, however. There are medical risks during the fast, and there is the risk of going back to your bad old habits afterward because you got so darn hungry during the fast. There has to be medical clearance before fasting and supervision during it. We have seen short-term fasting used as a successful way to initiate long-term healthy weight loss, but on the whole we don't recommend it. Fasting has so little to do with the behaviors of long-term weight control that it usually amounts to a very temporary fix.

Support Groups

There is no doubt that peer support helps. Sometimes it can be found in your own household. (Indeed, if you don't have the support of those living with you, your attempts at weight control are going to be much more difficult.) Formal, outside-the-home, regular support groups on the Weight Watchers model are also useful. Supervised by trained leaders, they can be effective in doing just what their name implies—supporting your personal efforts.

Diet Pills

The question of diet pills is highly controversial. For centuries, there have been diet pills and potions that range from useless to dangerous. Amphetamines ("uppers") and thyroid pills (when you don't have a documented thyroid problem) are the classic examples of dangerous approaches to dieting. But in recent years there has been some scientific evidence that medications such as fenfluramine and phentermine or dexfenfluramine can be used safely and effectively, at least for short periods of time. We don't have a problem with these as an adjunct to learning good dietary behaviors, *if they are prescribed by a competent professional with adequate follow-up.* But please heed our warning to beware of people who want to push all sorts of expensive, secret-ingredient pills.

Behavior Modification

Behavioral modification is a term that can be very general or very specific. As we have said, there is no way you will lose weight without modifying your behavior. So in common use, behavior modification means just what it says: changing the way you behave. More technically, a range of psychological/behavioral techniques have been developed over the years, many of which have been scientifically proven successful. Examples of behavior modification for weight loss might be to concentrate on putting your fork down on the plate between bites, to consciously take smaller bites, to stretch a meal to at least 30 minutes, or to force yourself to go out for a walk at just that moment in the late afternoon when you usually give in to a snack. The theory is that if you can recognize and pinpoint a specific moment when your behavior needs changing and can work out a way to keep bringing that need for change to the front of your mind, you can successfully modify behavior. This formal approach to behavior modification ought to be done with the help of a qualified professional.

The Interaction of Diet with Oral Hypoglycemic Medications and Insulin

If you are already on medication or insulin for diabetes when you begin to take your healthy eating and activity plan seriously, you need to be aware that your dosage requirement may go down very quickly. The amount of hypoglycemic pills or insulin you take when eating 1,600 calories per day may be too much if you cut to 1,200 calories per day. The result could be hypoglycemia (Chapter 5); it usually won't be severe, but it may make you feel suddenly weak, shaky, and sweaty.

You will need to monitor your blood sugar to know if you're low. If you notice a trend toward low blood sugars, adjust your medication or insulin downward and get in touch with your health care professional. The worst-case scenario would be for you to have to eat extra calories to keep up with your medication or insulin and not lose weight until the doses have been decreased appropriately.

Weight Gain with Insulin

The question of weight gain with insulin is a tough one, if you are overweight to begin with. The fact is that people who go from poor blood sugar control to good control by using insulin have a strong tendency to gain weight. The only scientifically proven reason is an obvious one: people in poor control are losing calories as sugar in their urine, so they have that much negative calorie balance. When they get into good control, they hang onto those calories, storing them as fat. There may be other explanations. Many people report increased appetite when they start insulin. But for whatever reason, if you have a weight problem, when you start insulin you have to be especially aware of controlling what—and how much—you eat.

Does this mean that it is better not to use insulin in Type II diabetes? Yes and no. We much prefer to control Type II diabetes with diet and exercise and, if necessary, pills. But if those preferred approaches have been used to their maximum effect and blood sugar control is still poor, then we definitely feel that the risk involved in poorly controlled blood sugars far outweighs (so to speak) the probable weight gain.

We feel the same about the often discussed theory that high insulin levels are a risk and that therefore you should avoid using insulin. While it is a *theory* that high insulin levels may be a risk, it is a *fact* that high blood sugar is a risk. Without question, we think insulin has to be used to control Type II diabetes if all other approaches have failed.

A Cautionary Tale of the Misuse of Dieting

Arthur is highly motivated, intense, and intelligent in everything he does. He was shocked to discover he has Type II diabetes, because he has always been a regular jogger and always maintained normal body weight at 174 pounds. After he learned to monitor his blood glucose, he was even more shocked to see his glucose gradually increasing. So he jogged more. And he dieted more, afraid to eat carbohydrate because it would increase his sugar level and afraid to eat fat because he didn't want to have heart problems. His weight went down to 157 pounds, which left him feeling even more fatigued. We started Arthur on insulin, making sure he didn't give up his exercise. We taught him a healthy diet, with adequate calories to maintain his normal body weight, which was 174 pounds. He regained his strength and energy, and kept on jogging.

If you are not overweight, then for you, weight reduction is not the answer to blood sugar control. Trying to eat a lot less to force your sugars down, avoiding the need for medication or insulin, is not the way to go. The chances are that your pancreas just isn't up to the job and that it needs help, first with pills and then, if necessary, with insulin. Understand that this isn't your failure, it's the fault of your pancreas. Believe us, you will feel much better when you get the medications you need.

Because the most common cause of Type II diabetes is the insulin resistance from being overweight, this chapter has stressed control of body weight. A generally healthy diet is the start, and we emphasize that a healthy diet is not a bad diet, not a bland diet, and not a boring diet. Once you start experimenting with the sorts of low-calorie meals that can be found in many cookbooks, you will see that there is a whole world of healthy dining out there, and you only have to learn to eat well and eat healthy.

If you need to turn your body weight curve downward, that will require some extra thought and effort. Especially if you are a person who has always been overweight, your goals should be realistic, taken a step at a time.

A final word of support and encouragement: don't let an occasional slip cause you to fall. No one we know is perfect (except that wise guy who said he thought he was wrong once, but found he was mistaken). We are especially worried about the high-achieving, compulsive, and intelligent person who tries to do everything perfectly. He or she easily falls into the "all or none syndrome," following a healthy diet perfectly for a while but then becoming so upset over a small lapse or two that the diet is abandoned. There's an old saying: "Don't let the perfect be the enemy of the good."

So take heart. Even a modest weight loss, successfully maintained, will have dramatic effects on your diabetic control and your overall sense of well being. You can do it.

Chapter 8

Dietary Health for Type I Diabetes

- *"The other night I ate this huge meal: a big steak, salad with a decadent blue cheese dressing, a potato with lots of sour cream. I took extra insulin, and it turned out that I had taken too much. I went low afterwards! What happened?"*

- *"I have the same breakfast every day—cereal, milk, and a banana— but every day my sugar at lunch is different. How come?"*

- *"I think my diabetes is getting worse. I eat better—more carbohydrate, less fat—and I need more insulin. Is that bad?"*

- *"Now that I have a handle on the carbohydrate content of my food, I'm doing so much better."*

With Type I diabetes, sometimes it seems that no matter what you do, your sugars bounce. And sometimes, that's true: we will never explain each blood sugar exactly. But you *can* learn to control some of the variables in life, and diet is one. With Type I diabetes, though, it's not easy. Because your own pancreas isn't helping out by making its own insulin (as it does in Type II diabetes), you have to think carefully about just what you're eating and how much insulin you need for the circumstance. (The answer to the first quotation given above, as you will see, is that this person ate a very high-calorie, high-fat meal that did not have much carbohydrate. The insulin dose was too much for the carbohydrate in the meal.)

In this chapter we'll take a look at the food–blood sugar connection in Type I diabetes. We will review what in your diet affects blood sugar most and outline some dietary strategies to bring about stability.

Type I Diabetes and the Effect of Diet

The person with Type I diabetes learns quickly that he or she must watch both the timing and the content of meals. Why the timing? Because once you inject that insulin in the morning, it's going to peak and drive the blood sugar down at a particular time. You have to eat to keep the sugar from going too low at these times. If you are on the run all day, you might find it helpful to pack your lunch and snacks.

> *Donna had only one problem time in her diabetic control. As a busy professional with kids at home, she would take her 6 units of regular insulin and 10 units of NPH upon arising and then race out of the house with a cup of coffee plus or minus a bagel. She found that sometimes if she didn't get lunch by 11:30, she'd break out in a clear insulin reaction. Donna finally figured out that she was low on the mornings she ran out minus the bagel, and fine when she left home bagel in hand. But to make sure, she decided to add a glass of milk and some crackers at 10:30. After that she could go out with the office gang for their usual 12:30 lunch date.*

Timing is crucial, and so is the amount of food you eat. Remember that you need insulin to allow the cells to use (metabolize) the food you eat. When your body doesn't make the insulin, you have to inject just the right amount to keep your blood sugar from going too high or too low over the next few hours. This is called "covering" the meal.

Remember also that it is perfectly normal for the blood sugar to increase some after a meal. For a person without diabetes, it may increase some 20–40 mg/dl. So anytime you measure your sugar one to two hours after eating, it's likely to be higher than before the meal. You might prefer not to make it *too* high, but we are less interested in controlling the immediate after-meal rise (except in the case of pregnancy) than we are in seeing that it comes back to a reasonable range within two to four hours.

Determining the right amount of insulin needed to cover a particular meal is like shooting in the dark unless you have some idea how different kinds and amounts of food will affect your glucose. Fortunately, a lot is known about this; in Chapter 6 we described some of it. Because a finely tuned diet is so important in Type I diabetes, we will review the highlights in this chapter.

Carbohydrates

The carbohydrate in your diet, more than any other foodstuff, determines how much your blood sugar will increase after a meal. That's because, as we have mentioned, carbohydrates are all made up of little sugar molecules stuck together. You eat the carbohydrate, the digestive system breaks it into single sugar molecules, which are absorbed into the bloodstream, and your sugar level goes up. If you have the right amount of insulin, the sugar will be cleared from your blood into the cells of the body and burned normally.

So carbohydrates—whether bread, pasta, candy, peas, rice, shredded wheat, milk, apples, or orange juice—all end up as sugar when absorbed into the bloodstream. This isn't bad; a considerable amount of carbohydrate (50%–60% of your total calories) is good for you. But you ought to learn to recognize portions, to count carbohydrates, so you can control your calories and use the right amount of insulin.

Our dietitian starts the lesson by holding up three cubes of sugar in one hand and a piece of bread in the other—and then drops the bombshell information that they represent approximately equal amounts of carbohydrate. That's just the start of carbohydrate counting (see below), but it makes the point that carbohydrate is the main factor in blood glucose control. Eat more carbohydrate, and you need more insulin; eat less carbohydrate, and you need less insulin. There has to be a balance.

Protein

Protein affects blood sugar much less directly than carbohydrate. It is broken down into amino acids, and later the liver can convert some of the amino acids into glucose, in a process called "gluconeogenesis." (Gluconeogenesis helps hold the blood sugar normal during fasting. Amino acids are released from the muscle protein and converted to glucose.) Just how much protein turns to glucose varies depending on the type of protein eaten and how much insulin is circulating. But in general protein will not significantly affect the blood sugar level unless it is taken in a large quantity (more than 4 ounces). Even then, the effect will not occur until some hours after the meal. Protein (like fat) does slow the absorption of carbohydrate somewhat.

Fat

At first glance, fat can be confusing. It's loaded with calories—more than twice the calories (ounce for ounce or gram for gram) of protein and carbohydrate—but fat has very little direct effect on the blood sugar. You could eat a pound of lard (not that you'd want to!), and your blood sugar would hardly move. For this reason we don't recommend including the fat content of your meal in the calculation of how much insulin you will need.

But don't misunderstand. We are not recommending a high-fat diet. Lots of fat may lower your insulin requirement a bit, but it will increase your risk of clogging up your arteries and suffering a heart attack or stroke. Fat will also rapidly increase your weight.

As we mentioned in Chapter 6, fat slows the absorption of the carbohydrate taken with it. The blood sugar rise from carbohydrate will be delayed, with the amount of delay related to the amount of fat consumed. In our experience, unless the fat intake is very high, there is no need to adjust the timing of the insulin. For the occasional high-fat meal, some people find that taking some insulin before the meal and some after is effective in preventing both a postmeal low and a later high.

Dietary Strategies and Insulin Therapy

To repeat, consistent timing and consistent content are important. By content, we mean consuming about the same grams of carbohydrates, protein, and fat (but especially carbohydrate) at each meal every day. Most people can do pretty well, and be perfectly happy, with essentially the same breakfast each day. That's real consistency. Some even carry it through lunch, "brown bagging" or choosing the same sort of soup and sandwich every day. But often by lunchtime, and almost always by supper, consistency breaks down. It's just too hard from day to day to eat exactly the same meals. Nor do we think you should try to eat the same foods, except perhaps at breakfast, because it gets pretty boring.

Learning an exchange system is the time-honored approach to maintaining consistency while varying your diet. The best way to do this is to work with a dietitian to figure out a meal plan using exchanges. Then all you have to do is put together the pieces at each meal. The grams of each food are already figured in. Remember, blood sugars reflect the carbohydrate intake more than the intake of fat and protein, so it's important to measure starch, fruit, and milk exchanges carefully.

If it is done skillfully, the carbohydrate counting system, while slightly more elaborate, is quite a bit more accurate than the exchange plan.

The Carbohydrate Counting System

Carbohydrate counting is a way of quantifying carbohydrates specifically. It measures the *amount* of carbohydrate, not the kind. Using this system, you can eat varied foods from day to day, provided the total grams of carbohydrate for that meal are the same. For example, one day you may decide to have cereal, milk, and a banana for breakfast, for a total of 60 grams of carbohydrate, while the next day you might have a piece of coffee cake and juice, for the same 60 grams of carbohydrate.

To use this system you have to learn to recognize portions of the foods you normally eat and how many grams of carbohydrate each contains. A dietitian can get you going with food models and perhaps a listing of the carbohydrate content of the foods you like. Practice for a while, just as you would for a piano recital or a spelling test. Pretty soon, you'll be rattling off the carbohydrate content of foods like a pro.

Still another level of carbohydrate counting would incorporate what is known as the *glycemic index*. Under controlled conditions dietary researchers have measured exactly how high a given quantity of each carbohydrate will raise blood glucose. The index relates everything to bread. For example, if 15 grams of some carbohydrate raises blood glucose slightly higher than 15 grams of bread, that carbohydrate has a high glycemic index. Other carbohydrates that, gram for gram, don't raise the blood glucose as much as the bread have a low glycemic index.

Frankly, we find the glycemic index to be too detailed for practical use. We are very happy if someone can accurately assess the grams of any carbohydrate in a meal. If they also learn that certain foods tend to raise their blood sugar further, fine. But the full-scale use of a glycemic index to multiply the grams of carbohydrate by some factor just seems too much for daily life.

People using external insulin pumps or multiple daily injections of insulin can use the carbohydrate counting system to add a level of flexibility. They learn to equate one unit of insulin with a specific number of grams of carbohydrate and, in effect, to vary the dose of insulin with a particular meal depending on the total grams that they plan to consume. Typically, as described in Chapter 14, we might teach a person to use 1.0 unit of Regular insulin for every 15 grams of carbohydrate in a meal, plus 1.0 unit for every 50 mg/dl she wants to decrease her blood sugar. This figure does not apply to everyone. You could require more insulin if you are resistant to insulin or less if you are particularly sensitive to insulin.

What's the downside of carbohydrate counting? By focusing on the carbohydrate content only, you may forget other aspects of good nutrition. Going overboard in the meat category, for example, won't affect your blood sugar much but could put you over the recommended daily 15% protein and 30% fat. And if, in your newfound freedom with food, you consume excessive calories, you may soon find yourself with a weight problem.

Balancing your insulin dose with food intake can be complicated, but it is a necessary skill to learn for good management of Type I diabetes. It is important to work with a good health care team. You may want to learn exchanges, or you may want to go all the way with carbohydrate counting. Either way, once you get used it, the system will become part of your life. Think about all the important and trivial things you routinely think about and do in the course of a day: How much travel time do I have to plan to get to that appointment? Do I have enough cash to do those errands? Adding an awareness of how much carbohydrate is in your meal becomes just as much second nature as any other routine calculation you do in your head.

The reward for paying attention to diet in Type I diabetes is immediate and gratifying: you feel better, with less worry and less bothersome insulin reactions. A side benefit of a good diet is that you'll live longer, too.

Chapter 9

Special Considerations
in Nutrition Therapy

- *"First diabetes, then high blood pressure. Now I know I won't be able to eat anything."*
- *"I don't think that dietitian knows what she's talking about. My triglycerides are high, and she told me to cut down on my carbs and increase the monounsaturated fat. That doesn't make any sense. Triglycerides are fat, right?"*

No one diet can fit every situation or every person. This is why, in all our discussions of diet, we emphasize *individualization*. Ethnic and personal preferences are one consideration. Italians don't eat the same foods as people from Ireland; African Americans tend not to eat the way Asian Americans eat. And one member of a couple may love a particular food that his or her spouse just can't abide. But individualization is most important when a person has more than one problem. This is not uncommon, especially in people with Type II diabetes, who very often have high blood pressure or high blood cholesterol.

By discussing special diets for special health needs in this chapter, we are extending the notion that all diets have to be tailored to the individual. If you are healthy except for having diabetes, then your diet is constructed in one way; if you have other conditions, they too must be taken into account. An individualized diet that considers all your health concerns does *not* mean that you "won't be able to eat anything." A skillful dietitian can work all sorts of interesting and good-tasting combinations into almost any dietary restriction. We only ask you to work with the professional, open up your mind and your tastebuds, and stick with it.

The specific special diets we describe here are for people with high blood pressure, kidney disease, high blood fats, and food allergies. (Healthy eating during pregnancy is discussed in Chapter 31.) We know that you may have another problem not covered here; whatever it is, your best bet for getting sound advice on nutritional therapy is to meet with a registered dietitian.

High Blood Pressure

Why do we talk so much about high blood pressure and diabetes? Because any way you look at it, they are closely related. One reason for this is that Type II diabetes is associated with being overweight, and so is high blood pressure. Another could be that diabetes and high blood pressure are each linked to kidney problems. But for whatever reason, if you have Type I or Type II diabetes, you should be especially aware of blood pressure control.

There are three nutritional considerations in the treatment of high blood pressure (hypertension): reduce sodium intake, reduce weight, and watch for potassium imbalances in the blood that may occur as a result of the medications.

What, exactly, is sodium? It is a normal part of the blood, where it is found in a concentration very close to that of seawater. Sodium chloride (table salt), which is found in most salty-tasting foods, is the most common source of sodium. There are other salts, to be sure, such as potassium chloride (a "salt substitute"). Because the *chloride* content of sodium chloride is not important to blood pressure, we emphasize the low *sodium* part and encourage the use of such substitutes as potassium chloride if advised by your physician.

Why emphasize low sodium intake? Many people with high blood pressure are very sensitive to the salt they take in. A high-sodium diet raises blood pressure in these people. Conversely, lowering sodium intake significantly lowers blood pressure. The probable reason for this is that when the sodium intake is high there is a tendency to retain fluid. It may not be enough fluid to show up as ankle swelling, but it is enough to "overfill" the blood vessels and raise the blood pressure—much like putting too much air in a tire.

It is difficult to predict exactly who will be salt-sensitive, so the recommendation for anyone with mild to moderate hypertension is to keep sodium intake below 2,400 mg (2.4 grams) per day. Some people need even more stringent sodium restriction.

Making the switch to a low-sodium diet can be hard at first. The sodium content of foods is usually pretty clear from the taste if not from the label on the package. If you are following a low-sodium diet, you should avoid adding salt to your food from the shaker; you should also stay away from high-salt foods, such as most pretzels, potato chips, pizza, and soy sauce. You should talk to the dietitian about *your* most common sources of salt and target those for drastic reductions.

Nothing will taste right for a while. But after you get through the first few weeks, believe it or not, you get used to the low-salt diet. You may well find a series of new tastes you'd been drowning with salt (ask a good cook what he or she thinks of the guest who douses the entree in a heavy dose of salt!). After a while, an accidental brush with a high-salt food will actually be unpleasant. Trust us. You're not really physically addicted to salt. The craving will go away.

Losing weight, if you are overweight to begin with, will also help in controlling hypertension. The response of blood pressure to weight loss is variable, but almost everyone benefits to some degree. (See Chapter 7 for nutritional and behavioral interventions for weight loss.) Exercise is especially valuable in both weight loss and control of hypertension.

Blood pressure, like blood sugar, has to be watched regularly. The rare visit to the doctor's office may not be enough. Is there a nurse at your workplace who can check your pressure? A spouse or friend? Or can you learn to do it yourself? If you have been told your blood pressure is high or even "borderline," you should watch it regularly.

Quite often, weight loss and reduced dietary sodium will not adequately control hypertension. Medications are often needed. ACE inhibitors are now the favored treatment of hypertension for persons with diabetes (see Chapter 24). There are several other antihypertensive agents, each with its own efficacy and potential side effects.

Many of the antihypertensive drugs cause changes in blood potassium or sodium content, the so-called "electrolytes" that can easily be measured on a blood sample. So you may want to ask your doctor if your potassium level should be checked. If it is too high, you may need to work with your dietitian on controlling high-potassium foods. If it drifts low, as often occurs with the thiazide class of fluid pills, you will need a supplement of dietary potassium, usually in the form of a banana, potato skin, orange, or potassium pill. The fact is that these electrolyte imbalances and their dietary implications are hard to predict. You need to know whether you should change your potassium intake, and you should work with a dietitian in designing a plan to accomplish that.

Kidney Disease

People with diabetes are advised to avoid eating too much protein. The evidence is that too much protein is bad for the kidneys if they are failing, although we do not know whether a very high-protein diet hurts kidneys that are not showing signs of nephropathy. So, to be safe, the recommendation is for protein to make up 12%–15% of the total calories for the day—not too little and not too much.

If you do have protein in your urine—the earliest sign of diabetes affecting the kidneys—you'll be asked to reduce dietary protein to about 10% of total calories for the day. Your dietitian will help you identify exactly where your protein is coming from, but generally you'll want to cut down on red meats, fish, eggs, poultry, and dairy foods. Certain legumes are especially high in protein, such as green peas and dried beans and peas (kidney beans, black eyed beans, and so forth).

If your kidneys begin to fail (usually signified by increases in the BUN and creatinine measures on a blood test), the situation does get more complicated. Failing kidneys have trouble keeping the sodium, potassium, and magnesium levels in balance, and nutritional therapy may be called upon to help. Your kidneys may not be able to get rid of enough potassium, for example. Meal plans for people with failing kidneys should usually be low in foods that contain potassium.

Another potential issue is your kidneys' inability to get rid of enough phosphorus. High levels of phosphorus cause low levels of calcium, which in turn can cause problems with the bones. In this case, nutritional therapy is aimed at reducing phosphorus-containing foods, such as certain fruits and vegetables or dairy foods. Individual consultation is essential, because you will also want to take in enough calcium, perhaps including supplements such as Tums. Controlling dietary phosphorus and calcium definitely requires professional advice.

Does this sound complicated? It is complicated, because you must take into consideration not only the condition of your kidneys but the medications being used. It's not something you will be able to figure out for yourself, no matter how much reading you do. If your kidneys are failing, you have to be sure that your doctor checks your electrolytes and prescribes a diet that the dietitian can help you implement. Usually, at this stage of progressively failing kidneys, it takes a kidney specialist to sort it all out. Otherwise, you will not know just what you should and should not eat.

Dyslipidemia

Several different problems are grouped into the diagnosis of *dyslipidemia*, which means abnormal levels of fat in the blood. They are discussed more fully in Chapter 24. Hardening of the arteries is the dangerous aspect of dyslipidemia: high fats in the blood increase the chance of accelerated hardening of the arteries, with resulting heart attacks, stroke, or circulatory problems in the feet. All dyslipidemias are not same, and all dietary modifications should not be considered equally. Even doctors may become confused by the subject, because it is quite complicated. So we will not attempt to help you become an expert in blood fats. Here, we will break the topic down into two basic problems, each with a different meaning for dietary treatment: high cholesterol and high triglyceride/low HDL cholesterol.

We discuss dietary changes, but if dietary changes do not normalize your blood level of cholesterol and triglyceride, you should consider pharmacologic approaches. Cholesterol-lowering and triglyceride-lowering drugs are now readily available and have relatively few adverse side effects.

High Cholesterol

This actually refers to high total cholesterol and high LDL cholesterol (popularly known as "bad" cholesterol, since increased LDL is what increases the risk of atherosclerosis; see Chapter 24). The total cholesterol can be measured whether or not you are fasting (no food for 12 hours), but it is usually measured when fasting.

When is a blood cholesterol level too high? Strict guidelines have been established and accepted by various professional associations. These guidelines are so strict that almost half of all Americans are classified as having high cholesterol. The rationale for this is that more than half of Americans die of heart disease, and if we were all to lower our blood cholesterol level, we'd live significantly longer, on average. A person who is at high risk because of other factors, such as family history, should try to maintain an even lower blood cholesterol content than other people.

If your total cholesterol or LDL cholesterol is high, the first thing to think about is diet. The first thing to do in changing your diet is to lower your total fat intake, especially saturated fat. Remember that saturated fats, in general, are animal fats and dairy fats. The tender steak is not tender because it comes from a tender cow, it's tender because it is high in total fat and saturated fat. Hamburger meat, unless specially ground from trimmed meat, is likely to be high in saturated fats.

Read product labels. Other sources of high saturated fats include palm, coconut, and palm kernel oils. In choosing milk, recognize that while low-fat or 2% milk is lower in saturated fat than whole milk, the only really fat-free milk is skim milk.

Monounsaturated fats, mentioned in chapter 6, are definitely in vogue now. If you can increase their content in your diet, all the better. But not a lot of foods are high in monounsaturated fats. Olive oil, canola oil, some nuts (such as almonds, pecans, and cashews), avocados, olives, and sesame seeds are all high in monounsaturates. Since none of these is likely to be a major ingredient in your diet, increasing the proportion of total calories derived from monounsaturates to 20% or so may be very hard.

What about the polyunsaturated fats that have been so popular for lowering cholesterol? There's no doubt about it, polyunsaturates, found in safflower oil and some margarines and fish oils, are effective in lowering total and LDL cholesterol. But they sometimes also lower HDL cholesterol, which is not desirable. So the polyunsaturates are not as highly recommended now as they were in the past. But if your HDL cholesterol is fine, then they can still be effective in lowering the LDL cholesterol.

A tricky little subplot has developed of late in the saturated/unsaturated fat story: *partially hydrogenated, hydrogenated,* and *trans-fatty acids* are all terms used on labels to disguise the fact that these are *saturated fats.* So be on the lookout for these words when you read labels, and be wary when the fats don't add up. The label may read: "Total Fat: 11 grams; Saturated Fat: 4 grams; Unsaturated Fat: 3 grams." Wait a minute! What happened to the extra 4 grams of fat? It probably consists of "trans-fatty acids," and that's not good. Take time to read the ingredients to figure out if partially hydrogenated or hydrogenated fats are listed.

What about dietary cholesterol itself? A lot of foods have a little cholesterol, but just one commonly eaten food has a lot of cholesterol: egg yolks. In the American diet, the number of eggs you consume, at about 275 mg cholesterol per egg yolk, will determine your total cholesterol intake. A whole lobster comes close to one egg in cholesterol content, and a crab has about one-third the amount of cholesterol. But, really, how many crabs and lobsters do you eat every day, even if you live in Maryland and vacation in Maine? Even 3.5 ounces of cheddar cheese, which has a bad reputation, contains only about one-third the cholesterol of an egg. In the end, the cholesterol content of your diet is likely to come down to how often you eat eggs. So, for the sake of your heart, how about switching away from that daily egg for breakfast and moving on to cereal?

The National Cholesterol Education Program Step II diet guidelines define the dietary recommendations for lowering cholesterol: less than 7% of total calories from saturated fat, less than 30% of calories from total fat, and cholesterol intake less than 200 mg per day.

High Triglyceride/Low HDL Cholesterol

The relationship between high triglyceride levels and low HDL cholesterol is difficult to explain, especially because we have only theories about why it happens. But as a rule, when your blood triglyceride is high, your HDL cholesterol (the "good cholesterol") is low, and the combination is dangerous. Triglyceride levels in the blood over about 200 mg/dl carry some increased risk of accelerated hardening of the arteries, but the risk is not very high unless it is combined with low HDL cholesterol. Tests for both triglyceride and HDL cholesterol have to be done at least 12 hours after eating.

How do we treat high triglyceride/low HDL-cholesterol? The first step is to be sure your diabetes is under control. It is remarkable to see how, when the blood sugar comes down, the triglyceride also comes down. But dietary treatment can be tricky. If the triglyceride is very high—say, over about 700 mg/dl—then you probably have to hold back your fat intake, because the severe high triglyceride can cause pancreatitis. With triglyceride levels that are not so high—say, 250–500 mg/dl—there is controversy about what diet is best. Some people seem to respond to a *low-carbohydrate* diet, even if it is high in fat. Others feel that reduced fat is the answer, or substitution of unsaturated fats for saturated fats.

For persons with high triglycerides, increasing the monounsaturated fats to 20% of total calories (a hard thing to do, as described above) and holding saturated and polyunsaturated fats to less than 10% of calories each may be beneficial.

Food Allergies

What do food allergies have to do with diabetes? People with diabetes are no more likely to have food allergies than anyone else. But allergies can make following a diet much more difficult, and misconceptions about what constitutes an allergy can further complicate life with diabetes. The problem is that you already have restrictions on what you eat, so adding food allergies or perceived food allergies into the equation may be an important consideration.

An allergic reaction to food is a response to food that can start immediately after ingesting a food or some hours later. The allergic response does not occur in the gastrointestinal tract: it is not abdominal upset or pain. It is either a skin response or a whole-body response. In mild forms, allergies usually cause some degree of itching, hives, swelling around the eyes, mild wheezing, or a rash. But they can be extremely serious and even fatal if the person has an *anaphylactic reaction,* such an extreme allergic reaction that he or she is in immediate danger of dying if not properly treated.

A food allergy is not just a dislike for a certain food. If you hate lima beans, you have a food aversion, not an allergy. A food allergy does not mean getting cramps or diarrhea from a food. Even lactose intolerance—a common cause of severe diarrhea and stomach upset after eating lactose-containing foods, such as milk—is not an allergy; it is the inability of the intestine to digest lactose. The lactose-containing foods cannot be properly absorbed and used.

If you think you are allergic to a certain food, the best thing to do is not to eat it at home or in a restaurant, at least until you check it out with your doctor. If the signs do point to an allergy, you should avoid the food completely. Sometimes you have to be very careful to determine whether or not a given dish contains the food you are allergic to. A physician friend knew that he was allergic to shellfish. He did his best to avoid them. But at a restaurant he ordered a fish chowder after being assured that it contained no shellfish, only to find out after he ate it that it had traces of crabmeat. His allergic reaction was so severe that he was in the hospital for three weeks.

Be aware that food allergies do exist. If you have one or more such allergies, be sure your dietitian knows it. Your special diet will have to be even more special.

Having not just diabetes but diabetes plus (fill in the blank) can be challenging. Special dietary modifications may well be indicated, and if so you will probably not be able to figure it all out yourself. So put the challenge to your treating physician and a professional dietitian. Ask them just what you can eat and how you should structure your diet. Work with the dietitian to get as many as possible of the foods you like into your diet, and be willing to try some interesting alternatives.

Changing your diet may mean tossing aside a family tradition of using fatback to season your vegetables; it may mean ending your serious love affair with high-salt pizza. But you will find that food selection targeted to your health needs as well as your tastebuds will keep your system in balance and keep you feeling better and living longer.

Chapter 10

Exercise and Diabetes

- *"I've been a couch potato for 25 years, and now, just because I got diabetes, you tell me I'm supposed to start exercising!"*

- *"When I first began walking, I couldn't make it to the corner without stopping to catch my breath. Now I walk for 40 minutes, and when I get back I feel better than I did when I left."*

- *"I never could stick with an exercise program until someone suggested I ride my stationary bike while I watch television. Now I kill two birds with one stone: I stay fit while I keep up with my soap operas."*

- *"I used to like racquetball as a kid. And you know what? I still do. Picking up the old racquet got me back into exercise."*

Exercise has to be a central part of your diabetes treatment plan. Increased activity provides a wide variety of physical, mental, and even social benefits. And it does all this without the side effects of medication. Still, we're very aware that most people don't want to exercise. Our goal is to help you develop an exercise plan you can not only live with but positively enjoy.

If you follow guidelines specifically tailored to your own condition and your own goals, you can exercise safely regardless of your age or physical condition. In this chapter, we'll take a close look at the benefits as well as the cautions of exercise for a person with diabetes. We'll also help you develop your own exercise plan, help you get started, and discuss rules for safe exercise when you have diabetes. Finally, we will offer some suggestions to help you stick with your exercise plan, to keep you from relapsing to that couch potato state.

Benefits of Exercise

The benefits of exercise are real and substantial:

—Improved blood sugar control
—Weight loss or weight management when combined with a good meal plan
—Reduced risk of heart disease
—Lower blood pressure
—Reduced need for insulin or pills to control the blood sugar

You'll feel stronger and healthier, look and feel better, have less stress, and feel much better about yourself. What more could you ask?

If this list sounds too good to be true, we can just point out that every bit of it has scientific evidence to back it up. So don't ask whether exercise is good for you: it is. We urge you to get started *now*.

Getting Ready

If you haven't exercised in years or you are considering a dramatic increase in the amount or intensity of your exercise, talk it over with your health care provider first. If you take insulin, ask whether you should decrease your dose on exercise days. If you are over 50, obese, or have a history of heart disease, your health care provider may want to check your cardiac status. Finally, if you have complications of diabetes, such as proliferative retinopathy or neuropathy, you should talk to your health care provider about the effect of exercise on these conditions, as well. (See the section on exercising safely below.)

If you are reasonably healthy and if you use your head, you needn't be frightened about starting to exercise. Start slowly, build up gradually, and go for it. Once you've made the commitment to exercise, you should give some thought to the kind of activity to start with.

What activities do you like?   Your chance of sticking with activities you enjoy is good; your chance of sticking with activities you hate is poor. How can you tell which exercise activities you might enjoy? Maybe you're already doing something you like, but not doing it often enough. Maybe you used to enjoy a particular activity and you can pick it up again, like the former racquetball player quoted above. Maybe there's a sport you've always wanted to try because it looks like fun. Or maybe you want to spend more time with your best friend. Exercise can even be a great way to meet people. Whatever you choose, it should be something you *want* to do.

Do you prefer to exercise by yourself or with other people?   Some people like solitude and opportunity for contemplation or don't want the hassle of always scheduling someone else into the exercise time slot. Some people are embarrassed at the start by how out of shape they are and so avoid exercising with others (this won't last). A work or school schedule may also make exercising alone the best choice. But other people find that company helps them stick to their commitment and makes exercise more fun. Company can also make some outdoor activities, like walking or running, safer. Naturally, the choice of exercising alone or with a partner is not a lifetime decision. You can vary your pattern depending on circumstances and your disposition.

Do you like competitive sports?   Anything from bowling to swimming can be undertaken in a hotly competitive or totally noncompetitive mode. Which approach do you prefer?

What facilities do you need?   If you like the idea of an aerobics class, what's available? What will it cost? If you're planning to swim, where's the pool? If you'd like to ski, how far away are the slopes, and what will you do for exercise when there's no snow? Whatever activity you are considering, you'll need to think through these issues of where, when, how, and how much. There is a very strong relationship between how *convenient* exercise is and how *often* and how *consistently* it is done.

Will you be better off exercising at home, outdoors, or in a specific facility?   Some people say they can complete their entire exercise routine at home—using an exercise bike, walking, or jogging—in the time it would take them to get to the local health club. If finding time to exercise is a problem for you, this might be the way to go. Other people like the social atmosphere and the wide range of activities and equipment available at an exercise facility. You'll want to think seriously about what's going to work best for you. You may want to pay a visit to a health club, if you think you might enjoy it. Most clubs offer one-time visits or short-term trial memberships free or at very low cost.

How intense an exercise program do you want?   The intensity of exercise that is best for you depends on your age, physical conditioning, and motivation. Exercise intensity can be estimated by the pulse rate (which is the same as heart rate) you reach while you are exercising and how long you exercise. Begin by determining your maximal heart rate, which is approximately 220 minus your age. For example, if you're 50 years old, your approximate maximal heart rate would be 220 minus 50, or about 170 beats per minute.

Low-intensity exercise might involve 10–20 minutes of activity at a heart rate of about 60% of your maximal heart rate (102 beats per minute, in the example given above). At the other end of the spectrum, very high-intensity exercise could include 60 minutes at a heart rate of 80% maximal (about 140 beats per minute in the example). Your exercise will likely fall between these extremes. To determine your heart rate while you are exercising, stop several times to check your pulse rate. If you are exercising at a very low level of intensity, your heart rate may be about 60% of maximum for 10–20 minutes; if you are exercising at a high level of intensity, your heart rate may go up to 80% or even 90% of maximum for an hour or more.

If you find the prospect of intense exercise daunting, you should know that even brief, infrequent, low-intensity exercise is better than none at all. In fact, you can improve your blood sugar control and overall health with activities that aren't really exercise at all. For example, you could walk a flight or two of stairs rather than taking the elevator or escalator. Or you could park a block or two from the store rather than seeking the closest parking space. When you are home, you could turn on your favorite music and dance for 10–15 minutes. Take your age into account. Walking the dog may be great for a 70-year-old but not enough exercise for a 30-year-old.

If you are looking for higher levels of fitness, your exercise plan needs to be more ambitious. At the same time, make sure that it is realistic. Setting your goals too high will almost certainly lead to frustration or injury, and ultimately you probably won't stick with your exercise plan. Start where you are. If you are already fairly active, add a little to your current regimen or make exercise a more regular part of your routine. If you are basically sedentary, start with a modest regimen, maybe walking a few blocks several times a week. (See Table 9 for exercise guidelines from the American Diabetes Association and Table 10 for a list of activities and an account of how much energy you expend when engaging in them.)

Getting Started

You're convinced of the benefits of exercise, you have selected an activity you think you will enjoy, and you have encouragement to get started from your health care provider. Now what? Getting started is one of the hardest parts of exercising (sticking with it is another). Most people have lots of excuses (some people call them "reasons") for not exercising regularly. Let's look at some of the most common ones.

I can't find time.   We hear this one often, and for good reason. Exercise

Table 9.   American Diabetes Association Guidelines for Exercise

General guidelines:
- Use proper footwear and protective equipment.
- Avoid exercise in extreme heat or cold.
- Inspect your feet daily and after exercise.
- Avoid exercising during periods of poor blood glucose control.

Specifically for those with Type I (insulin-dependent) diabetes:
- Exercise is recommended to improve your cardiovascular fitness and psychological well-being and for social interaction and recreation. Safe participation in all forms of exercise, consistent with your lifestyle, should be the main goal. Participation in competitive sports is possible if you so desire. You need to self-monitor your blood glucose so that necessary adjustments can be made in diet or insulin dosage.

Specifically for those with Type II (non–insulin-dependent) diabetes:
- Exercise should be part of your diabetes therapy, in addition to appropriate diet and medications, to improve your blood glucose control, reduce your risk of cardiovascular complications, and increase your psychological well-being. An exercise stress test is recommended if you are over 35 years of age. If you take oral hypoglycemic medications or insulin, you need to self-monitor your blood glucose level. Your exercise program should include moderate aerobic exercise (50–70% of VO_2 max)[a] for 20–45 minutes at least 3 days per week. Always perform low-intensity warm-up and cool-down exercises.

[a]VO_2 max measures an individual's limit for exercise: it tells how fit the person's heart and lungs are.

does take time, though probably not as much as you think. As we've mentioned, 30 minutes of low-intensity activity three times a week represents a good basic exercise routine. Think about how you might fit this into your busy schedule. If all else fails, you might try exercising while you watch television or read a book or newspaper.

If you are serious about establishing and sticking to your exercise program, you need to set a schedule and keep to it. Make an appointment with yourself to exercise, just as you would schedule any other essential activity in your life. Think about the time of day you are most likely to exercise. Think about what obligations might interfere with your plan. (If you have a fixed obligation most evenings, don't plan to exercise in the evening.)

I'm too old and out of shape.   Recent studies show that it's never too late to start exercising. Many of the physical consequences of aging are primarily the result of inactivity. People in their 80s and even in their 90s show

Table 10.   Energy Expenditure Associated with Common Exercises

Activity	Calories Burned Each Minute	Calories Burned in an Hour

Light housework
  Polishing furniture
  Light hand-washing of dishes,
  clothes, windows, etc.
	2–2½	120–50

Golf, using power cart Level walking at 2 miles per hour	2½–4	150–240
Cleaning windows, mopping floors, or vacuuming Walking at 3 miles per hour Golf, pulling cart Cycling at 6 miles per hour Bowling	4–5	240–300
Scrubbing floors Cycling at 8 miles per hour Walking at 3½ miles per hour Table tennis, badminton, and volleyball Doubles tennis Golf, carrying clubs Many calisthenics and ballet exercises	5–6	300–360
Walking at 4 miles per hour Ice or roller skating Cycling at 10 miles per hour	6–7	360–420
Walking at 5 miles per hour Cycling at 11 miles per hour Water skiing Singles tennis	7–8	420–480
Jogging at 5 miles per hour Cycling at 12 miles per hour Downhill skiing Paddleball	8–10	480–600
Running at 5½ miles per hour Cycling at 13 miles per hour Squash or handball (practice session)	10–11	600–660
Running at 6 miles per hour or more Competitive handball or squash	11 or more	660 or more

SOURCE: Adapted from H. Rifkin, ed., *The American Diabetes Association Guide to Good Living* (New York: American Diabetes Association, 1982).

marked improvements in mobility, strength, and endurance when they engage in regular exercise.

We have heard countless stories of people with diabetes who begin to exercise and go on to reach amazing heights. One woman was diagnosed with diabetes at the age of 30. A classic couch potato, she decided to take up running. The first day she couldn't make it to her corner mailbox. But she stuck with it and within a year she could run a mile without stopping. At this point she really got the running bug and began to train harder and enter local weekend races. Eight years after her diagnosis, this woman completed a *100-mile* race! We aren't advocating this level of exercise but we do believe that anyone at any age can enjoy the benefits of a healthy, active lifestyle.

Exercise hurts. If you do it right, exercise shouldn't hurt. Sure, you may get winded and your muscles may stiffen up a bit. Working up a sweat and getting winded are part of exercise. But the expression "no pain, no gain" is just plain wrong unless, perhaps, your goal is to be a professional athlete. (See below for a discussion of how to keep exercise safe.) Remember, you are trying to develop an exercise program for life. If you are pushing so hard that it hurts, you need to ease up. Rethink your exercise program and consider switching to a less stressful activity, or check with your health care provider.

Exercise is boring. For some people this is a real problem. If you are one, there are several things that might help. First, try to combine exercise with things you like to do, such as walking in a pretty place or watching a good movie on videotape while you do aerobics. As we said, you might find an exercise partner or take up a competitive sport. We all have days when we just don't feel like exercising. If you have a partner whom you can't let down, you'll be more likely to get out there and exercise, even if you don't feel like exercising.

Another way to avoid boredom is to cross-train, or vary your exercise routine. If walking is your main activity, consider an occasional swim, a bike ride, or an evening of dancing. Cross-training not only cuts boredom, it also gives you a more balanced workout and reduces your risk of overuse injuries.

I just can't maintain my motivation. Maintaining your motivation will be less of a problem if you are doing an activity you like or love. But if you can't find an exercise you really enjoy, you're more likely to stick with your exercise program just briefly, then lose focus.

There are several ways to avoid this pitfall. First, set goals. Those who succeed *plan* for success. Consider writing an exercise contract with yourself. This kind of formal planning may be a big help. Your contract can be a simple one that you draft in a few minutes. It might look something like this:

Exercise goal for week of: July 3
Activity: Walking 12 blocks in 30 min.

Exercise goal for week of: July 10
Activity: Walking 15 blocks in 35 min.

Exercise goal for week of: July 17
Activity: Walking 15 blocks in 30 min.

An added benefit of a weekly contract is that it keeps you from getting discouraged by the inevitably slow progress you will make toward your long-term goals. To maximize your motivation, have both short-term and long-term goals.

Notice that the contract states goals in terms of behavior. It's better to set behavioral goals, because behavior is something you can control. In contrast, if you set a goal of losing 1 pound a week, you might do everything you could to make it happen and still not succeed. Besides, if you meet your exercise (and diet) goals, you will reach your weight loss goals, as well.

Another way to maximize motivation is to recognize that no one is perfect—not even your most physically fit friend. There will be days, and even weeks, when you don't meet your goals. The key to coping is to see these rough spots as lapses, not failures. You've simply had a bad day or week (even world-class athletes have slumps). You can put the lapse behind you and get back with the program. If you take the opposite tack and tell yourself you've failed, you create a self-fulfilling prophecy: your motivation evaporates and you continue to slide.

So be good to yourself. Give yourself credit for your hard work and accomplishments. And pay attention to how you feel when you work out regularly. Most people tell us they feel better: stronger, healthier, more energetic, and more confident. Don't lose sight of these benefits, especially if you feel your commitment beginning to flag. That's when you most need to accentuate the positive.

Exercising Safely

We have talked about the importance of not trying to do too much too soon when it comes to exercise. This is not a book on sports medicine, but we can still tell you that pulled muscles and strained ligaments are a definite complication of taking up exercise directly from the couch potato position. So start slowly and work out regularly. If a muscle pull occurs, back off.

There are also some cautions about exercise that apply specifically to people with diabetes.

Exercise and Blood Sugar

Exercise will affect your blood sugar levels, but the effect may be less predictable than you might expect. You probably think of exercise as lowering blood sugar, and this is often right, but not always. You will need to learn your own responses. As you become familiar with how exercise affects *your* blood sugar, you will learn how to reduce your risk of hypoglycemia or hyperglycemia.

With Type II diabetes treated by diet alone or with pills, it is likely that moderate exercise will have a hypoglycemic effect. As discussed in Chapter 5, the effect may last quite long—in the range of 6–12 or even 24 hours. When you start to exercise, you will probably need to make changes in other parts of your diabetes regimen: you may need less insulin or oral hypoglycemic medication, for example, or you may need more food (see Table 11). Timely self-monitoring of blood glucose is the key to making these adjustments safely and effectively. If you don't check, you'll never know why you feel different.

Especially with insulin-requiring diabetes, you may notice some sur-

---

Table 11. Strategies to Avoid Hypoglycemia and Hyperglycemia with Exercise

1. Eat a meal 1–3 hours before exercise.
2. Take supplemental carbohydrate feedings during exercise at least every 30 minutes if exercise is vigorous and of long duration.
3. Increase food intake for up to 24 hours after exercise, depending on intensity and duration of exercise.
4. Take insulin at least 1 hour before exercise. If less than 1 hour before exercise, inject in a nonexercising area.
5. Decrease insulin dose before exercise.
6. Alter daily insulin schedule.
7. Monitor blood glucose before, during, and after exercise.
8. Delay exercise if blood glucose is over 250 mg/dl (over 14 mM) and ketones are present.
9. Learn individual glucose responses to different types of exercise.

SOURCE: Ed Horton, "Exercise," in H. E. Lebovitz, ed., *Therapy for Diabetes Mellitus and Related Disorders* (Alexandria, Va.: American Diabetes Association, 1990), p. 110.

prising effects of exercise. For instance, the same amount of insulin may lower your blood sugar more than it used to. This may be especially noticeable the day *after* exercise. Exercise also increases the rate at which insulin is absorbed from your injection site, so your insulin may start to work more quickly than normal. This is particularly true if you injected your insulin in a part of your body that you are exercising vigorously. On the other hand, very strenuous exercise can increase the amount of glucose released from the liver into your bloodstream, so sometimes your blood sugar level actually *increases,* especially right after exercise.

In sum, when you exercise, you have to watch out for both hypoglycemia and hyperglycemia. Try to sort out for yourself what a given type of exercise does to your sugar level. Just be aware that the effect could depend on a combination of exactly how much exercise, how vigorous the exercise, when you took your last insulin shot, and when you ate last. Sorting it all out can be complicated.

Effect of Exercise on Long-Term Complications

Exercise does not cause long-term complications; on the contrary, there is evidence that it may help prevent them. But several complications, if they are in a relatively advanced stage, may be aggravated by exercise. Heavy lifting and other strenuous activity should be avoided if you have serious (proliferative) retinopathy or have had multiple bleeds in your eyes.

If you have significant peripheral neuropathy, you are at increased risk for soft tissue and joint injuries, since you are less likely to feel the trauma. You have to be much more careful of footwear. Take measures to avoid blisters or foot trauma and inspect your feet especially carefully. You may want to choose low-intensity exercise, such as walking, using a stationary bike or low-intensity rowing machine, or swimming. If you have autonomic neuropathy (see Chapter 27), your capacity for high-intensity exercise may be reduced due to a decrease in your maximum heart rate and your cardiac capacity. In this case, select a lower intensity exercise.

Even after kidney or pancreas transplantation, exercise is important. Prednisone, the drug people take to prevent organ rejection, causes weight gain, muscle wasting, and weakness. Aerobic exercise and resistance or strength training are the best ways to fight these side effects of prednisone.

Exercise during Pregnancy

Exercise during pregnancy helps you stay fit, control your weight gain, increase your strength and stamina, and reduce back pain. Exercise can also help you control your blood sugar levels, which is especially important during pregnancy. If you already exercise regularly, you can probably continue with your routine as long as you take special precautions. Don't do exercises that involve straining, holding your breath, or making jerky movements or that cause rises in your core body temperature above 100 degrees (such as exercising in extreme heat or taking saunas or whirlpool baths for longer than 10 minutes).

If you did not exercise regularly before pregnancy, this isn't the time to start a *strenuous* new program. Low-intensity activity, on the other hand, might be a wonderful idea. Check with your health care provider to discuss the best plan for you.

Exercise for Older Adults

Physical abilities inevitably decline with age. Even the serious athlete loses speed and fast reflexes. For recreational athletes or "weekend warriors," much of the decline is a result of simple inactivity. So increased activity, in the form of sensible exercise, can provide older adults with the same benefits it offers younger people.

Older adults with diabetes should have a pre-exercise physical examination and work out an exercise prescription with their health care provider. Once you begin exercising, you'll need to keep certain precautions in mind. Starting slowly and building up gradually is especially important. Not letting your heart rate rise above about 60% of maximal is also a good idea. You may want to stay away from exercises that require fast movements and quick changes of direction, because coordination and reaction time can slow with age.

Even so, there are many activities to choose from. Consider walking, for instance. Many senior citizen groups organize "mall walks" or neighborhood walks. These can be a great way to meet other people. Water exercises are another favorite of many older adults because these activities place so little stress on the joints and feet. Aqua-aerobics, water walking, and swimming are all excellent ways to stay fit. Bicycling is another great form of exercise, whether you do it outdoors or on a stationary bike in the comfort of your own home. Check with your local Y, health clubs, community colleges, and local recreation centers to find out where there are outdoor trails and tracks or indoor facilities in your area.

If you have difficulty with balance and standing, chair exercises can help you improve your strength, coordination, and flexibility. You can gain these benefits in as little as 30 minutes a day, and you can watch television or listen to music at the same time.

For older people, one special alert is chest pain. *Angina* (also called *angina pectoris*) is a characteristic kind of chest pain that usually occurs when exercising and is suggestive of heart trouble. It is usually described as a heaviness, squeezing, or tightness that occurs beneath the breastbone and may go into the back, jaw, or left arm, stopping within a minute or so after you stop exercising. If you have any sort of chest pain, be sure to stop exercising right away and have it checked out by your doctor.

Exercising to Lose Weight

Exercise helps you lose weight because it burns calories. But it's hard to exercise enough to lose much weight unless you also make some changes in your eating habits. Recall that to lose 1 pound of fat through exercise, the average person has to burn about 3,500 calories. This could require walking or running 6 miles or swimming for an hour, every day for a week. Another way to achieve this would be to cut your caloric intake by about 500 calories a day by skipping a second portion of fatty meat five days of the week and to walk 30–45 minutes four days of the week. The point is, exercising *and* holding down the calorie intake is clearly the way to go unless you can maintain a very heavy exercise schedule.

If you haven't been exercising and you are quite a bit overweight, even low-intensity activity, such as walking around the block, may be difficult. If so, start very slowly. Walk for 5 minutes, then rest for a few minutes, then walk another 5 or 10 minutes. Add a few minutes to your total walking time every couple of weeks, and eventually you will be able to complete an entire 30–45-minute workout without stopping.

The key to effective weight loss through exercise is to focus on duration, not perspiration. It's better to go *longer* than *harder.*

Some people worry that exercise will lead to weight *gain* rather than weight loss because it will make them hungrier or will "increase their muscle mass." While it's true that extended exercise (or any exercise that leads to hypoglycemia) can produce a need to eat, most low-intensity exercise has the opposite effect: it makes dieting easier. If you really train hard, especially if you lift weights, the increased muscle mass may compensate for loss of weight in fat. But don't worry about it: you'll feel and look much better.

So use exercise as an adjunct to dieting, and both will be more successful.

Do yourself a favor and exercise. It doesn't have to be anything major at first. In fact, it shouldn't be. Start very easy, with something you like (or think you might like), at a level you find comfortable. Even walking one block can be the beginning of something wonderful, if you stick with it and build up gradually as your fitness improves. We like this advice: "Ask your doctor before you *stop* exercising." You will discover that exercise is a veritable fountain of well-being, offering all the benefits we've described in this chapter. And it's yours for the taking.

Chapter 11

Treating Type II Diabetes with Oral Hypoglycemics

- *"I want to take pills for my diabetes. I don't want to take insulin."*

- *"The pills used to be perfectly good for me, but now they aren't as effective. This worries me."*

- *"Whenever a doctor says I should take a pill, I want to know what it could do to me. I read the insert that comes with the bottle, and then I get agitated. How should I interpret what's said in the insert?"*

- *"I'm always hearing about new pills for diabetes. What's really new? What's proven? What's good for me?"*

During World War II a French army doctor wrote back from the front to tell a colleague about a strange observation he had made. When he treated soldiers' combat wounds with the new sulfa antibiotics, some of the soldiers acted as if they had taken too much insulin. His colleague tried to duplicate the finding in dogs and demonstrated that their blood sugar level did indeed go down when they were given sulfas. He then removed the pancreas from the animals and found that the sulfa drugs had no effect on blood sugar in the dogs that lacked a pancreas.

That discovery marked a change in the treatment of diabetes. Other medications and herbs had been shown to have small effects on blood glucose, but the sulfa derivatives, called *sulfonylureas*, have a major effect in lowering blood glucose and have become a mainstay of the treatment of Type II diabetes.

In over 50 years of use, pills for treating diabetes (the *oral hypoglycemic agents*) have undergone some changes, and new agents have come along. Used in the right setting, they are outstanding in their effectiveness. Many people with diabetes are treated successfully with them. But like all medications, they have limitations and side effects. In this chapter we review the principles for using oral hypoglycemic agents and then take a closer look at the specific drugs.

How the Oral Hypoglycemic Agents Work

Two fundamental features of oral hypoglycemic agents are that *they are not insulin* and *they cannot take the place of insulin.* The French researchers demonstrated this when they removed the pancreas of the dogs and discovered that the sulfa drug no longer lowered blood glucose. This meant that the drug needed an intact, insulin-producing pancreas. This is true of all pills used to treat diabetes: the person has to be making at least some insulin from his or her own pancreas. So far there has been very little success in giving insulin itself by mouth. Because insulin is a fragile chemical that is immediately destroyed by the stomach acids if given orally, it must be given by injection instead.

The practical implication is that oral hypoglycemic agents will not work when the person has Type I diabetes. They often do not work, either, when Type II diabetes has progressed to the point where the person is secreting very little insulin from the pancreas.

How, then, do the oral hypoglycemic agents work? One class of oral hypoglycemic agent, the sulfonylureas, act primarily by stimulating insulin secretion from the pancreas (Figure 11). They are like a booster, giving the pancreas an additional push. They are effective because they not only help the

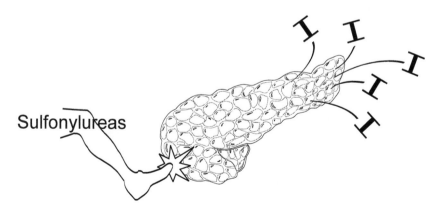

Figure 11. Sulfonylureas lower blood sugar by causing the pancreas to make more insulin. In effect, they give the pancreas a kick to work harder.

pancreas put out more insulin throughout the day and night but also help it respond appropriately to meals.

Another class of oral hypoglycemic agent, of which metformin is a member, has a different mechanism of action. It acts not by pushing the pancreas to put out more insulin, but by assisting the action of the insulin that is secreted on the body's tissues (Figure 12). As discussed earlier, insulin resistance (lessened effect of insulin) is a major problem in Type II diabetes. Although some uncertainty about its mechanism still exists, metformin seems to help overcome that resistance. As far as we know, like the sulfonylureas, it is not effective if there is no pancreatic insulin secretion.

A third type of pill, called acarbose, slows the absorption of carbohydrates from the intestine (Figure 13). The effect is to reduce the rise in blood sugar after a meal. Gastrointestinal side effects, especially gas, seem to be a problem with this agent.

A new class of pills for diabetes is exemplified by the drug troglitazone. It has a mechanism of action that is different and potentially very useful: troglitazone specifically enhances the action of insulin. Since insulin resistance is a basic problem in Type II diabetes, this could be a great addition to its treatment. Troglitazone may also allow reduction of the insulin dose in people who do take insulin. It is a drug to watch and to use as it becomes generally available.

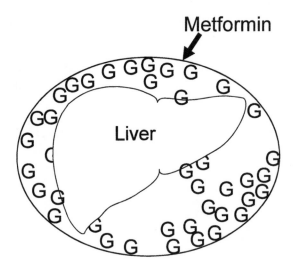

Figure 12. Metformin lowers the blood sugar indirectly by decreasing the amount of sugar released from the liver.

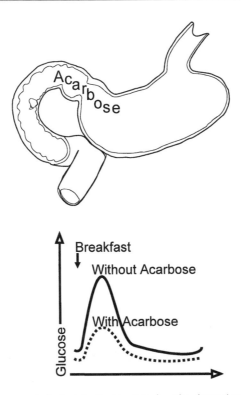

Figure 13. Acarbose works in the intestinal tract to slow the absorption of glucose into the bloodstream. Because of this, it helps to keep the after-meal blood sugars from going too high.

How to Use Oral Hypoglycemic Agents

As noted, the oral hypoglycemic agents are useful only in treating Type II diabetes; they are not useful in treating Type I diabetes. Nor are they used in treating gestational diabetes mellitus (GDM), because of the possibility of causing injury to the developing fetus. Sometimes when it is not clear whether the correct diagnosis is Type I diabetes or Type II diabetes, the oral agents may be given a trial use.

For best effect, the oral hypoglycemic agents should be taken regularly every day, not taken irregularly or started and stopped according to blood sugar. A wide range of doses is available, so if blood sugars are running too high or too low, the dose can be changed. These medications are not meant to be used just when the person is feeling bad or just when the blood sugar has already been too high. They can be stopped and restarted later, but this should be done in consultation with the health care professional, not on a whim.

Of course, you should not use a medication if you have an allergic reaction to it. An allergic reaction is typically characterized by a rash all over the body, hives, or difficulty breathing. A true allergy to other sulfa drugs, such as the antibiotics often used to treat urinary tract infections, may signal an allergy to the sulfonylureas also. If you are allergic to sulfas in general, discuss this with your doctor before beginning a sulfonylurea for diabetes. Also, if you should have significant stomach symptoms, such as nausea or heartburn, while on the medication and you cannot reach the health care professional for a discussion, you should not restart the medication on your own. Wait until you can talk it over with your health care provider.

Perhaps the most important thing to know about using the oral hypoglycemic agents is that *they are not a substitute for diet and exercise.* People who think they can give up efforts to follow a healthy diet and get regular exercise when they take their pills will be sorely disappointed. Type II diabetes is fundamentally a condition treated with diet and exercise, whether or not the person also needs oral hypoglycemic agents or insulin.

When the Oral Hypoglycemic Agents Don't Work

Since their introduction in the 1950s it has been known that in some people with Type II diabetes, the pills work for a while and then lose their effectiveness. Others may continue to respond to pills indefinitely, especially if they follow a pretty good diet, exercise, and control their weight. Needing the pills to control your diabetes does not mean that you will end up needing insulin. (Chapter 3 describes how to tell when your treatment is and is not working.)

The general understanding is that the oral agents no longer work if the pancreas grows progressively weaker and less able to secrete insulin. It is not clear whether this natural deterioration of pancreatic function is speeded up or slowed down by pushing the insulin secretion along with the sulfonylurea, but it doesn't make a lot of difference. Most people would prefer to try using the pills rather than moving directly from diet to insulin, even if their response to the oral hypoglycemic agents only lasts a few years.

Experience with these agents in the United States is limited, but it is likely that adding a different class of oral hypoglycemic agent (for instance, adding metformin to the treatment regimen of a person who is slipping out of control on sulfonylureas alone) will be effective, at least temporarily. Another trend that has become more popular in recent years is *combined therapy*—

that is, the use of insulin and sulfonylurea. The approach is called *BIDS therapy* (bedtime insulin, daytime sulfonylurea). It may be tried when the morning (fasting) blood sugar is elevated, while blood sugars during the day are in a better range, using sulfonylurea alone. The point is to use an injection of intermediate-acting insulin at bedtime to suppress the liver's sugar production overnight and count on the sulfonylurea to control blood sugar during the day.

The Risks of Oral Hypoglycemic Agent Use

There are many ways to find out about the pills that have been prescribed for you. The patient package insert (PPI) gives detailed technical information but is written in very dry language. It also is likely to include every side effect ever reported, making little distinction between what is common, what is rare, and what is probably not due to the drug at all. The PPI can be scary reading.

Pharmacies often provide computerized printouts that use more readable language. But again, since part of the printouts' purpose is to protect the providers from lawsuits, they may list problems that are very rare or not caused by the drug at all. And all these official sources will counsel you, when any doubt at all exists, to "contact your doctor," as though she or he were just waiting at the other end of the telephone line, 24 hours a day, to answer your most technical question.

Every now and then, a patient will read the PPI for sulfonylurea or metformin very carefully or will get a tip from someone he or she knows and come in asking how we could possibly give them something that causes death from cardiovascular disease or lactic acidosis. Does use of an oral hypoglycemic agent increase one's risk of death? The Food and Drug Administration (FDA) insists that a warning be put in every PPI of sulfonylureas and metformin. The facts behind these warnings, however, are complicated and somewhat uncertain.

In the 1960s and 1970s a large trial was carried out comparing a sulfonylurea (tolbutamide or Orinase) and a metformin-like drug (phenformin) to insulin or diet alone. The study was called the University Group Diabetes Program (UGDP). There were slightly more deaths among people taking the two oral hypoglycemic agents than among the people in the other groups. Reams of commentary have been written discussing the UGDP and whether its findings were "real." The FDA could not agree on whether sulfonylureas were safe. In the end, they were not banned but were made available only with the frightening warning in the package insert.

The case against phenformin was considered stronger. It clearly (though rarely) caused a very dangerous and sometimes fatal complication called lactic acidosis. The FDA therefore decided to ban phenformin and metformin (a similar drug), although metformin does not appear to cause lactic acidosis. Only in 1995, after more than 20 years' further experience throughout the world and careful trials in the United States, was metformin deemed to be safe and made available in this country.

Most specialists in diabetes, including ourselves, have carefully reviewed the UGDP study and concluded that it was not valid. Admittedly, we cannot point to a single fatal flaw in the study, but some very serious questions have been raised. We think that when all factors are taken into consideration, the evidence is overwhelming that the sulfonylureas do not cause death from cardiovascular disease. Although we strongly support carefully conducted research, the UGDP would not be the first case of a research study coming up with a result that is later proven to be wrong.

Specific Oral Hypoglycemic Agents

In this section we will describe in more detail the oral hypogylcemic agents that are available, so you can look up the one you take and get a good idea of what to expect. We are not trying to be comprehensive or to replace the printed material you get with each prescription. But we will try to sort out the most significant differences and distinguish the more common and the rarer side effects.

Sulfonylureas

These are the class of pills most often used to treat diabetes. Indeed, these were the only pills available from the 1970s to 1995 (when metformin and acarbose were approved by the FDA). The sulfonylureas have been used for more than forty years and are effective in treating many people with Type II diabetes who do not respond adequately to diet and exercise alone. They act by stimulating the pancreas to make its own insulin. If the pancreas is too weak to make much insulin, the sulfonylureas are not effective. And even if they work for awhile, these agents may not be effective permanently, since everyone's pancreas tends to weaken over the years.

There are six specific sulfonylurea drugs available in the United States (Table 12), and they are divided into first-generation and second-generation drugs. There are some differences among these various sulfonylureas, but the similarities are much greater than the differences. They all act by the same

Table 12. Sulfonylureas

Generic name	Brand name or names	Maximum daily dose	Comments
First generation (the older drugs)			
Acetohexamide	Dymelor	1500 mg.	Has slight diuretic effect.
Chlorpropamide	Diabinese, Glucamide	750 mg.	Sulfonylurea most often associated with "alcohol flush" when alcoholic beverages are consumed. Has very long duration of action; has antidiuretic property.
Tolazamide	Tolinase	1000 mg.	Has slight diuretic effect.
Tolbutamide	Orinase	3000 mg.	Usually prescribed to be taken 2 or 3 times a day.
Second generation (more recently developed drugs)			
Glipizide	Glucotrol	40 mg.	To be taken on an empty stomach; food delays absorption.
Glipizide-extended release	Glucotrol XL	20 mg.	Do not break tablet; may be taken once a day.
Glyburide	Diabeta, Micronase	20 mg.	
Glyburide-micronized	Glynase	12 mg.	Not equivalent in action to Glyburide.
Glimepiride	Amaryl	8 mg.	

Note: All sulfonylureas work by stimulating the pancreas to produce more insulin. They may also make the body use insulin more effectively. As a consequence of these actions, low blood sugar (hypoglycemia) is a side effect of taking these drugs.

The liver metabolizes sulfonylureas, and the kidneys eliminate them; therefore, the sulfonylureas should be used more cautiously in people with liver or kidney impairment and those with a sulfa allergy. Sulfonylureas should *not* be used during pregnancy.

basic mechanisms, they share some of the same side effects, and there is little evidence that if you fail to respond to one sulfonylurea, you will respond to another.

First-generation sulfonylureas. The so-called first-generation sulfonylureas have been used since the 1950s. Tolbutamide (Orinase and generic forms) is the oldest. It has the shortest duration of action because it is in-activated by the liver. (Drugs that are excreted by the kidneys have a longer duration of action than do those inactivated by the liver.) Because tolbu-tamide is short-acting, it has to be taken three times a day to be effective over a 24-hour period. Also, it is not the best choice in the presence of significant liver disease.

Chlorpropamide (Diabinese and generic forms) is at the other end of the duration of action spectrum. It is excreted by the kidneys into the urine, so one pill lasts a full 24 hours. It is not the drug of choice if the kidneys are not functioning normally. Because of its long duration of action, chlorpropamide is a notorious cause of prolonged hypoglycemia, a side effect that may occur again hours after being treated once.

There are two other peculiarities of chlorpropamide. First, about 15% of people when they are taking chlorpropamide react to alcohol with a characteristic flush of the face. This side effect, appropriately called the *chlorpropamide-alcohol flush,* is specific to chlorpropamide, and changing to another sulfonylurea usually solves the problem. Second, chlorpropamide causes some people to retain water, which lowers the sodium concentration in the blood. This is usually insignificant but occasionally causes a more se-vere drop in serum sodium level. Taking the drug does not cause ankle swelling (edema).

The other two first-generation sulfonylureas, acetohexamide (Dymelar and generics) and tolazamide (Tolinase and generics), have intermediate du-rations of action and can be taken once or twice daily. They are inactivated and excreted by both the liver and the kidneys.

Second-generation sulfonylureas.   The second-generation sulfony-lureas, glyburide (DiaBeta and Micronase) and glipizide (Glucotrol and Glu-cotrol XL), became available in the mid-1980s. They are taken at much low-er doses than the earlier sulfonylureas (1.25–40 *mg* rather than 0.10–3 *grams*), but they act in very much the same way as the earlier sulfonylureas. Glyburide has an intermediate duration of action and is taken once or twice daily, while glipizide has a shorter action, requiring twice-daily doses. Glu-cotrol XL is a form of glipizide with a long (24-hour) duration of action. Glimepiride (Amaryl) is another sulfonylurea with long-acting properties, taken once a day.

There are some relatively minor advantages to the newer sulfonylureas, such as less frequent or less serious interactions with other medications the person may be taking. Otherwise they are essentially the same as the drugs in the first generation.

Side effects of sulfonylureas. The most common side effect of the sulfonylureas is hypoglycemia. In a sense, this is not a side effect at all but just an extreme of the intended purpose of the pill. Since most people who start taking sulfonylureas have significant hyperglycemia (high blood sugar), it is not common for them to overrespond to the pills and actually go too low. But it can happen, especially if the diabetes is mild and the person's eating habits are erratic.

As mentioned, chlorpropamide (Diabinese or generic forms) may cause more problems with hypoglycemia because the pill lasts longer in the blood.

If you think you may have hypoglycemia due to sulfonylureas, it is important to document it. Check your own blood sugar at the time you are having symptoms (see Chapter 5 for a description of symptoms). Remember that fatigue, hunger, sweating, and nervousness are not always due to hypoglycemia. That's why we want you to prove to yourself that your sugar is actually low (for example, less than 60–70 mg/dl) when you are having symptoms and not automatically assume that you are hypoglycemic.

If hypoglycemia does occur, the treatment is to eat some carbohydrate right away. If it happens with any regularity, then the dosage has to be reduced or the medication stopped altogether.

Other side effects are much less common, but they do occur. Gastrointestinal side effects, such as nausea, heartburn, or a full feeling in the stomach, occur in less than 2% of people taking these drugs, and these symptoms may go away spontaneously. If they persist, a lower dose may help. Abnormal tests of liver function may occur, and rarely the liver abnormalities are severe enough to cause jaundice, in which case the drugs should be stopped right away. Significant anemia is even rarer but has been reported, as have other rare side effects. If there is evidence of liver problems or anemia, be sure the condition is evaluated carefully because it may or may not be due to the sulfonylureas.

True allergy to sulfonylureas occurs in less than 2% of people and usually results in a faint red skin rash on the torso or over the entire body. People who are allergic to other sulfa-containing drugs, such as sulfa antibiotics, are more likely to be allergic to sulfonylureas. But you should be sure to distinguish true allergy from other side effects or unrelated problems. Drug allergies, like food allergies, usually start with a widespread skin rash, which may progress to hives, swelling around the eyes or in the joints, or even wheezing and severe difficulty breathing. This is very different from milder problems, such as a full feeling in the stomach, headache, or diarrhea, which are usually better described as an *intolerance* than as an *allergy*. It is important to know if you are truly allergic because allergies can be serious; however, you don't want to deny yourself a useful medicine because you mistakenly consider yourself to be allergic to it.

As with most drugs, a serious overdose can be very dangerous. The effect would be to cause severe hypoglycemia, possibly with lethargy, changes in speech, inability to think clearly, or even seizures and coma. This is not likely to occur if someone takes a relatively mild overdose (such as double the usual dose one day), but it could certainly occur, for example, if a child were to take a handful of pills.

Metformin

Metformin became available in the United States in 1995, although it had been used around the world for over 30 years. (As mentioned earlier, the University Group Diabetes Program study caused enough concern to hold up approval of the drug for use in this country for all these years.) Metformin is usually taken two or three times a day, in total doses of about 1–2.5 grams daily in two to three doses, preferably before meals. It is available in 500 mg and 850 mg tablets.

Metformin's mechanism of action is not fully understood. The one area of agreement is that it does *not* cause the pancreas to secrete more insulin. Instead, it appears to act at two sites: it increases insulin's effect in tissues throughout the body (especially muscle), promoting more effective use of sugar by the tissues, and it helps insulin suppress new sugar production by the liver. There is even some evidence that metformin slows down absorption of carbohydrate from the intestine. In all these ways metformin acts to lower blood sugar, and it definitely needs to have insulin around to have an effect. Because metformin does not depend on stimulating pancreatic insulin release, it can be considered a supplement to, or substitute for, the sulfonylureas.

Can metformin also help the action of insulin given by injection, maybe allowing a reduced insulin dose or more effective blood sugar control even in insulin-dependent diabetes mellitus? It's a good thought, but we know of no evidence that metformin actually benefits people who use insulin injections.

Side effects of metformin.   One consequence of metformin in many people is weight loss or at least less weight gain. This effect, of course, may be very useful in treating Type II diabetes, since most people with Type II diabetes are overweight. Some people taking metformin find that their food has less taste. That may be why they eat less and lose weight. The weight-reducing effect of metformin is inconsistent and needs further study.

The most common side effects of metformin are gastrointestinal, consisting of nausea, abdominal discomfort, or diarrhea. They may occur in as many as 30% of people taking the drug, but they are less of a problem when the dose is started small and gradually built up. Usually this side effect gradually goes away, and it generally does not cause people to stop taking metformin.

We have said that lactic acidosis does not normally occur due to metformin, and this seems to be true *unless* you have certain conditions that predispose you to building up lactic acid in your blood. These conditions include congestive heart failure or severe vascular (circulatory) disease and kidney or liver disease. In these cases, metformin is not recommended. Also, if you are undergoing an X-ray dye study or surgery, you should not take metformin for 24–48 hours beforehand.

Acarbose

Acarbose is one of the so-called alpha-glycosidase inhibitors. These agents act by blocking the enzymes in the intestine that break down the long chains of sugar in complex carbohydrates into their sugar building blocks, which are absorbed into the blood. The effect of blocking this breakdown is to slow the absorption of carbohydrate, as sugar, into the blood. In this way, acarbose reduces the after-meal rise in blood sugar. It does not depend on insulin for its effect. In fact, acarbose itself is barely absorbed into the blood at all; its real action takes place locally, in the intestine. It is taken immediately as you begin a meal. The downside of acarbose is that it causes increased gas production in the intestine in as many as three-fourths of users. This side effect can be reduced by starting at a low dose and building up gradually, but it does reduce the acceptability of acarbose as a medication for everyone.

Troglitazone

Another very promising medication is troglitazone. By acting to reduce the body's resistance to insulin, it could be very useful in the treatment of Type II diabetes. Trials are under way to find out if using troglitazone in conjunction with insulin injections will allow reduction of the insulin dose. If it remains as free of side effects and toxicities as initial studies suggest, troglitazone could be a major addition to the treatment of diabetes.

There are now four kinds of oral hypoglycemic agents available in the United States: the sulfonylureas, metformin, acarbose, and troglitazone. All are used to treat Type II diabetes; none has been proven effective in treating Type I diabetes. They are not effective if people do not also follow a reasonable diet. The sulfonylureas act by stimulating the pancreas to secrete insulin, and they certainly have the longest and most successful track record. As the pancreas ages, however, there are lessening returns from the sulfonylureas, and sulfonylurea failure is common. Metformin has been used around the world for more than 25 years but became available in the United States only in 1995. It acts by enhancing the effect of insulin. Acarbose acts by slowing the absorption of carbohydrate in the gut. Troglitazone acts specifically by sensitizing the body to insulin. With combinations of these three kinds of pills, it may be possible to put off the time when insulin is needed to treat Type II diabetes or even avoid ever needing insulin. But the bottom line is blood sugar control, and if the time comes when the pills are not working well enough, it is important to go ahead and take some insulin to treat your diabetes.

Chapter 12

Treating Diabetes with Insulin

- *"I'll do anything except take that needle."*

- *"I don't think of insulin as a drug. I think of it as a little replacement hormone—perfectly natural."*

- *"I don't want to take insulin. My grandmother took it, and she had her leg cut off."*

- *"I feel so much better since I've been on the insulin, I can't believe it. My golf game is even better. I wish I had started taking it sooner."*

Like most scientific advances, the "discovery" of insulin involved a series of steps, beginning with the demonstration in the 1890s by the German physiologist Oskar Minkowski that an antidiabetic chemical is present in the pancreas. In 1901 a Johns Hopkins pathologist, Eugene Opie, showed that this material came specifically from the beta cells in the islets of Langerhans in the pancreas. And then the race was on to see who would isolate this antidiabetic material in a form that could be used to treat diabetes. Frederick G. Banting, Charles A. Best, James B. Collip, and John J. R. MacLeod are credited with the discovery of insulin in 1921 in Toronto. They worked with tenacity, repeating their experiments and purifying the extract to the point that in less than a year it could be used to treat dying children. We highly recommend Michael Bliss's book *The Discovery of Insulin* (University of Chicago Press, 1982); the following account of the events surrounding this dramatic episode in medical history is based on that account.

Before the availability of insulin, treatments for people with Type I diabetes were unpleasant and ineffective. Exercise and a low-carbohydrate, semistarvation diet were all that could be offered. As doctors and families stood helplessly by, patients would lose more and more weight, dying within a year of the first diagnosis. One of the first people to be given "Banting's extract" (as it was called) was a terminally ill girl named Elizabeth Hughes, who was 14 years old and weighed just 52 pounds in the winter of 1921. She received the new extract over several months on the ward of the Toronto General Hospital, while those around her witnessed a "miraculous" transformation: Elizabeth blossomed into a healthy 109-pound young woman. (She lived into her 70s.)

Scientific egos and jealousies flared within the researchers' little circle, as the world learned about the miracles happening at Toronto General. A Nobel Prize was certain to be given to two of the four researchers, and full-blown battles ensued about who deserved it most. If the truth be told, at least four other investigators, working independently, had also prepared pancreatic extracts that lowered blood sugar levels in animals or humans. But Banting, Best, Collip, and MacLeod pushed their discovery to the point of practical therapy, an achievement that has been called no less than the beginning of modern medicine. For perhaps the first time, it gave health care providers the ability to treat people who would otherwise certainly have died. The 1923 Nobel Prize was awarded to Banting and MacLeod, who promptly split their cash awards with their allies, Best and Collip.

How Insulin Works

Harold is a professional athlete. For him, getting diabetes was a huge pain. He counts on physical fitness for a living and wants to concentrate on his sport, not his blood sugar. For several years, he was adequately controlled on oral hypoglycemic agents, but over the past 18 months, the glycohemoglobin results were going up, and although he did not test as often as we would like (no doubt fearing the high numbers), his symptoms were unmistakable. He could not complete a day's workout without a few bathroom breaks, was always thirsty, and often felt excessively tired. Finally, we convinced Harold to take a shot of insulin at night, while continuing his pills during the day. The result, Harold told us, was spectacular. All of a sudden, he felt like himself again. He gained back some needed weight, improved his strength, and felt altogether better. He is the source of the last quotation given at the start of this chapter—another therapeutic success on insulin.

No one can live without insulin. If your own pancreas doesn't make enough, you have to take extra. Elizabeth Hughes described insulin as "unspeakably wonderful." She could not have understood exactly how it works, but the evidence was there even with that early use: insulin relieved her of her insatiable thirst and constant urination (by lowering blood glucose); it gave her back her body strength (by promoting muscle development); and it allowed her to gain her normal adolescent fat stores (by promoting the storage of calories as fat). Let's look at these actions of insulin individually.

Many people think of the glucose (sugar) in their blood as coming only from their diet. In fact, it comes from two sources—the diet and the liver. The carbohydrate you eat raises the sugar directly, and the liver makes "new glucose" from storage forms (glycogen) or from protein. The liver action is why, if you don't have enough of your own insulin, the blood sugar tends to rise overnight, even when you aren't eating.

Insulin lowers blood sugar by both increasing the removal of glucose from the blood and reducing the production of glucose by the liver. To dispose of the carbohydrate you eat, insulin opens the body cells' doors to glucose that is circulating in the blood. The sugar enters the cells and is used as the cells' fuel for energy. Insulin shuts down the liver's production of glucose, especially overnight. This is why we sometimes start people with Type II diabetes on one shot of insulin at night, continuing the pills during the day.

Insulin also builds muscle. It actually delivers the building blocks of muscle protein, the amino acids, to the muscles. Without insulin, muscles melt away as the amino acids are drained into the liver and inappropriately used for glucose formation. With insulin, the amino acids are put back in the muscle where they belong, and muscle strength increases noticeably.

Finally, insulin signals the body to store extra calories as glycogen and fat, two efficient storage forms to be used by the body during unanticipated fasts. Lack of insulin explains ketoacidosis as well as uncontrolled weight loss. Restoring insulin causes the body to rebuild fat.

Since insulin is at the center of so many of the body's chemical reactions, it is no wonder that it is required for life itself. Various other body functions, such as the complicated hormonal changes involved in women's menstrual cycles, are also dependent on the presence of adequate levels of insulin. The hormone is present in some of the most primitive and ancient of living organisms and is the most finely tuned of all the body's hormones. It is, in truth, a miracle of nature, a central regulator of all the body's complex chemical pathways.

Given all these wonderful effects of insulin, why does just hearing the simple words, "You need insulin," elicit such a flood of emotions, all negative? The reason, of course, is that it has to be given by injection.

What People Think about Taking Insulin

The thought of taking several injections every day is not a happy one. People worry about needles, syringes, and pain. They wonder whether the need for insulin means that their diabetes is worse. They ask whether they will have to stay on insulin for the rest of their lives. As you think these thoughts, keep in mind that you are not the first person to wonder, to resist, to be afraid, and to ask hard questions. Any question that you have about insulin use deserves an answer. Consider how the following people with diabetes responded to their need to use insulin.

> *When six-year-old Amanda was diagnosed with Type I diabetes, her parents thought her life was going to be ruined by endless pain from countless injections. They were amazed when, no more than two months later, Amanda was drawing up the syringe and plunging it right into herself, as proud as she could be and without a whimper.*

> *When Elmer, a man with Type II diabetes, was told it was time for him to start using insulin, his first thought was of a relative who took insulin and developed complications of diabetes. He mistakenly blamed the complications on insulin rather than on poorly controlled diabetes.*

> *Jesse thought that taking insulin meant his diabetes was "worse" and would therefore cause more complications. No one told him that insulin was being prescribed precisely to help him avoid complications.*

> *Bell was afraid that she would go into coma with insulin, because she didn't know that severe hypoglycemia is preventable.*

> *Steve associated the needles and syringes with drug abuse. He was terrified that someone would see him taking an injection and assume that he was a junkie.*

All these people hated the idea of taking insulin. What's remarkable to those of us who care for literally thousands of people with diabetes is that we find very, very few who do not accommodate themselves successfully to insulin injections. Like teenage boys learning to shave, after an initial struggle taking insulin just folds itself into the daily routine. Virtually everyone ends up taking the situation in stride.

Is the diabetes "worse" if you need insulin? In a sense it is, since the need for insulin by injection means that the pancreas is not able to do the job, despite whatever pills, diet, and exercise you have been using. But in a truer sense, diabetes is "worse" only to the extent that its *complications* are worse.

Think of how you feel and how well you live when you take insulin, check your sugars, eat your healthy diet, and exercise regularly. Then think about how well you would live if you were suffering severe complications of diabetes. We know you'll conclude that it is the complications, not the treatment, that is "worse."

Is insulin treatment forever? Most often it is, but not always. In Type II diabetes, weight loss and increased activity improve the body's response to insulin. For some people, this may mean reducing the insulin dose, even to the point of stopping it altogether. Sometimes as little as 10 pounds makes a big difference. But even with this possibility, our usual answer to the question, "Will I always have to take insulin?" is "Take it one day at a time."

Deciding to Take Insulin

When your health care professional recommends insulin, it is only reasonable to expect that she or he will explain the whys and wherefores. If the two of you agree on some definite improvements you can make in your self-care before committing to insulin use, then it's certainly worthwhile to give those changes a try and see how they affect your blood sugar levels. But even when you are armed with a plan, it is essential to set a target date by which your blood sugar will have gone down. One month is reasonable. Twelve months is too long to have out-of-control diabetes.

If you need insulin, don't prolong the negotiations with your doctor: "I'll start the insulin after I get done with this work assignment (or this party, or the visit from my mother-in-law)." "I'm not sure I want to do it right now, but definitely by next winter." "How about if I cut my calories down to 900 and run a mile after every meal?" We've heard them all! When insulin is needed, don't kid yourself by procrastinating.

Principles of Insulin Use

Exactly what insulin regimen and what doses will work for you depend on lots of different factors:

—How old are you?
—What do you weigh?
—How closely do you follow your diabetes?
—What are the goals you are trying to achieve?
—Perhaps most important of all, what kind of diabetes do you have?

These and many other considerations will be worked out between you and your health care professional. But the fundamental differences between Type I and Type II diabetes are especially important when it comes to insulin treatment.

As you recall, with Type I diabetes you have virtually no insulin left in your pancreas, while with Type II your pancreas still does make some insulin. This means that for Type I diabetes, the insulin injections have to "do it all." The doses tend to be more complicated and fine tuned. For Type II diabetes, insulin injections are just giving the pancreas a helping hand, and while more insulin may be needed, the doses usually aren't so complex. Let's consider each situation individually.

Type I Diabetes

With Type I diabetes insulin treatment is always required. Usually, it should be started as soon as the diagnosis is made. There is even some evidence that controlling the blood sugar very well and very quickly may have later benefits by "protecting" beta cells in the pancreas, although this is not proven.

Many people with Type I diabetes have a "honeymoon" during which their pancreas seems to recover. It may start within a month or so of the first diagnosis and last a few months to a year. During the honeymoon, the need for insulin drops dramatically or even disappears. Commonly, the diabetes is very stable, and blood sugar levels are relatively easily controlled. You can be tricked into thinking that the diabetes is going away, but it is more accurate to think of the honeymoon as a final burst of activity from the remaining beta cells in the pancreas. Research is focusing on how to prolong the honeymoon period in hopes of preventing damage to the remaining beta cells. In the future, Type I diabetes may be prevented by learning what the body is trying to tell us with the honeymoon period. In the meantime, we look on it as an opportunity to learn good diabetes self-care while things are a little easier.

In treating Type I diabetes, replacing the function of the pancreatic beta cells is no easy task. You need *some* insulin all the time, much more at mealtime, and never too much. Getting this right requires a complicated schedule of injections, preventing gaps in insulin levels and matching the input of carbohydrate taken with meals. Most people with Type I diabetes learn by necessity to fine tune their diet, insulin, and exercise patterns. They learn that inattention to details may have consequences, such as hypoglycemia, that they very much want to avoid.

Type II Diabetes

Why is insulin sometimes used to treat people with Type II diabetes, when Type II is also called non–insulin-dependent diabetes? The answer (discussed more fully in Chapter 2) is that the pancreas of some people with Type II diabetes does not produce enough insulin to control the blood sugar, so that insulin injections are needed. The old name, non–insulin-dependent diabetes, was misleading.

If you were to ask a room full of diabetes professionals *when* insulin should be used in treating Type II diabetes, you would start a discussion lasting well into the night. There's just not much agreement on this issue. Our own practice, simply put, is to start insulin when your own pancreas cannot make enough. You will know this by the following signs:

—The blood sugar levels are too high.
—You are losing weight uncontrollably.
—You are thirsty and urinating too much.
—Other treatments—diet, exercise and pills—are no longer working.

People often ask for one last chance. They want to exercise even more or eat even less. Sometimes this is reasonable, and more attention to self-care will work. But often the insulin-producing beta cells of the pancreas just wear out, and no amount of diet, exercise, or pills will be enough. Insulin is what you need.

Since people with Type II diabetes continue to make insulin in their own pancreas, the job of achieving good control of blood sugar levels with injections is usually easier than in Type I diabetes. Only one or two injections a day often work just fine. Sometimes insulin can be used along with the pills. Usually, though, the total amount of insulin needed is much greater than in Type I diabetes (often 50–150 units per day, especially for larger people). This high insulin requirement has nothing to do with how "bad" the diabetes is; it has to do with how well—or poorly—your body responds to insulin (how "sensitive" it is to insulin).

There are some experts who believe, with partial evidence, that insulin can do harm and, in particular, that it can worsen hardening of the arteries. But the research is inconclusive, and the much better established fact is that high blood sugar is bad for you. So we conclude that blood sugar control is most important, even if it requires large amounts of insulin. Other health problems, such as high blood pressure or high cholesterol, should be treated vigorously without allowing blood sugar to go out of control.

Pregnancy

If you develop diabetes during pregnancy (see Chapter 31) and diet alone is not normalizing your blood sugar, then insulin must be started for the well-being of the developing fetus. Oral medications for diabetes are not to be used when a woman is trying to become pregnant or is pregnant. Insulin use is usually temporary in gestational diabetes. After delivery, most women with gestational diabetes will return to a nondiabetic state and can stop taking insulin, although there is a much higher chance that they will develop Type II diabetes later in life. Naturally, if a woman has Type I diabetes before pregnancy, insulin is continued during pregnancy. And occasionally, Type I diabetes will start during pregnancy. In that case, the diabetes would continue after pregnancy and would continue to require insulin.

Surgery and Other Stressful Situations

People who have previously been well controlled on diet or diet and oral medication may need insulin to control the blood sugar during periods of stress, such as surgery. This is another case, though, in which insulin treatment may be temporary. When the stress is over, the person may no longer need insulin.

Adverse Reactions to Insulin

Like Elizabeth Hughes, and contrary to what you anticipate, you too may describe insulin as being "unspeakably wonderful." On the right dose of insulin, the bothersome symptoms of high blood sugar disappear, and your overall sense of well-being improves. But for all its wonderful qualities, insulin use has some unpleasant aspects beyond the needle stick. We'll consider some of the adverse reactions to insulin and give suggestions for dealing with them.

Hypoglycemia

This is by far the most common downside of insulin therapy. It happens when the amount of insulin taken is too much for the amount of food ingested, exercise undertaken, or starting level of blood sugar. Even with generally good blood sugar control, you will miss the mark periodically and have hypoglycemia; it can usually be easily treated by eating a sweet or a snack. If you are having frequent low blood sugars—daily or more often—you may need to adjust your insulin dose downward. You definitely want to avoid insulin reactions that are severe enough to cause confusion or loss of consciousness. Telephone or visit your health care provider if you are concerned about frequent lows.

Weight Gain

Achieving better blood glucose control on insulin means that your body is now working more like the body of a person without diabetes and is properly using the foods you eat. When your blood sugar was high, some of the calories you ate were spilled into the urine as sugar. This drain of calories made losing weight relatively easy. In good control, that isn't happening anymore. Instead, any excess calories you consume (beyond what you burn by just living and breathing plus exercise) are stored away as fat. That's right, *fat*. On your waistline, your hips—wherever you don't want it. So with good blood sugar control, you become like most people without diabetes: you have to watch your calories closely or your waistline grows. But there are some things you can consider doing to avoid the weight gain that so often comes with insulin treatment.

Be sure that your insulin dose is not causing frequent hypoglycemia, driving you to eat snacks continuously. To control weight, you may need to limit your calories (this is best done with the assistance of a dietitian) or increase your activity. Keep in mind that if you diet strenuously, you may have to cut down how much insulin you take.

Needle Phobia

Insulin needles are vastly improved over what they were like in the past. The point of the needle is beveled so that it is very sharp, and the gauge or diameter of the needle is fine. Also, the needle itself is coated with a slippery layer of silicone. Sharp, fine, slippery needles pierce through the skin and slide through the tissue easily, with little or no pain.

Of course, knowing this and being able to inject yourself without getting nervous are two different things. As we said, almost everyone eventually gets used to it. But in the beginning, some people have to push themselves. Try thinking ahead ("If I just get it done, I can go on with breakfast"). You may have to make a more concerted effort to visualize a relaxing place, such as a beach at sunset, to prevent that cold sweat. If you continue to suffer with the injections and are unable to get the needle in quickly, with a dartlike motion, you may consider purchasing a device designed to do that step for you. A nurse educator can explain the options. But almost without exception, people on insulin find that injections become easier with time.

Insulin Allergy

Fortunately, as a direct result of using human insulin, allergy is a much rarer problem than it used to be. It is so rare nowadays that we are surprised when we see it. Being uncomfortable taking insulin, being sensitive to it, or even getting a bruise at the injection site, is *not* an insulin allergy. With an insulin allergy, either there is redness around the site of insulin injection, often with some itching (this is called *local allergy*), or there is a reaction involving several body systems (a *systemic allergy*).

A local allergy is rarely severe and is not a reason to stop insulin use. A systemic allergy is much rarer and more severe. It includes hives, rashes on the skin in places away from where you inject insulin, and sometimes facial swelling or wheezing. Since there are many causes of such allergies, you should not assume that just because you take insulin, you are allergic to it. You may be allergic to pollen, a specific kind of soap, nuts, shellfish, or any number of other things. Check the situation out with a good allergist, and don't be too hasty to stop the insulin, since you may make things a lot worse by doing so.

Insulin Edema

Infrequently, pronounced swelling, or edema, will occur with the initiation of insulin therapy. This occurs more frequently when blood sugars were very poorly controlled before the insulin was started. It resolves in a matter of weeks with a low-sodium diet and short-term use of a diuretic (fluid pill), such as furosemide.

Living with insulin therapy makes your life different. There are routines to follow, supplies to juggle, and monitoring to see if everything is in balance. But it can also make your life a lot better when symptoms of diabetes disappear and your risk of long-term problems is reduced. As one of our patients said, "Insulin is good stuff when you need it."

Chapter 13

Types of Insulin

- *"I'm on Humulin insulin. Is that the same as NPH?"*

- *"What's the truth about how to store and handle insulin? Where should you keep it—in a refrigerator? an ice pack? on a shelf? in a box?"*

- *"I don't understand the insulin peak. Is it always the same? Does it mean that my sugar goes up or down?"*

- *"How do I know if my insulin needs to be adjusted, how do I do it, and should I talk with my doctor every time I change it?"*

In the last chapter we described the incredibly exciting events surrounding the discovery of insulin. But diabetes was far from cured when insulin became available. In fact, early insulin preparations were crude at best, sometimes entirely inactive at worst. The insulin was extracted from cow and pig pancreases, was impure, and often caused allergic reactions. Furthermore, because it was originally a weak form of what we now call Regular, the person with diabetes had to inject large volumes three to four times a day, and pits often appeared at the injection sites.

The manufacturing of insulin has come a long way. Today, insulin is well standardized, pure, and of uniform potency. Most insulin used now is identical to that produced by the human pancreas. Allergies and other adverse reactions are much less common than they were in the past. But along with these enormous improvements in insulin has come increased complexity in what's available. Add to this the current trend toward improved blood glucose control, and you can see that there's more opportunity for confusion than ever before.

In this chapter, we will explain the characteristics that distinguish different insulin preparations. We will discuss specifics of insulin storage and handling, insulin injection technique, factors that affect insulin absorption, and how to adjust your regimen safely and rationally.

Key Characteristics of Different Insulin Preparations

There are several characteristics of insulin that you should be aware of:

—The source (cow, pig, or human)
—The formulation (lispro, Regular, NPH, Lente, Ultralente)
—In some countries, the concentration (U-100, U-80, U-40)
—The different brand names put on each kind of insulin by different companies

Several companies produce and market insulin, and each has different brand names. Table 13 summarizes the characteristics, but here we'll consider them one at a time.

The Source

Since there are lots of cows and pigs, and both species have large pancreases, the Eli Lilly Company set the standard for insulin preparation in the 1920s by extracting beef and pork pancreases. These "animal source" insulins were purified and refined over the years, and remained the only source of insulin until the early 1980s. In truth, purified beef/pork insulins worked very well in the past, and they still do.

"Human insulin" was the first major commercial product developed by recombinant DNA technology. It does not come directly from humans but is made by changing the genes of certain bacteria so that the bacteria are "programmed" to make insulin that is precisely like human insulin. Human insulin, compared to animal-source insulin, causes less antibody response, since it is the same as insulin produced by the normally functioning pancreas. It works slightly more rapidly than beef/pork insulin, but the difference is rarely significant. When introduced in the early 1980s it cost more than beef/pork insulin but now costs about the same.

Brand names for human insulin include Humulin (by Eli Lilly) and Novolin (by Novo-Nordisk). These brand names refer only to the *source* of the insulin (beef/pork or human), not to its formulation (Regular, NPH, and so forth). Most people who have always taken beef/pork insulin want to know if they should switch to human insulin. The answer is usually yes, if only because the manufacturers are phasing out beef/pork insulin, and soon it will

Table 13.   Characteristics of Insulin

Characteristic	Example	Effect
Source	human (made by bacteria)	less allergy, less antibody
	beef/pork	somewhat more allergy, more antibody
	purified pork	less allergy and antibody than beef/pork
Concentration	U-100, U-40	How much insulin per ml (100 or 40 units). A unit of insulin is the same regardless of the concentration.
Preparation	lispro	fastest time of action
	Regular	fast time of action
	Semilente	fast time of action
	NPH	intermediate time of action
	Lente	intermediate time of action
	Ultralente	long time of action
Mixtures	70/30	70% NPH, 30% Regular
	50/50	50% NPH, 50% Regular
Brand[a]	Eli Lilly	human Regular insulin
	Humulin R	human NPH insulin
	Humulin N	human Lente insulin
	Humulin U	human Ultralente insulin
	Humolog	lispro insulin
	Iletin	beef/pork, pure beef, or pure pork insulins
	Novo	
	Novolin L, N, R, 70/30	human Lente, NPH, Regular, 70/30 insulins
	Insulatard NPH	pork NPH
	Velosulin	pork Regular

[a]Other company brands exist.

not be available at all. In truth, there is no other real advantage to switching.

How should you go about switching? Talk it over with your doctor. You should get a new prescription, so you don't get a wrong insulin preparation altogether. But ordinarily you can switch beef/pork insulin for human insulin, unit for unit. If you took 33 units of beef/pork, take 33 units of human insulin. Some specialists recommend cutting down the dose by 10% or so; we do not find that this is necessary.

Human insulin developed a reputation in the media for causing more hypoglycemia or less awareness of hypoglycemia. After reviewing the literature, we do not think this is true. The scientific evidence supports the equivalency of human insulin and beef/pork insulin.

Insulin Units

Insulin is measured in *units*. In manufacturing, insulin is calibrated so that a unit has a particular "biologic effect"—it lowers the blood sugar a certain amount, whether it is human insulin or beef/pork insulin. Many people ask us exactly how much a unit of insulin will lower *their* blood sugar. Unfortunately, we can only guess. The figure will vary enormously from person to person (see the discussion of insulin resistance in Chapters 2 and 7), and of course any insulin effect on lowering blood glucose will be counteracted by eating carbohydrate. On the other hand, *you* can probably get a pretty good feel for how much a unit (or 5 or 10 units) lowers your blood glucose, if you pay close attention and test your glucose level.

Insulin Concentration

The *concentration* of insulin in the United States is almost always 100 units in one milliliter (ml), called U-100. In other countries, U-40 is often available, meaning that the insulin has 40 units in a milliliter. Think of a teaspoon of blue dye put in a half glass of water—it will make a certain shade of blue. The same teaspoon of blue dye in a *whole* glass of water will make a fainter blue. Likewise, U-40 insulin is more dilute than U-100. One unit of insulin is still one unit of insulin; it is just more dilute in U-40 preparations. The easiest thing to do when you travel outside the United States is to take along U-100 insulin. But one friend of ours accidentally lost his bottle of insulin down the toilet on a flight to France. In Paris, he couldn't find a pharmacy with U-100 insulin. So you never know when an understanding of insulin concentration will come in handy! Remember this: take U-40 insulin with a U-40 syringe; then take your usual number of units.

Insulin Syringes

Syringes come in several sizes. If you take relatively large doses, say 75 units in a shot, you will use a syringe that can hold a full milliliter, or 100 units of U-100 insulin. By filling the syringe to the 75-unit mark, it will be three-quarters full. For lower doses, such as 15 units, there are smaller syringes, holding a maximum of 30 or 50 units. The numbers printed on the side of the syringe are bigger when the full syringe holds only 30 or 50 units, so you can be more accurate. With these half-ml or third-ml syringes, you still draw up insulin to the mark that corresponds to 15 units, if that is the dose you want. So don't be mixed up by the size of the syringe—always pull up the insulin to the mark that represents your own desired dose.

Insulin Durations of Action

Here, the plot thickens. You will almost certainly be using different kinds of insulin—Regular, NPH, and so forth. Each has a different *duration of action*. We explain the differences between lispro, NPH, Regular, Lente, and Ultralente insulin below. But, first, let's consider some key terms: *onset, peak,* and *duration of action*.

When insulin is injected beneath the skin, it is not effective at that very instant, any more than your blood sugar jumps up the very moment you put a piece of bread in your mouth. It takes some time for insulin to be absorbed into the bloodstream and to reach the cells where it acts. The step that takes the longest is the absorption of insulin from beneath the skin into the bloodstream. This time between the injection of insulin and the start of its action to lower the blood sugar is called the *time of onset*. Even with the fastest acting insulin, the time of onset is at least 10 minutes; more often, it is at least 30–45 minutes.

The *peak* of insulin action comes when, after injection, the insulin reaches its maximum activity. If you inject, say, 5 units of insulin and don't eat, this would be the time when the blood sugar is lowest, before the insulin effect begins to wear off.

The insulin's *duration of action* refers to the time between the start of the effect of the insulin injection and the end of the effect, when the insulin is no longer driving the blood glucose down.

A word of caution is needed here. Everyone talks about these features of insulin—the onset, peak, and duration—as though it were true for everyone. We even present representative curves. But in real life, the duration of action varies substantially from person to person and from injection to injection. The curves in Figures 17, 18, and 19 represent only one typical action curve for each type of insulin. Curves of action may be quite different for you. The most common difference would be for a person who has taken insulin for many years (say, over 20) to have a much longer duration of action of insulin. You can find out for yourself about how quickly a particular preparation of

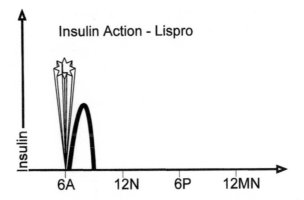

Figure 14. **Lispro insulin** is an insulin analog. It has a rapid onset of action—about 15 minutes. It peaks in 1.5 hours and lasts about 3 hours in the body.

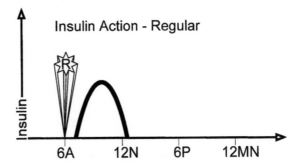

Figure 15. **Regular insulin** is referred to as a short-acting (clear) insulin because it lasts only about 5 to 6 hours. It starts working about 45 minutes to an hour after injection and peaks in about 2 hours.

insulin acts in you. If you take NPH at 6 A.M., do you notice a tendency to go low by 10 A.M. or not until 2 P.M.? You can reduce the injection-to-injection variation, for instance, by always injecting into the abdomen or by trying to inject to the same depth each time. But you can't eliminate the variation.

Types of Insulin (Lispro, Regular, NPH, Lente, Ultralente)

To categorize insulins in terms of their time and action characteristics, consider three types: short-acting, intermediate, and long-acting. Any of these

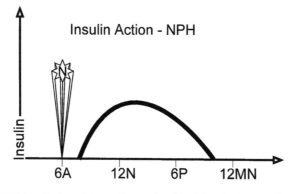

Figure 16. NPH insulin is an intermediate-acting (clear) insulin. It generally starts working about 1 to 3 hours after injection, peaks at about 8 hours, and lasts about 20 hours.

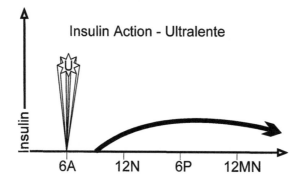

Figure 17. Ultralente insulin is the longest-lasting insulin available. It starts working about 2 to 4 hours after injection, peaks at about 16 hours, and lasts about 32 to 36 hours.

types can be available from a human or an animal source, in any concentration. So, for instance, you could have Regular U-100 beef/pork insulin, or you could have Regular U-100 human insulin. You may well use any or all of these types.

The *shortest* acting insulin is called lispro (brand name Humalog, Eli Lilly). It became available in 1996 and represents a new use of recombinant DNA technology to modify the insulin molecule so that it is absorbed more quickly even than Regular insulin. The idea is to take lispro insulin just before a meal rather than 30–45 minutes before the meal.

Regular, or R, insulin is easily recognizable not only by the R on the bottle but also because it is clear. Regular insulin is unmodified human or beef/pork insulin. Its typical onset is within about 45 minutes, its peak action is at about two hours, and its duration of action is about four to six hours (see Figure 17). We have much more experience using Regular insulin than lispro. For decades Regular has been used to "cover" meals. This means that when a person is about to eat a meal, he or she injects Regular 30–45 minutes before the meal. One of our patients calls it the "breakfast killer."

There are two *intermediate*-acting insulins: Neutral Protamine Hagedorn (NPH or N) and Lente (L). The absorption of NPH from the injection site is slowed down by the addition of a protein called protamine. The absorption of Lente insulin is similarly slowed by a change in crystal size. The intermediate-acting insulins start working about one hour after injection; peak, on average, at six to eight hours; and last a total of about 12–18 hours (see Figure 18). They are identifiable not only by the N or L on the bottle but also by the fact that they are cloudy. The insulin is actually in the cloudiness, which settles to the bottom when the bottle is allowed to stand still. Therefore, you must invert or roll these insulins before you inject them in order to mix the insulin into the solution.

NPH or Lente insulin is typically given in the morning, to provide some insulin effect through midday and afternoon, covering lunch, or in the evening, to control the blood sugar through the night.

Ultralente is the *longest* acting insulin because it has the largest crystal size. It has a slow onset, peaks at about 8–12 hours, and lasts for as long as 36 hours (see Figure 19). Like NPH and Lente, Ultralente must be mixed before injection. Ultralente is often used to provide a steady flow of insulin, supplemented with Regular insulin at each meal. Given the new ability to modify insulin's structure, new longer acting insulins may soon be developed.

Insulin Mixes

Several insulins are marketed now that are premixes of NPH and Regular. The most commonly used mix is called 70/30, because it contains 70% NPH and 30% Regular. We find these mixes useful for premeal dosing if people cannot mix their own insulin reliably. Since the 70/30 mix contains so much Regular insulin, it is not a good idea to use it if you are not about to eat.

Handling Insulin

Insulin is special stuff that needs and deserves to be treated with care. How, exactly, should you handle it? Opinions and even official recommendations have flip-flopped over the years. The fact is that insulin is a fragile protein. It can be damaged by very vigorous shaking or by extremes of temperature. You need to keep the following cautions in mind:

THINGS TO AVOID	EXAMPLES
Excessive physical trauma	Vigorous shaking when preparing injection; very bumpy car rides or sports activities
Excessive heat	Sunny windowsills in summer; closed cars in the sun in warm weather; unprotected sun exposure on the beach
Excessive cold, freezing	Cold car in winter; freezer compartment in refrigerator

Insulin lasts for weeks to months at room temperature and even longer at refrigeration temperature. There is no reason to worry, then, if a bottle has been kept at room temperature rather than cooled, even for days. For travel, we recommend that you keep insulin in a handbag or carrying bag to avoid extremes of temperature. Keep your spare unopened bottles in the refrigerator for long-term storage. For trips to the beach or a cold ski slope, temperature-regulated cases may be required. Desert-dwelling Arabs are taught to bury their insulin deep in the sand to keep it cool, which seems a good idea.

Travel can present special challenges in caring for your insulin. If you fly, keep it (and the rest of your diabetes supplies) in your carry-on luggage, for two reasons. First, cargo holds of aircraft (and boats, trains, or cars, for that matter) may be subjected to extremes of temperature that can ruin the insulin. Second, it has happened that the traveler goes to London while the luggage goes to Hong Kong. Don't get stuck without your insulin. Keep it close at hand.

Can Insulin Go Bad, and How Do I Know?

Yes, insulin can go bad—due to mishandling or for unknown reasons. The best indication is when it isn't acting normally (your blood sugar level stays high for no good reason).

Some low-dose insulin users notice that their insulin seems less effective when they get close to the end of the bottle. Their blood sugars trend higher. This could be related to how many times the stopper of the insulin bottle has been pierced. If it is happening to you, start a new bottle of insulin when it gets down to about one-third full. Just throw away the ineffective insulin.

Another clue that your insulin has gone bad is that it looks different. If supposed to be clear, it gets cloudy; if normally cloudy, you notice clumps, even after you have rolled it between your palms. Don't take chances with bad insulin: replace the bottle right away, and save yourself the aggravation of uncontrolled blood sugars.

Drawing Up and Injecting Insulin

First, you have to get the insulin into the syringe, then you have to inject it through the skin into the fatty tissue (*subcutaneously,* abbreviated *SC* or *SQ*). Let's consider six easy steps to the perfect insulin injection:

1. To get started, it's just as well to wash your hands and check that the spot that you are going to inject is reasonably clean. Frankly, infections from insulin injections are very rare, but if you are especially dirty, wash up.
2. Next, clean the rubber stopper of the vial (bottle) with alcohol.
3. If you are using intermediate (NPH or Lente) or long-acting (Ultralente) insulin, mix it up by rolling or rotating the bottle (see Figure 18a). Do not shake the insulin bottle, since that could damage the insulin and introduce air bubbles into the solution. (Injecting air bubbles will not cause you any harm, but you will not be getting your full dose of insulin.)
4. It is easier to withdraw insulin from the vial if you inject air to replace the insulin you plan to take out. Otherwise, a slight vacuum gradually builds up in the vial. So open the syringe, say, to the 10-unit mark if you are going to draw up 10 units, and inject the air into the vial just before you withdraw the insulin (see Figure 18b).
5. Then, turn the bottle upside down with the needle still through the septum, so that the tip of the needle is covered with insulin (or else you will be drawing up air).
6. Pull down on the plunger, drawing insulin into the syringe—more than you plan to use (see Figure 18c). Give the syringe a few taps with your finger to get the bubbles to go to the top, and push the bubbles back

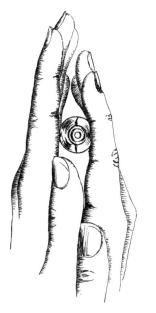

Figure 18(a). If the insulin to be injected is a cloudy solution (NPH, Lente or Ultralente), roll the bottle between the palms to get the white stuff evenly distributed.

into the bottle. Also push the extra insulin out of the syringe, back into the vial, until the syringe is cleanly full (no bubbles) to the right point on the syringe (say, the 10-unit mark.) Then pull the syringe out of the vial.

Now for the injection.

1. Pinch up the skin in the chosen area (choice of a site is discussed below), and poke the needle in at right angles (perpendicularly; see Figure 18d.) Some people have the mistaken notion that if they put the needle in slowly, it won't hurt. In fact, the trick is to get the needle in fast, past the nerve endings, before they have a chance to know what hit them.
2. Push down the plunger and withdraw the needle. It's done. Some people recommend pulling back the needle a bit to see that you aren't injecting directly into a vein, but in our experience this is not a real problem. If you see a spot of bleeding, you will avoid a small bruise if you keep some pressure on the spot for a minute or so.

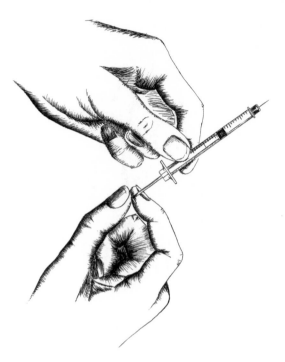

Figure 18(b). Pull the plunger down to the number of units to be taken and inject this air into the bottle.

So there, you've done it! It really isn't that hard, and you don't need to memorize the steps, because after two or three tries they will become second nature. But there are a few more fine points people often ask about.

Mixing insulins   Frequently, a short-acting insulin will be mixed with a longer acting insulin in the same syringe (for example, 10 units NPH plus 5 units Regular). Draw up the short-acting (Regular) insulin first (5 units), and then the 10 units of NPH (filling the syringe to a total of 15 units.) This keeps the additive (protamine) of NPH from contaminating the Regular insulin. And when you mix insulin, it makes sense not to draw up too much and reinject it into the bottle, since you will be reinjecting the mixture.

Reusing syringes   Studies and anecdotes from our patients suggest that syringes can be reused safely in most cases, recognizing that the duller they get, the more they will hurt. This is not true for people with compromised immune systems, however: those who are HIV-positive or who are taking immune-suppressive drugs for a transplant or an illness such as lupus. Never even think about sharing a syringe with others.

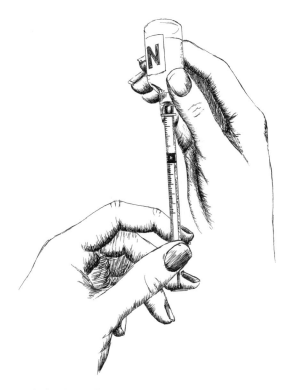

Figure 18(c). Turn the bottle upside down and withdraw the insulin by pulling down on the plunger. You may need to push the insulin back into the bottle to eliminate any air bubbles that may have gotten into the syringe. Pull the plunger down to the number of units to be taken.

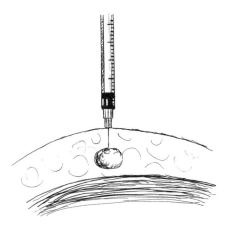

Figure 18(d). Pull the needle out of the bottle. Inject the insulin by inserting the needle quickly into pinched up fatty tissue, at a right angle (perpendicular) to the skin. Push down on the plunger to expel the insulin into the tissue.

Disposing of syringes   We recommend that used syringes be placed in an opaque container that is thick or hard enough to prevent needles from piercing through. (Why opaque? So that drug abusers don't see a supply of syringes and swipe them.) Ask your local health department how to dispose of the full containers. There may be local regulations.

Dispose of lancets used for blood sugar testing in the same way. Obviously, you must be especially cautious not to put trash collectors and other people at risk; follow "universal precautions." Everyone should consider their used syringes and lancets potentially infectious.

We recommend *against* breaking the tip off your needles, unless you have a device that cuts the tip off and contains the needle inside. We hear too many reports of lost needle tips reappearing accidentally in a foot.

Sites for Insulin Injection

This topic is full of confusion and varying opinions. Arms or legs? Abdomen or limbs? To rotate or not? First of all, let's consider the basics.

Insulin, as we noted, is injected into fatty tissue beneath the skin (subcutaneously). Ideally, it is injected at exactly the same depth each time and near little blood vessels that can absorb it. But this ideal cannot be achieved to perfection. You should therefore try to maintain a technique that holds variations to a minimum. What you want is consistent, reliable absorption of insulin.

Standard spots for the injection of insulin include the outside or front of the thighs, the upper- outer part of the buttocks, the outside of the upper arm, and the abdomen (an inch and a half or more away from the belly button).

But all sites are not created equal. Insulin absorption is fastest from the abdomen, slower from the arms and legs, and slowest from the buttocks. You can take advantage of this. If your blood sugar is high, for example, inject into your abdomen to get it down more quickly.

It is a good idea to "rotate" injection sites, but think about how this should be done. The best way, if you feel up to it, may always be to inject in the abdomen, rotating around to different parts (upper right to upper left to lower left to lower right, farther from and closer to the belly button, and so on.) Many people, however, don't want to inject only into the abdomen.

If you rotate from limb to limb, with or without the abdomen, work out a schedule in which you *inject in the same area at the same time of day.* Maybe you can take your morning shot in the abdomen, suppertime shot in the arm or leg, and bedtime shot in the buttocks.

Factors That Affect Insulin Absorption

The site of injection is not the only thing that affects insulin absorption and its time of action. Be aware that other factors determine how fast insulin action takes place. For instance, exercise can increase insulin absorption, especially if the insulin was injected into a limb being exercised and if you exercise within 45 minutes of injection. So, avoid the leg if you're about to go running and avoid the arm if you're pitching a ball game.

Overuse of an injection site can also affect absorption. Repeated injections can toughen up the tissue and slow down absorption. That's why, in moving your sites around, you should not only change from one large area to another, but also keep injections within an area (like the front of the thigh) at least an inch and a half apart.

Insulin Regimens

Your *insulin regimen* is the plan you have for the types of insulin you take and the timing and doses of each injection. It is based on your type of diabetes, physical needs, blood sugar goals, and lifestyle (especially eating patterns and activity). Because it involves so many variables, your regimen should without question be initiated and fine tuned in regular consultation with a health care professional knowledgeable in the modern use of insulin. We want you to be able to modify your regimen on a day-to-day basis (see below), but you need to start by discussing it with your care provider.

There are as many insulin regimens as there are people using insulin. We'll mention some of the concepts involved and give some examples.

Insulin Added onto Oral Medications

> *Sonya has Type II diabetes. She was on maximal dose oral medication for diabetes, but her blood sugars were high and she was bothered by severe fatigue, blurry vision, thirst, and frequent urination. She found that her morning blood sugars were not good (in the 200–250 mg/dl range). She agreed to try some bedtime insulin while continuing her oral diabetic medication.*

This "combination therapy" is worth a try, especially if the goal is to reduce the morning blood sugar so as to give the pills a better chance to work during the day. Insulin is best given at bedtime; in fact, the regimen is often called BIDS (bedtime insulin, daytime sulfonylureas). It works by counting on the insulin to hold the liver's output in check.

Twice-a-Day Insulin

Ted is a large man with Type II diabetes. He did fine for quite some time on one shot of insulin before breakfast, 15 units NPH and 5 units Regular. But he began to notice that he was getting up frequently at night to urinate large amounts. When he tried monitoring his blood glucose four times a day for awhile, he made an amazing discovery: his morning sugar was okay at 100–130 mg/dl, the lunchtime figure was fine at 85–110 mg/dl, and the figure before supper was okay at 120–150 mg/dl. Ted's bedtime sugar, however, was 190–260 mg/dl! His doctor suggested a presupper insulin dose of 8 units Regular and 4 NPH, and this solved the problem.

Ted's problem was that he ate a large supper and had no insulin to cover it. The presupper dose did the job because it contained quite a bit of Regular, covering the supper well, and some NPH to last into the night.

Three Shots a Day, Three Opportunities to Adjust Insulin

Maggie is a 29-year-old woman with Type I diabetes. She wanted to intensify her insulin regimen to control her blood sugars tightly before attempting to become pregnant. She had been taking two shots a day of a fixed dose of NPH and Regular insulin: before breakfast at 7 A.M. and before supper at 6 P.M. Her blood sugar control was somewhat erratic, and she was most bothered by middle-of-the-night insulin reactions. With the help of her diabetes nurse educator, she decided to take only Regular insulin before supper and only NPH at bedtime (11 P.M.). She also learned to adjust her doses further, according to her needs at the time.

The three-shot regimen provided several advantages for Maggie. First, it eliminated the middle-of-the-night low blood sugars because the NPH was peaking closer to morning; taking it at 6 P.M. caused a peak action at 2 A.M. The presupper Regular covered her evening meal nicely and was pretty much worn out before the NPH kicked in overnight. Also, three injections provided Maggie with three opportunities to adjust her insulin for variations in control. She learned to take a bit more Regular if her supper was going to be bigger, a bit less if her sugar was low going into supper.

An Intensive Insulin Regimen: Long-acting Insulin with Short-acting Insulin at Every Meal

William has Type I diabetes. He was doing all right with his three-times-daily insulin regimen, but he found that he had to time his meals carefully by the clock.

*Every day at noon, he knew he had to eat something or he'd go low; late in the af-
ternoon, he felt the same way. So William decided that he would like to try a regimen that is more intensive but offers the best flexibility while maintaining excellent control. We suggested that he use Ultralente instead of NPH and take it in the
morning and at bedtime, with a dose of Regular before each meal or snack. With
four shots a day, varying the amount of Regular according to his estimated need
for each meal, the regimen worked well for William.*

Ultralente is used to provide a relatively stable background level of insulin—although it does not provide a truly constant "basal rate" of insulin.
But by using Ultralente with shots of Regular before each meal, it is possible
to mimic fairly well the action of a normal pancreas, which produces a low
level of insulin between meals and a much higher level each time the person
eats carbohydrate. The intensive regimen that William adopted requires considerable attention on his part and a good knowledge of how much carbohydrate he eats at each meal and how much Regular insulin is needed to cover
that carbohydrate.

When people are sufficiently interested and involved to take three or four
injections a day, to vary their dose of insulin, and to be aware of their carbohydrate exchanges, we think they should also be introduced to the option of
external pump therapy (see Chapter 14).

High-dose Insulin in Type II Diabetes

*Ethan's Type II diabetes was controlled with pills, but he is now on the maximum
doses and his sugars are in the 200s. He and his doctor have agreed that insulin
treatment should be started, and he is given a prescription for a fairly average starting dose, 15 units of 70/30 insulin. It doesn't work. His sugars even increase to the
200–300 mg/dl level. The insulin dose is gradually increased, but only when he
gets to 65 units of insulin every morning do his sugars come under control. Before
long, Ethan needs an additional 30 units of NPH at bedtime.*

One of the cardinal characteristics of Type II diabetes is insulin resistance, meaning that dose requirements are usually high (see Chapters 2 and
7). It is not really surprising, then, that Ethan needed such a large dose of insulin to establish control.

The following points summarize our overall guidelines concerning insulin regimens:

—We do not think of one regimen as intensive and another as not intensive. We prefer to start with a fairly basic regimen and then "intensify" it until we have reached the number and kinds of insulin injections needed to control the diabetes well. The bottom line is how well your diabetes is controlled, not how many shots you take.

—A basic principle is to use Regular or lispro insulin to cover meals (to hold the blood sugar in control as food is absorbed) and longer acting insulin to cover between meals and overnight. Regular insulin should be taken at least a half-hour before a meal, so that it is active as the meal is absorbed.

—The first dose of insulin in the morning should usually include some Regular or lispro (to cover breakfast) as well as some NPH, Lente, or Ultralente.

—In the evening, Regular or lispro insulin should be used to cover supper. NPH or Lente insulin taken at suppertime may cause middle-of-the-night lows, so these are often better taken at bedtime.

Insulin Adjustment

Insulin doses need to be adjusted often, even daily, since very few people keep a lifestyle that is exactly the same, day in and day out. We believe that people with diabetes should understand enough to modify their own doses, safely and reasonably, on a daily basis if necessary. You can't call your health care professional for every larger or smaller meal you eat, every cold you catch or period of stress that you undergo. Furthermore, with the availability of self-monitoring of blood glucose, people can keep better track of their own management than ever used to be possible.

Here are some suggestions for how you can modify your own insulin regimen:

—*Look for trends.* Don't worry excessively about a single surprising blood sugar. For instance, if a sugar reading is low once before lunch, it probably doesn't mean much, but if you check it three or four times and find that it is *usually* low before lunch, this is a trend. Act on it.

—*Be aware of changes in diet and changes in body weight.* If you make a real effort to eat less and lose weight, there is a good chance that your insulin requirement will decrease significantly. If you gain weight, you will probably need more insulin.

—*Find the high and low blood sugars.* If you lead a reasonably consistent life, it is likely that you will be highest and lowest at a particular time of day and that certain situations or meals will have a consistent effect. For instance, your level may go lowest before lunch (sometimes having insulin reactions, sometimes just being in the 60s–70s), and it may rise after supper. A particular kind of meal, exercise, or alcoholic drink may cause you to go low or high. Chinese food and hidden sugar in pasta sauces or bagels are common offenders.

When you are looking for these trends, try to keep other factors constant; otherwise, the trend will not be easy to spot. For example, you won't notice the before-lunch trend if you eat a different kind of breakfast every day.

If your first morning (fasting) blood sugar is high, find out why. Consistently high blood sugars before breakfast can be caused by a variety of factors. The most common is a lack of insulin coverage overnight: whatever doses you are on are not lasting overnight. A second possibility is the "dawn phenomenon," referring to a period around dawn in which blood sugar has a natural tendency to rise. A much less common cause of high fasting blood sugar is the rebound, or so-called "Somogyii" phenomenon. In this case, you actually dip low during the night and then rebound high by morning. The "Somogyii" pattern is often talked about by doctors, but recent studies show that it rarely occurs.

Travel Tips

Insulin adjustments are sure to be necessary when you travel across more than three time zones (either across the United States or across the ocean). Look at the length of day and duration of your insulin. Traveling from west to east, the day is shorter, so you should eliminate or reduce your long-acting insulin shot (NPH or Ultralente) and cover blood sugars and meals with only short-acting insulin. This prevents you from overlapping injections of long-acting insulin as you start living in the new time zone, having lost some hours of the day. Traveling from east to west makes a longer day. In that case, you do not need to eliminate the long-acting insulin but will probably need to supplement it with an extra injection of short-acting insulin if you have any extra meals or if the blood sugar rises too high between injections. You can obtain pamphlets from the American Diabetes Association that provide many additional travel tips.

Self-Adjusting Your Insulin Doses

Self-adjustment is a tricky subject, because it varies so much from person to person. As a rule, we encourage thoughtful, safe self-adjustments of insulin dose. But we recognize that it all depends—on how sensitive you are to insulin, how much you've been taught, and, frankly, whether you know what you're doing.

A reasonable rule of thumb is to change your basic insulin regimen by no more than about 10%–20% at a time and not to change more often than every three or four days. If you're taking 12 units NPH at night and it isn't enough (your fasting blood sugar stays high), try taking 14 units for a few days; if you're going low at lunch with 8 units of Regular in the morning, try 6 units and see what happens. If 40 units of insulin in the morning isn't enough, try 44 or 46. However, if you've had an alarming problem, such as a severe insulin reaction in the middle of the night, you may need to change more abruptly, and you should call your health care professional.

> *John was on an insulin regimen that consisted of 10 units NPH and 5 Regular in the morning, 5 Regular before supper, and 10 NPH at bedtime. There was only one problem: he often forgot to take the bedtime insulin and sometimes, when he "felt high," would increase it to 20 units NPH. John couldn't understand why his fasting blood sugar was so unpredictable. And when he started the day with highly variable blood sugars, he tended to stay variable all day.*

John's problem, of course, was that his bedtime dose was varying way too much, from none to 20 units (varying his total daily dose from 20 to 40 units.) Now he concentrates on always taking the bedtime insulin and varying it by perhaps 5 units if he is high or low at the time.

Sliding-Scale Insulin

The sliding scale is a common and effective way to adjust insulin doses with every shot. In essence, the sliding scale recognizes that you need more insulin if you go into a meal with a blood sugar of 180 than if your blood sugar before the same meal is 80. Your health care professional will work out the sliding scale. The doctor or nurse will write down what dose to take for each blood sugar range, such as 4 units for 60–120, 6 units for 121–180, 8 units for 181–250.

A more elaborate way to adjust your insulin dose is to consider not only your blood sugar at the time but also what you are going to eat. A formula is developed to calculate how much insulin you need to lower your sugar to a certain target level, plus what you need to cover the carbohydrate you are about to eat. Whether you are using a formula or a sliding scale, be absolutely certain you understand what it means. If you have "math panic" and can't handle arithmetic, or if you find the notation confusing, tell your health care professional.

We find that sliding scales are effective, and we believe that in many ways they represent the best approach to diabetic control, since they strive to match the dose to the actual requirement at the time. But there are some pit-falls to avoid when using a sliding scale:

—It depends on regular glucose monitoring before meals. Otherwise, you don't know how to adjust the insulin dose.

—Usually, the Regular insulin is the one that is adjusted to cover the next meal. Sometimes, NPH can also be adjusted.

—The blood sugar going into a meal is not the only thing that determines your insulin requirement. Other factors include, as we mentioned, the size of the meal, previous or planned exercise, stress, or illness.

—A sliding scale used before meals is not likely to be correct for bedtime. For example, if you are to take 7 units of Regular before supper for a blood sugar of 180, chances are you should not take that much at bedtime, since you won't be eating. The sliding scale at bedtime, if you use one, should call for much less Regular insulin than you take before a meal.

—The sliding scale is never to be considered carved in stone. It may be too much or too little, and it may be wrong only at one end of the sugar spectrum. For instance, your sliding scale may say to take 12 units for a sugar over 250, but each time you do this you end up with an insulin reaction later. Your scale needs to be reduced at this high end, say to 8–10 units maximum. Or your scale says to take 2 units before a meal if your sugar is under 100, but when you do this you find that your next reading is always over 200. In this case your scale is too low at the low end, and you should take 3 or 4 units for the lower sugar range. With some thought, you will find that you can make these small adjustments in your sliding scale.

Insulin types, doses, and regimens can be the most confusing aspect of diabetes self-care. Still, if you put your mind to it, it is no more complicated than driving a car or setting a digital watch, much less programming a VCR. In this chapter, we have broken down the elements of insulin use: the kinds of insulin, the various dosing regimens you might want to consider, and how you may want to think about self-adjustments.

When dealing with insulin, there is no substitute for a good relationship with a knowledgeable health care professional. Experienced professionals may disagree with some of the guidelines we have presented, and they may be right in your case. There may also be more than one way to reach the goal of good control. So it is essential that you and your treating team work together. We firmly believe that the key to using insulin right (and to most other aspects of diabetes care) is a good relationship between the person with diabetes and the health care professional.

Chapter 14

External Insulin Pumps

- *"My husband has diabetes, and the pills don't work any more. I want him to get a pump so he doesn't have to stick himself with needles."*

- *"I've heard that some people get better control by using the pump. I want to try it."*

- *"I lead a stressful and inconsistent life. People tell me that I should try an external pump. Why?"*

- *"I've got a good hemoglobin A1c, but it's because I balance my highs with awful lows. Is there a way to even things out? I want to feel better."*

One of the newer approaches to insulin delivery is the use of external insulin pumps. People often want to know if using a pump will make their life easier, give them better control of their diabetes, or make them feel better. In this chapter, we will demystify the technology of the external insulin pump, discuss its advantages and disadvantages, and describe how it works. Then you can decide if you want to try "pumping."

External insulin pumps are another way to deliver insulin. They are about the size of a pager and are worn on the belt or in the clothing, with a thin plastic tubing coming from the pump to a needle (or to a soft flexible catheter called a *cannula*) that penetrates the skin, usually in the abdomen (Figure 19). The needle or cannula must be changed every two to five days. The pump is in place 24 hours a day unless it is taken off, for example, for swimming. *Implantable* insulin pumps are entirely different, being surgically implanted under the skin. Implantable pumps are at present only available in research studies, as discussed in Chapter 33.

All insulin pumps used to treat diabetes today are "open loop." This means that *they do not measure blood sugar.* An external insulin pump can't

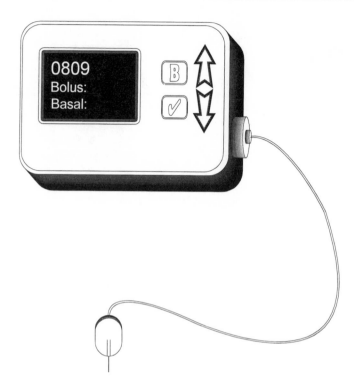

Figure 19. An external insulin pump is about the size of a pack of cards. It has an internal reservoir of insulin, and a computerized mechanism to deliver insulin through the tubing to the insertion site in precise quantities.

think for itself. It has no way to know how much insulin you need. You still have to measure your own blood sugar and tell the pump what to do.

The Basics of Pump Use

Insulin is delivered continuously from a syringe or cartridge in the external pump to the inserted needle or cannula in the skin. There are two basic rates of delivery: *basal rate,* which is a slow, continuous trickle, meant to meet your insulin needs when you are not eating, and *bolus rate,* which is a much higher flow rate, delivered for a short time before you eat a meal. Only short-acting insulin is used with an external pump, because there is no need to have insulin absorbed more slowly from the skin (Figure 20).

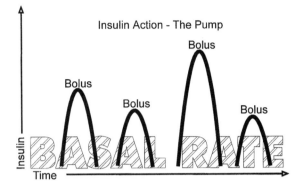

Figure 20. Insulin action of the pump. The insulin pump delivers insulin in two ways. The first is in the form of a continuous trickle (the *basal*), to meet the body's background need for insulin. The second is the *bolus*, a larger amount of insulin, delivered all at once to meet the body's need for more insulin at mealtime.

Basal Rate

Over 24 hours the basal flow of insulin usually accounts for about 40% of the total daily insulin requirement. For instance, if you take a total of 50 units of insulin a day, in the neighborhood of 20 units of that would be basal, amounting to just under 1 unit per hour. When the basal is right, your blood sugars should stay fairly stable overnight and when you go longer than usual between meals.

Bolus Doses

Bolus doses of insulin are taken all at once or within a few minutes. For example, it may take two minutes to deliver a 6-unit bolus dose. The person using a pump just presses a couple of buttons. Bolus insulin has two uses: to correct the blood sugar when it is higher than the target level and to cover food to be eaten. Pump users learn how much their blood sugar will drop from 1 unit of insulin without food and how much insulin is needed for a given amount of food.

Advantages and Disadvantages of External Insulin Pump Use

Jeanine is a successful young lawyer. She has had diabetes since childhood but never found the timing of her day uncontrollable until she became a litigator. Now, lunchtime break is up to the judge, the jury, the opposing lawyers, and innumerable other factors over which she has no control. An external insulin pump has turned out to be a good answer. She just continues on basal rate until lunchtime comes along, whether it is 11 A.M. or 2 P.M.

Flexibility

People on conventional insulin injections learn not to eat lunch very late, or else they will go low. But the basal and bolus functions of an external insulin pump usually result in more flexibility of lifestyle. With the external insulin pump, people like Jeanine can choose when to give their lunchtime bolus. If the basal rate is approximately right, they will not be going low even if lunch is late.

Safety

You may have heard that pumps can "run away" and start giving you a whole lot of insulin at once. This is not true. Current models are programmed so that they cannot overdeliver insulin by mistake. Some can even be set with maximum bolus and basal rates so that the user can't tell the pump to deliver an excessive amount, either accidentally or on purpose. There are other safety features: alarms that signal the presence of high pressure in the tubing (a consequence of a clog or other flow obstruction) or that the reservoir is empty. Finally, there are alarms to let you know that the batteries are low. A pump is a machine, so it can break down, but there are safeguards in place to minimize the risk of that happening.

Improved Control?

Does an external pump give better control? This is a good question, because it is not inevitable or automatic that starting a pump improves control. The pump user has to be aware of what his or her blood sugar is, how much carbohydrate is being eaten, and what basal and bolus doses are right. But external insulin pumps do have an advantage in that the pattern of insulin delivery more closely mimics the pattern of insulin secreted by a functioning pancreas. The insulin trickles out between meals and comes out in a big spike to cover the meals. In our experience, for most people, this pattern of insulin delivery does improve overall control of blood sugars and does reduce the uncomfortable swings.

That's the good news. But there are some pitfalls that a pump user must guard against.

Skin Complications

The risk of skin infection is greater with the pump than with injection therapy. With an injection, you stick the needle in and then remove it right away. Bacteria don't have much chance to get into the opening. But with the pump, disposable parts (the needle or cannula, tubing, and reservoir) stay in place much longer (two to five days), giving bacteria more opportunity to infect the site. Some people are more susceptible to infection than others, so they need to do more elaborate skin preparation and change the needle insertion site more frequently. A man with hair on his belly is especially at risk. But almost everyone gets a local infection (something between a pimple and a boil) at one time or another. These infections usually go away on their own once you change the site of needle insertion. Infrequently, an oral antibiotic or even drainage by a doctor is needed.

Diabetic Ketoacidosis

People on external pumps must understand that there is a risk of ketoacidosis (see Chapter 23) if the delivery of insulin stops for any reason. In all cases, this should be preventable if the person is involved in good self-care. The most frequent cause of flow interruption is a pump that has been allowed to run dry—and that is totally preventable! Other causes may be that the needle falls out of the skin, the reservoir is improperly placed in the pump, or insulin clogs up the line. Whatever the reason, since only short-acting insulin is being delivered and only at a very slow rate, if it stops, the body will become completely insulin-deficient within a few hours. This is one step away from ketoacidosis. Regular monitoring of blood sugar and attentiveness to symptoms should allow pump users to become aware of an infusion problem before it gets out of hand.

Cost

A drawback of pump therapy is the cost of the pump and supplies. In 1996 insulin pumps cost about $4,000, plus the continuing cost of supplies, which is quite variable. Of course, there are costs involved in taking three or four injections a day. But we prescribe insulin pumps when we are convinced that the therapy will definitely improve the patient's health and well-being. In the well-selected cases, the pump should be covered by insurance, just like other medically indicated devices or therapies. Why? For one thing, the well-being of the person with diabetes is essential. Pumps are *not* convenience items but a way to improve the medical care of a person with a very serious and disabling disease. Second, the major expenses caused by diabetes are long-term complications, hospitalization, and time lost from work, not the cost of insulin pumps.

This said, any person considering a pump should check with his or her insurer *before* purchasing it. Just as you wouldn't want to pay out of pocket for an appendectomy, you don't want to spend your own money for your external pump.

Is Pump Therapy for You?

The desire for more flexibility, better control, or an improved sense of well-being are usual reasons for starting insulin pump therapy. Perhaps you are tired of never being able to get on track with your irregular work schedule, you want good control for a healthy pregnancy, or you would just like to smoothe out the bumps in your control, because feeling poorly all the time is driving you crazy. These are all good reasons for considering an external pump.

The decision to use an external pump depends on several factors. Before we recommend the use of external pumps, we consider the medical issues:

—Does the prospective pump candidate understand diabetes pretty well? Pump therapy won't work if a person really can't distinguish an insulin reaction from the flu, a carbohydrate from a fat. So we want the person to have a good basic education in diabetes.

—Does the person test his or her blood sugar regularly and frequently? Without such monitoring, external insulin pumps are too dangerous. We want to see the person testing blood sugar regularly for at least a few months, to confirm that he or she is serious about it.

—Can the person accept the technology of an external pump and the mechanics of dealing with it? Every now and then, a person will come along who talks about using a pump but wouldn't feel comfortable changing a lightbulb without someone else's help. Usually, these people are relieved when we suggest that perhaps external insulin pump therapy is not for them.

—Are the individual's expectations reasonable? If a person has never even tried to follow a diet, has very late-stage complications, or thinks that the pump will solve all his or her problems, then some reality testing is more valuable than starting this therapy.

The most important thing for you to do is carefully question your own motives. Ask yourself some questions. This is not a decision that your cousin or best friend or a pump salesperson can make for you. Work through the issues by yourself, and then perhaps talk them over with someone close to you (as well as with your doctor). It's important to take an honest look at your state of mind about the whole thing.

Do you personally think that pump therapy will work for you? It won't work if you're doing it just to get your mother, husband, or doctor off your back. It won't work if you're skeptical or have too high expectations. And it won't cure all your problems. With the additional flexibility comes a heightened responsibility for the components of diabetes control. You may be used to your doctor telling you exactly how much insulin to take and when. Although you will have guidelines and education, with an insulin pump many of the decisions related to diabetes control will be left up to you.

Are you committed to regular testing of the blood sugar? Generally, we recommend that pump users test their blood sugar before each meal and at bedtime. Not only is it necessary to get the feedback needed to properly adjust pump rates, it is also necessary to avoid ketoacidosis should the pump stop.

Are you worried that the pump will get in the way when you want to play sports, go swimming, or have sex? Some prospective pump users do have concerns about "being hooked up to something all the time." Some adjustments have to be made, but most people find that they can do everything they were able to do before the pump. It is even possible to go off the pump for an hour or two, or even longer, if you slip in an injection of Regular insulin.

Are you ready to be connected to a device that lets people know you have diabetes? For some people, this is a real and deep-seated concern about being hooked up to a pump. True, the pump can be hidden under clothing, but you know it's there, and at some point others will also. More people may find out that you have diabetes. Is that okay with you? Answering this question may mean exploring your feelings about having diabetes.

Is there a health care provider nearby who can help you? This should not be an issue that stops people from using the pump, but in some locales it probably is. More and more endocrinologists are becoming familiar with pump use, so seek one out if you are interested.

These are not easy questions to answer, and we certainly don't present them in order to be negative. We think that pumps are a terrific advance for many people. There are resources to help you. Talk to health care professionals who are familiar with pump therapy. Other pump users can also be an excellent source of information. Your health care provider may be able to put you in contact with some experienced pump users. Also, many areas have an insulin pump support group led by a diabetes educator. It can really help to talk to people who are already using pumps. We regularly hear the testimonials: "I worried about sleeping with it, too, but in two years the needle has never come out while I was sleeping and has never waked me up." "Even after pregnancy, the pump has been great, and I just can't imagine being without it now."

Finally, in considering whether pump therapy is for you, take a look at the equipment itself. Watch a demonstration, check out the important features. Pump company representatives can show you the operation of their specific pump in detail if you don't have an experienced diabetes educator readily available.

Starting an Insulin Pump

Starting an insulin pump can be exciting, but it can also be scary. Some pump users say that starting an insulin pump is "like learning about diabetes all over again." There may a new angle to food: "How much insulin is that plate of pasta worth?" The pump can give a new slant on interpreting blood sugars: "My blood sugar is 164 but I bolused 4 units just 2 hours ago. Should I bolus some more?" It's a lot easier to take another small bolus by pressing buttons than it was to get out all the equipment and take an injection. And the pump provides another tool to keep from "bottoming out" with exercise: "How much should I reduce my basal to keep from going low with aerobics?"

Starting an insulin pump requires support, equipment, education, and testing. Support refers to the team of professionals who will assist you with getting started and becoming comfortable with pump therapy. Usually this means a diabetologist, a nurse educator, and a pump company trainer. We usually ask that our patients see a dietitian as well before beginning on a pump. Now is a good time to review what is meant by healthy eating; the dietitian will also help you develop some tools to use in determining the composition of various foods. As you start pump therapy, keep in frequent contact with the team. The time spent in the short term is worth it in the long term. As your questions are answered, you will gain the confidence needed to take on the responsibility of a new management approach.

Your team will help you take the first step in starting pump therapy: choosing equipment and being trained in its use. Our advice is to find out from your doctor or educator what pumps they are familiar with and whether they recommend a specific brand or model. Once you have a pump, you need to learn the technical steps for operating it: setting the clock, filling the reservoir and tubing, inserting the needle and taping it into place, changing sites of needle insertion, setting the basal rate, programming a bolus, and so on. We prefer that our patients learn how to do these things before they get started on actual insulin delivery; that way, learning the mechanics doesn't get in the way of learning how to use the pump for blood sugar control.

Some educators like to have the future pump user practice with a saltwater solution (normal saline) in the pump so that learning can take place without the pressure of making mistakes with the insulin (usual insulin injections are continued during this "saltwater training" period). In our area of the country, the pump company provides a very good initial training in use of the pump, followed by reinforcement and further practice with the educator.

The next step is to get started with insulin in the pump. In the first few days the goal is to estimate beginning basal and bolus rates and, with testing, to make modifications until the blood sugars are reasonably well controlled. While you are beginning on a pump you may stay in the hospital or at home, keeping in close (at least daily) contact with the health care team. Whether you stay in the hospital or at home depends on the lability of your blood sugar control before the pump, whether you live alone, and whether you have other health care problems. Two essential components in the first few days of using a pump are frequent blood sugar testing (before and after meals, at bedtime, and at 3 A.M.) and frequent contact with the pump team.

Initially, a safe basal rate (or series of rates) will be determined. If the basal rate is right, your blood sugars should stay relatively stable when you are not eating and when you are not especially active. If the basal rate is too high, with long intervals between meals your blood sugar will trend down; if the basal rate is too low, your blood sugar will trend up. There may be a need for several basal rates. For example, you may need a higher rate of flow in the early morning hours (the "dawn phenomenon"), a low rate at night, and somewhere in between the rest of the time. Ordinarily, the basal rate does not require much adjustment after the first few days of use. You can just program the pump to deliver the same set of basal rates day after day. You may, for instance, need 0.4 units per hour all night, 1.0 units per hour from 4 A.M. to 8 A.M. (dawn hours), and 0.6 units per hour during the day.

Recall that the bolus dose has two purposes: to correct the blood sugar when it is higher than target and to cover food to be eaten. To make corrections in the blood sugar, you need to know how much your blood sugar will drop from 1 unit of insulin. Generally, a person with a large total daily insulin requirement (for example, over 60 units per day) can expect his or her blood sugar to drop less from 1 unit of insulin than a person with a small total daily insulin requirement (under 30 units per day). For many people, the drop in blood sugar per 1 unit of insulin remains consistent throughout a 24-hour period. For some people, however, it may vary throughout the day. For example, 1 unit of insulin may bring a certain person's blood sugar down 40 points in the evening but only 25 points in the morning.

We estimate the amount of insulin needed to cover food primarily from the *carbohydrate* content of the food. Again, higher dose insulin users need more insulin to cover a given amount of carbohydrate than those with lower insulin requirements.

The total bolus is the sum of the insulin needed to correct blood sugar and cover the carbohydrate (see below). Bolus insulin is taken by pressing a series of buttons on your pump. Some people who are still new to pump therapy fall into the trap of expecting the blood sugar to respond immediately, because they are able to give the bolus so quickly and easily with the pump. Ideally, the bolus should be taken well in advance of the meal, however, so that the insulin starts to work at about the same time that the blood sugar starts to rise. A little more lead time is helpful if the blood sugar is higher than target (see Table 14). Remember, Regular insulin peaks at about two to three hours and lasts about four to six hours. When you test your blood sugar, take

Table 14.   Lead Time for Bolus Related to Blood Sugar Level

Blood Sugar at Time of Bolus	Before You Eat
Less than 70 mg/dl	No lead time required.
70–100 mg/dl	Wait 15 minutes.
100–200 mg/dl	Wait 30 minutes.
200–300 mg/dl	Wait 45 minutes.
Over 300 mg/dl	Check site, infusion line, and pump; wait 60 minutes.
Over 300 mg/dl with nausea	Take insulin by injection; check urinary ketones; check site, infusion line, and pump; recheck blood sugar in one hour.

NOTE: These lead times assume that you are using Regular insulin in your pump. If you use lispro insulin, the lead time will be shorter.

into account when you bolused last, to keep from overtreating the blood sugar and hitting a bad low.

In the first few days of pump therapy, you and your pump team will be studying your blood sugars closely and making adjustments in both basal and bolus dosing. You will work together to reach a goal of a predictable blood sugar pattern: blood sugars starting at a certain level before the meal, elevating after the meal, and returning to target level four to six hours later. Of course, daily living with a pump will bring into play all sorts of factors that will cause the blood sugar to fluctuate in predictable and unpredictable ways. Your pump team will help you learn how to use the pump in your daily life.

Using the Carbohydrate Counting System

Let's assume that one unit of insulin lowers your blood sugar 50 mg/dl, and one unit of insulin covers 15 grams of carbohydrate.

Example 1. Your blood sugar is 198. You plan to have 2 cups of cereal, $\frac{1}{2}$ cup of skim milk, and a 9-inch banana for breakfast. You calculate your bolus as follows:

—The nutrition information on the cereal box shows that there are 48 grams of carbohydrate in the cereal.
—One-half cup of milk is half of a milk exchange, or 6 grams of carbohydrate.
—A 9-inch banana is two fruit exchanges, or 30 grams of carbohydrate.
—Your total insulin requirement *for the food alone* is

$$48 + 6 + 30 = 84 \text{ divided by } 15 = 5.6 \text{ units}$$

—Plus, you have a blood sugar target of 100 and calculate the insulin needed to correct your blood sugar as follows:

$$198 - 100 = 98 \text{ divided by } 50 = 2 \text{ units}$$

—Your total bolus is

$$5.6 + 2 = 7.6 \text{ units}$$

Example 2 You are on the road and decide to stop at a deli for lunch. You do not have your blood glucose meter with you. You order a sliced turkey sandwich on rye bread and french fries. You can "eyeball" your insulin requirement by estimating your exchanges.

—Two pieces of rye bread equals two starch exchanges, or 30 grams.
—Ten french fries equals one bread exchange (plus some fat) and there appear to be about 30 fries in your order, so you figure there are about 45 grams of carbohydrate in the fries.
—Because you do not know your blood sugar and do not have any reason to think that you are high or low, you bolus for the food alone:

$$30 + 45 = 75 \text{ grams divided by } 15 = 5 \text{ units}$$

—Alternatively, if you think more easily in terms of exchanges, you figure one unit for each starch exchange, for a total of 5 units.

The exchange lists for meal planning found in Chapter 6 are helpful references for determining the carbohydrate content of your food.

Advanced Use of an Insulin Pump

Changing the Basal Rate

In some situations you may need to change your basal rate temporarily. During exercise and after exposure to hot outdoor temperatures (such as a day at the beach), you may want to decrease the basal rate or actually stop the infusion of insulin temporarily. Ordinarily, we recommend that you *do not stop the infusion of insulin for more than a few hours, unless you plan to supplement with an injection of Regular insulin.* (Remember, insulin deficiency can result in a matter of hours if the infusion of short-acting Regular insulin is stopped.)

Stress, whether physical (an illness or injury, for example) or emotional, may increase your basal insulin requirement. Some women find that in the days preceding their menstrual period their basal requirement is increased. Steroid medications, such as prednisone or cortisone (even if just injected into a joint), also markedly increase the insulin requirement.

A temporary alternative to increasing the basal rate is to take larger boluses based on blood sugar readings. Changing the basal rate is a slow way to change insulin delivery compared to changing a bolus. For example, increasing the basal rate from 0.5 to 0.8 units per hour for two hours only gives 0.6 units extra insulin—an amount more easily given as a bolus.

More about Boluses

Some people are bothered by symptoms of high blood sugar after eating a particularly high-carbohydrate meal, even if the insulin has a good head start. "I know my blood sugar is 250 right now but I guarantee by lunchtime it will be down to normal." Sometimes this effect can be blunted by splitting the intake of calories. That is, take most of the meal within 45 minutes of the bolus, but save one part for about 2 hours after the bolus, when you can eat it as a snack.

High-fat meals may also call for some changes in the bolus. As we have mentioned, although fat does not affect the blood sugar directly, it can slow the absorption of carbohydrate taken along with it. If too much of the bolus is taken all at once before a high-fat meal, the blood sugar may actually go low before the meal is absorbed. Pump users are able to compensate for this by giving part of the bolus before the meal and the remainder several hours later. Alternatively, part of the bolus can be given before the meal and the remainder given in the form of a temporarily increased basal over several hours following the meal. Some people, for instance, will smooth out the effect of an 8-unit premeal dose by giving it as a 6-unit bolus, then upping their basal rate, say, from 0.5 to 1.5 units per hour for the next two hours (delivering the extra two units).

With boluses, the first rule is to *be safe,* and being safe means not having a severe hypoglycemic episode. For example, it is not advisable to bolus for your supper at work and assume that the drive home will be the lead time for the insulin. What if you got stuck in traffic? Do you have sugar in the car?

Treating Low Blood Sugar

As with any type of insulin therapy, low blood sugar reactions should be treated immediately with fast-acting carbohydrate. An additional snack may be needed if low blood sugar occurs within two to five hours after a large bolus, since the bolus may still be acting. Stopping the basal rate will have very little effect. The more important thing is to eat carbohydrate.

Treating High Blood Sugar

If you have unusually high blood sugar, you will need to do some problem solving to determine the cause. The following are common reasons why the blood sugar may be high:

—*Missed bolus.* Check the pump to determine if you bolused with your last meal.

—*Insufficient bolus.* This commonly occurs when you eat unfamiliar food and you are not sure what's in it.

—*Prolonged use of needle insertion site.* With extended use, absorption at the needle insertion site may be hampered and insulin is less effective.

—*Illness.* Some people find that with illness there is a rise in blood sugar levels.

—*Pump malfunction.* If there seems to be a problem with the device itself—for instance, if the display doesn't respond when you push the button—contact the manufacturer. The company will help you with the problem or send you a new pump.

—*Empty reservoir.* If you're a careful driver, you wouldn't let your car run out of gas. Similarly, you should never allow your pump reservoir to run dry.

If you are not sure why the blood sugar is high, bolus some insulin to get it down. If there is no significant decrease in the blood sugar within one hour, change your syringe, tubing, and needle and check to see that the pump is delivering insulin out the needle tip. Then bolus again. Remember, since the pump uses only short-acting insulin, if there is an interruption in flow, within several hours you could develop ketoacidosis. If you are in doubt or if you have ketones in your urine, take an injection of Regular insulin right away.

Exercise

Learning your individual response to exercise and to different kinds of exercise is key in determining what adjustments to make in your pumped insulin dosing. Pump users have found several strategies helpful in preventing hypoglycemia related to exercise:

—Eat extra carbohydrate before you exercise. If exercise is prolonged, then take additional carbohydrate during exercise.

—Take a reduced bolus for a meal preceding exercise.

—Decrease the basal for two to three hours during and/or after exercise.

—Eat additional carbohydrate after exercise.

In the weeks and months after pump initiation, you will learn how to handle the many situations that arise in living with a pump: what to do with your pump when showering, how to tell your date what that funny-looking beeper is, where to put the pump during sexual activity, how to conceal it in a form-fitting ball gown or macho T-shirt. Although you may find solutions to these situations on your own, remember that there are resources out there to help: experienced pump users, your doctor, educators, support groups, counselors, and the insulin pump company. Pump therapy can be a great way to help your self-care.

Part III

Living with Diabetes

We once had three tough individuals in our diabetes self-management program at Johns Hopkins: a retired CIA agent, an ex-Marine, and a New York City cop. Not one of them was thrilled when our psychologist came in to talk about living with diabetes. The fact is that one had never even told his family, much less his friends or co-workers, that he had diabetes; another thought there was no way that anything emotional could affect him; and the third just plain didn't "believe in" psychology.

Rather than give up, the psychologist used his own skills to make a dent in these men's strong defenses. Gradually, he convinced them that there *is* a link—as Alan Alda once put it in a commencement address to the Columbia University College of Physicians and Surgeons—between the head bone and the heart bone. Emotions *do* play a role in the success of your self-care. In fact, emotions play a *huge* role.

In Part III we discuss these links between how you feel about diabetes and what you do about it. We even go further, considering how the world around you may react: your family, friends, employer, health care professional, and "the system" (meaning the organization that provides care and pays for it). Your interaction with the world around you, how you get help and support, is a key to successful self-care.

You can't do it without recognizing that emotions play a role, and you can't do it all by yourself—even if you're a CIA agent, an ex-Marine, or a New York City cop.

Chapter 15

The Emotional Side of Diabetes

- *"I don't have diabetes, I have just a touch of sugar."*
- *"I'd rather die than turn into a pincushion."*
- *"I guess it's time for me to stop fighting and accept my diabetes."*

Do you think much about the emotional side of diabetes? Many people think of diabetes strictly as a medical problem. The importance of the emotional side of diabetes, however, cannot be overestimated. If you ignore your own emotions, it will be really hard, perhaps even impossible, for you to take good care of your condition. Our goal in this chapter is to help you explore your feelings about having diabetes, so you can cope better. Coping well emotionally gives you a firm foundation on which to build your diabetes management plan.

Interest in the relationship between feelings and diabetes goes back centuries. In 1679 a British physician named Thomas Willis wrote, "The cause of diabetes is an emotional state I call 'profound sorrow.'" For centuries, researchers interested in the connection between emotions and diabetes followed Willis's lead, searching for psychological *causes* of diabetes. In the early decades of the twentieth century attempts were made to identify a so-called diabetogenic personality—a technical way of saying that diabetes occurred in people with a specific type of personality, which predisposed the person to develop the disease.

We now know that there are no psychological causes of diabetes, though we are learning more every day about the psychological *consequences* of living life with this disease, and how psychological stresses affect people's self-care. One of these consequences is a cluster of emotions many people experience as a part of living with diabetes. These emotions—denial, obsession, anger, frustration, fear, and guilt—all sound negative, and most of the time they are. But not always. Being emotional about serious illness is natural and normal, and it is inevitable when you live with diabetes. In some cases, the emotions can even be helpful or protective.

Denial

Many people are tempted to deny the diagnosis of diabetes, and even more do not fully acknowledge that they must live as if they have diabetes. Some people go on for years fighting the need for any change in behavior beyond taking their pills or their insulin shots. Others pretend not to see the relationship between how much they eat or how much they weigh and problems in controlling their blood sugar levels. Still others never "get" the connection between their out-of-control diabetes and symptoms such as constant fatigue, chronic infections, or painful neuropathy.

Almost everyone thinks it's bad to be in denial, especially if what you are denying is a serious but treatable condition like diabetes. This is partly right. It's not good to deny that you have diabetes, even subconsciously. It's not good to deny that you have to change your life to care for your diabetes. But there are times when a little denial can be a good thing. If you were constantly aware of every awful thing that could happen to you as a person with (or without) diabetes, you'd be a basket case in no time. Who is to say that anyone, with diabetes or not, won't be struck by a bus tomorrow?

Accepting the seriousness of your diabetes without becoming overwhelmed by it is a tough balancing act. If you slide to either extreme, you'll suffer. If you don't treat your diabetes with respect, your risk of short-term and long-term complications goes way up. But if you are preoccupied with your diabetes, the concern may take over your life. Either way, you won't do all you can to take care of yourself.

So denial is perfectly understandable. You already know that diabetes is a serious disease that anyone would be tempted to deny. But there's one big problem with denying diabetes: denial doesn't work in the long run. It has another downside: it is almost never complete. Even if you are great at denial, you are almost certainly carrying a burden of guilt, because you are aware to at least some degree that you are not taking proper care of yourself. You may keep that guilt buried deep inside yourself, but it still gnaws at you.

Are you in denial? Do you have symptoms that you prefer not to admit, even to yourself, are caused by diabetes, such as frequent urination, chronic exhaustion, infections, blurry vision, or pains in your feet? Do you avoid getting medical care for fear of what you will be told? Do you feel uncomfortable acknowledging to others that you have diabetes? Do you believe you can take care of your diabetes by medication alone? Do you tell yourself that your diabetes isn't serious? If you answered yes to any of these questions, read on. Almost everyone is in denial at least some of the time.

Dealing with Denial

Think about the proverbial ostrich. We imagine that it buries its head because it feels hopeless, convinced that there is nothing it can do to avoid disaster. People who deny they have diabetes or deny that they have to care for their diabetes often do so for the same reason. The key to pulling your head out of the sand and overcoming denial is to transform hopelessness into confidence. With confidence, you'll find that there's a lot you can do to improve your situation.

How can you build confidence? Three factors are crucial: an understanding of your diabetes and its treatment; skill in managing your diabetes from day to day; and skill in coping with the emotional side of your disease. The first two factors are covered elsewhere in this book. Here, we will focus on the emotional aspects. To illustrate how coping with the emotional aspects of diabetes builds confidence, let's take the example of exercise.

James's doctor tells him that he should start an exercise program. James's first thought is, "Here we go again—the same old thing. Like my dentist telling me to floss." James already knows the benefits of exercise: better blood sugar control, reduced weight, cardiovascular conditioning, and emotional well-being. But he also knows that he's 52 years old and hasn't exercised since he graduated from high school. The prospect is daunting, to put it mildly.

What can James do? He might begin by trying to break the problem down into a series of manageable steps. If you would like to implement an exercise program, or if you've been told that you should begin one, start by identifying any exercise you might be willing to try. That's all. You aren't making any commitments yet, just compiling a list. Let's say you come up with three activities that might interest you: dancing, bowling, and walking. Next, list what opportunities you have to engage in each of the activities you listed. Then, consider which are workable, given your schedule and your pocketbook.

Now you've taken three steps. Of course, you've taken all these steps in your head; you haven't moved a muscle yet. But that's fine, because you've made the task of actually exercising much more manageable. Now start planning your exercise program. Be sure to think about any support you'll need. Will you need (or want) to have company? Do you need coverage at home with children or other responsibilities? Be realistic but be determined. You can do it.

Keep on with this step-by-step approach, even once you have your exercise program under way. You may find that some of the choices you've made don't work. In fact, this is almost a certainty. So you need to identify what isn't working and set out a different approach. Each time you successfully take a step, the remaining problem is smaller and your confidence is greater. You're overcoming denial by proving to yourself that you can do it.

Obsession

Like being in denial, having some degree of obsession is a natural, normal response to life with diabetes. But obsession is the opposite of denial. People become obsessed with their diabetes regimen because they desperately want to believe that if they do everything perfectly, diabetes and its consequences can be perfectly controlled. Unfortunately, diabetes management is *not* a precise science, so a compulsive approach to diabetes can't provide the desired benefits. (Compulsive *behavior* is the result of obsessive *thinking*.) Leonard Pray, author of *The Journey of a Diabetic,* once wrote, "Don't try to be perfect. Try for good control, to be sure, but perfection lasts for a moment, and diabetes lasts a lifetime."

Perfectionism, the driving force for obsession, is not an effective long-term approach to anything, and living with diabetes is definitely a long-term proposition. Obsession is a set-up for disappointment; you may even reach the point where you are so discouraged that you say, "To hell with it, no matter how hard I try, nothing works." Obsession also tends to leave little room for the rest of your life, allowing diabetes is control you, rather than the other way around.

Overcoming Obsession

If you are sometimes obsessed with your diabetes, you might work on an emotional coping skill we call "letting go." Letting go preserves your precious energies for the battles you can win, rather than wasting them on those you cannot win. Letting go is a painful (and continuing) process, because it means accepting the loss of something precious. No one can do that without anger and tears, but letting go is an essential part of the process of living well with diabetes. Consider Ann, a highly intelligent, highly successful young stock-broker.

The world was Ann's oyster—until she got diabetes. Her response was typical Ann. She put tremendous energy into maintaining her blood sugar levels in the normal range, sticking to an extremely strict regimen. She ate her meals precisely on time, everything by the book. She tested her blood sugars six or more times a day and was undone by any readings over 120 mg/dl. Diabetes controlled Ann's life. In fact, she often felt as if she didn't have a life. Naturally, Ann couldn't maintain such an existence. But instead of easing up a bit, she would often swing to the opposite extreme, abandoning her entire regimen. "It's a busy time at work. I just can't do both work and diabetes." Like many intelligent, disciplined, and successful people, Ann took an all-or-nothing approach to her self-care. The result was not very successful.

Things began to turn around for Ann when she finally learned to let go of the fantasy of perfect control. She stopped draining her energy in this vain quest and focused instead on the realistic goal of good control. Once Ann made this shift, she was happier, and her family life and her work improved dramatically. Her long-term blood sugar control actually got better, compared with the fluctuating results of her old all-or-nothing approach.

Anger

Anger is another emotion all too familiar to people with diabetes. The primary source of their anger is the constant, unpleasant, nonnegotiable demands of life with the disease. Many people tell us they feel angry because diabetes is such an *imposition:* they are angry because of all the things they *have to do.* Others say they are angry because diabetes *deprives* them of so much: they are angry because of all the things they *can't do.* People are also angry because diabetes is forever. They are angry because *they*—rather than their parents, siblings, spouses, neighbors, friends, or strangers—developed diabetes. They are angry because they can't eat what they want, because they have to schedule and plan in ways no one else has to, because they feel like pincushions as a result of all the shots and blood tests. Sometimes people get angry about things that are not even true: misunderstandings about the meaning of a particular reading or laboratory result, or about the likelihood of developing complications, for example. Surely, there is no lack of things to be angry about.

A common target for the anger is health care professionals. Health care providers don't appreciate how difficult it is to live with diabetes, people say. "They don't care how I feel." "The nutritionist gave me a meal plan that has nothing to do with real life." "The nurse acted as though I were lying when I told her what I actually do." "The doctor was offended by my questions." "The doctor was too rushed to listen to me." We've already touched on the issue of your relationship with health care providers, and we'll go into more detail about this in Chapter 19. But we'll say here that anger rarely helps.

Another trigger for anger is the feeling that family and friends are unsupportive. Sometimes they minimize the demands of diabetes. At other times they may act like police, monitoring eating, exercise, and blood sugar results, as though you can't do it for yourself. This can make the person with diabetes feel like a prisoner, surrounded by guards rather than loved ones. We will discuss diabetes as a family affair in Chapter 16. Here again, anger is a negative emotion that rarely helps.

People with diabetes sometimes even focus their anger on other people who have diabetes. Listening to someone say that he has perfect control of his diabetes or that she finds her diabetes is no trouble at all to manage can be really irritating if your experience is not so positive.

Finally, angry feelings are often the result of extremes in blood sugar levels. We've heard countless stories from people who lose control emotionally when their blood sugars skyrocket or bottom out.

Away with Anger

As uncomfortable and sometimes destructive as anger can be, like denial and obsession it is a natural, normal emotion and one that is practically inevitable for people with diabetes. It is important to deal with these angry feelings effectively when they come up. The last thing you want is for anger to rule your life. Once again, the key is strengthening your emotional coping skills.

Let's say you are really angry that you can't eat all those delicious treats that you enjoyed so much before you got diabetes. It's all very unfair, and you have every right to be mad about it. You can even choose to stay mad about it for the rest of your life, but that's not a particularly smart choice. The real question is how you manage the feelings when they arise, how you work through them.

Start by asking yourself *precisely* what you are angry about. Is it that you can't ever have another treat? Or that you can't have as many as you used to? Or perhaps you can't stand seeing your co-workers devouring goodies at work. By specifying in your own mind what bugs you, you may find that so-lutions present themselves: have a small treat once a week, carry a snack that you can munch on at work when your co-workers pass around the cookies or candies. Even if you don't come up with a solution, at least the true mag-nitude of the problem will be clear: no, you can't eat everything you used to eat. Whatever the source of your anger, you can choose to deal with it directly rather than stewing about it.

It's all a matter of choice. Ultimately, everything you do (or don't do) is your choice. If this sounds strange, think again. Do you follow every recom-mendation others make about how you drive or how you exercise? Certain-ly not. You have veto power over the suggestions of others. You can stick to your diet or ignore it completely—or anything in between. In any case, *you* are choosing. Not your physician, spouse, or best friend, but you yourself.

Recognizing that you are always making choices can be liberating. If you aren't happy with one choice you made, you can make another one next time. It's up to you, and you usually do have second chances with your self-care decisions.

Frustration

People with diabetes feel frustrated that they have to keep diabetes on their minds every waking hour. They feel frustrated by the lack of freedom and flexibility. People are also frustrated by the relatively slow progress of science in its efforts to find a cure for diabetes. Ten years ago one of us gave a talk with the theme, "A cure for diabetes in ten years." Unfortunately, we could probably still use that theme today.

For most people, the biggest source of frustration is the unpredictable nature of their own bodies. You know: those times when you've done every-thing (or almost everything) right, and you get a blood sugar reading that makes no sense at all. The worst thing about frustration is that it may lead people to give up, to say, "To hell with it, it doesn't matter anyway." While un-derstandable, this reaction initiates a downward spiral. As one of our patients said, "When you take a 'to hell with it' attitude toward your diabetes, that's exactly where you go."

Defusing Frustration

How can you avoid "chucking it all" when you feel frustrated? Try some pos-itive diabetes self-talk. Imagine this scenario: your meter reads 287 (or any number that you would consider high). You might feel like saying, "I never do anything right!" or "That's it. I give up!" But try another approach instead. Try analyzing the situation: "That's really high. I hate it when I'm that high. Now, what could have caused that? Did I eat any differently today or skip my exercise? Is the sound of construction outside my office getting on my nerves more than I thought? It must be something." Perhaps you decide that there is no good reason for you to be high that day. So you look at your log of readings for the last three days and find that most of them were high, too. You consider the usual possibilities: bad insulin? sinus infection? stress at work? In the end you say to yourself, "Something is up, but I haven't a clue what it is. I'll try to get my level down right now and if I'm still high in a day or so, I'll call my doctor or nurse and see if two heads are better than one." You take some extra insulin, the sugar comes down, and the whole episode is forgotten.

It may take lots of practice before you can talk to yourself this way, accepting some blood sugar results without understanding them and without excessive frustration. But it's worth the effort. Constructive diabetes self-talk focuses you on solving a problem instead of beating yourself up. Besides, as everyone who has looked closely at their blood sugars knows, many highs simply go away before you ever really know why they happened in the first place. Why give yourself grief?

Fear

Diabetes is a scary disease, so it's probably inevitable for people with diabetes to feel fearful and to think more about death than the average person does. These worries are even more likely to plague you if you have older relatives with diabetes who did poorly. People tell us about many diabetes-related fears. Among people with Type II diabetes, one of the most common is the fear of having to take insulin. One man said, "I know my diabetes is out of control, but I'd rather take poison and die than go on insulin." Some fear insulin reactions. And just about everyone fears long-term complications.

These fears, which are all understandable, are a mix of fact and fiction. Starting insulin is hard for some people: insulin reactions are unpleasant, and there is some risk of long-term complications. On the other hand, going on insulin does not mean that your diabetes will have a worse outcome. On the contrary, the risk of complications goes way up if you need insulin but don't take it. Insulin reactions can be avoided or treated by detecting mild, early symptoms. And many, many people live long, healthy lives despite diabetes. So recognizing and dealing with your own particular fears can be liberating.

Facing Your Fears

Fear is sometimes a positive force. In moderation, it can motivate people. Realistic fear of complications can strengthen your resolve to take the best possible care of yourself. Fear of hypoglycemia can lead you to find effective approaches to keeping your blood sugars as close to normal as possible without putting yourself at risk.

The key to making your fears work for you instead of against you is to keep reminding yourself of the positive. The fate of older relatives or others who had diabetes ten or twenty or more years ago will not be your fate. For one thing, with advancing research and technology, the power to control blood sugars—minimizing highs and lows—improves every day. The better shape you are in now, the better shape you will be in when even more effective treatment, or even a cure, arrives. These are not just dreams. Progress in treatment has been dramatic over the decades and will continue to be so. Your fears are most likely grossly exaggerated.

Guilt

Many people with diabetes tell us they feel guilty. No question about it, there are plenty of opportunities to feel guilty when you have diabetes, what with all the things you are supposed to do and all the others you are not supposed to do. One of our patients provided a perfect description of these sentiments: "I know I don't go to the doctor as often as I should. I don't go because I always end up feeling so guilty. She asks me if I've been exercising, if I've been testing my blood, if I've been eating better and lost any weight, if I've stopped smoking. And for every question I have to give the same answer. 'No.' It's not like she's criticizing me on purpose; she's actually really gentle. Then she tells me that there's nothing she can do if I won't make the commitment to helping myself. I know she's right. What's wrong with me?"

Guilt is the one emotion that seems to have no positive side, and yet we see guilt all the time. Many patients come to our office with marginal notes in their diaries: "I cheated!!" "Really pigged out today!" "I was bad!" It might be natural and normal, but guilt is a paralyzing emotion. It gets you down on yourself, and when that happens, you're focused *backward,* on things you can never change.

Getting Away from Guilt

To avoid feeling paralyzed by guilt, you have to celebrate your accomplishments and downplay your deficiencies. Probably no one is as bad as their inner voice tries to tell them they are. So when you take any step toward healthy living, celebrate. You should pat yourself on the back because each step represents significant movement. The people who succeed in life with diabetes (and those who succeed in life without diabetes) are people who acknowledge and enjoy their accomplishments at the same time that they continue to strive for new successes.

At first you may find precious little to celebrate, but there's always something. To get started, try this: every night just before you fall asleep, tell yourself three things you did that day concerning your diabetes that you feel good about. They can be large or small: resisting a sweet treat at work, testing your blood sugar one extra time that day, talking openly to a friend about your diabetes, making an appointment for the eye exam you'd been putting off, walking even when you didn't feel like it, eating a healthy dinner. Celebrating your achievements will help you avoid focusing on the times you slipped up, and *that* will help you avoid that useless emotion, guilt.

As we've seen in this chapter, the seemingly negative emotions—denial, obsession, anger, frustration, fear, and guilt—are natural and normal. The important thing is how you deal with them. Positive thoughts and positive self-talk are the keys to coping successfully with the emotional side of diabetes. In the chapters that follow, we will talk about other opportunities to sharpen your self-talk skills.

Chapter 16

Families Who Live with Diabetes

- *"My husband tells me that ever since I got diabetes I'm mean as a junkyard dog, and I guess maybe he's right."*

- *"We have six people in the family, but since one of us got diabetes, it's tearing the family apart. We just don't know how to deal with it."*

- *"My husband will not take care of his diabetes, but when I say anything to him, he jumps right down my throat."*

- *"I was diagnosed four months ago, and the diabetes has actually brought my wife and me closer. We walk miles every day, and we talk and talk."*

Diabetes is a family affair. This is true in a scientific way, since diabetes is in part a genetic disease, and you are more likely to have it if another member of your family has it already. But even more important, the effects of diabetes are so powerful and pervasive that they touch everyone who loves, lives with, or cares for a person who has diabetes.

This chapter is for families with diabetes, whether the person who has the disease is an adult or a child. We discuss concerns that we hear from family members about how their loved ones manage the disease. We discuss how diabetes affects all the family, how simple caring can be misinterpreted, and how tensions can spread throughout the family unit. We hope those who have diabetes will read the chapter too, so they can learn more about what their families might be thinking and feeling. Our goal is to help everyone in the family to live better with diabetes.

We'll offer 10 suggestions we've developed over the years, five presented as things "to do" and five as things "not to do" (or to try not to do). Each is introduced with a real-life anecdote, some of which you may find familiar.

Think about these suggestions when the tension seems to be rising around diabetes-related issues in your family. We think they'll help.

Lesson 1: Don't Act Like a Police Officer

Sara was extremely frustrated because her husband Phil refused to care for his diabetes. His attitude was "if I die, I die." Earlier in their marriage, before Phil had diabetes, she had found his devil-may-care attitude attractive, but now all she could think of was that he was killing himself. Sara refused to accept Phil's fatalism. So she acted like a domestic police force, constantly bugging him to do the right thing: "Don't eat that, get off your duff and exercise, check your blood sugar, keep your appointments." All to no avail. Sara was beside herself because her love and concern for Phil were turning to anger and frustration. She couldn't control his diabetes, and their relationship was suffering as well.

Attempting to police someone's behavior rarely works. In fact, it usually has the opposite result, and it can ruin your relationship, whether the target is your spouse or your child.

We know that it's hard to follow this guideline. For one thing, the worrying and nagging are done out of love. We talk to many people who are frantic because they see their family members denying their diabetes and refusing to take responsibility for it. If they really didn't care what happened to someone, they wouldn't get so upset.

So let's consider how Sara can be more successful in dealing with Phil. First, she should recognize that she's frustrated because she *does* care, not because the man she loves is insufferably stubborn. Next, she has to accept the fact that her attempt to police his behavior does not work and will never work. The trick is not to give up caring, but to change the way that caring is expressed. Maybe Phil sees Sara's efforts as a challenge to his independence or his masculinity, or as accentuating his "differentness." Whatever is going on inside Phil's head, it's obviously enough to keep him fighting every effort on Sara's part. What a waste of energy for both of them!

So Sara needs to develop more effective strategies and rebuild their relationship. She might try gradually finding out from Phil if there is anything he *wants* her to do to help him with his diabetes. A flat "stay out of it" may be the first response, but over time the dialogue may begin. In the meantime, there are things she could try on her own, like keeping sweets and junk food out of the house, or buying his test strips and laying them out where they will be convenient for him to use, or offering to join him for walks, swims, or tennis games. These are positive, friendly gestures that he'll be sure to notice and that will make things easier without beating him over the head.

Sara can also make sure that her husband knows her feelings, her motivations. She can tell Phil that she loves him and wants to spend many happy, healthy years with him. She can tell him she feels scared when she sees that his diabetes is out of control. She can tell him she feels helpless, frustrated, and guilty about her inability to help him deal better with his diabetes. But she must be careful not to bring up all these deeply felt emotions in the midst of a quarrel, when voices are raised and these feelings are the last thing Phil wants to hear about. Better to tell him over a candle-lit dinner, when the feelings are positive.

Retiring from the role of household police officer is hard. It takes conscious effort, time, and patience. But it is the only approach that works.

Lesson 2: Don't Ignore Diabetes

Jim never quite faced up to the fact that his teenage son Josh got diabetes. His own upbringing had stressed rugged individualism and independence. Fall down? Pick yourself up and get on with it. Feeling sorry for yourself? Suck it up and do something useful. Deep inside, there was nothing Jim would have liked better than to be able to help Josh, to cure his diabetes or even just be able to communicate as father to son, "I feel for you. I want you to do well. I hurt for you." But it was beyond him, so Jim buried himself in his work and ignored Josh's diabetes.

In this case, as so often happens, the person trying to ignore diabetes is suffering inwardly much more than if his feelings were let out. Josh has probably experienced his father's standoffish approach before, and he probably doesn't even realize his father's deep hurt. The remedy lies in Jim's accepting the fact that his son has a difficult disease, talking about it at least sometimes, and making realistic accommodations when it comes to timing activities, dealing with emergencies, and the like.

The accommodations a family makes sometimes aren't easy. People may feel bored, irritated, or downright angry when the person with diabetes controls the action. Meals might have to be rushed or delayed and activities postponed or canceled to accommodate the demands of diabetes.

You can't ignore a loved one's diabetes, but neither can you deny the irritation you feel at the way the disease rules your life. So what can you do? For starters, face up to the fact that you do care and that whatever accommodations you are making for your family member's health are a lot more important than whether you eat an hour later or put chocolate syrup on the strawberries. And recognize that your own irritation has a positive side: it puts you and your loved one in the same boat. He or she is at least as irritated by the demands of diabetes as you are. Try staying on the same side of the fence, recognizing that you are both angry about the same thing: diabetes. You are not mad at each other.

Lesson 3: Don't Lead Your Loved One in the Path of Temptation

> *The Crosby family always had snacks around: potato chips, ice cream, chocolates. When son Saul came down with diabetes, it just didn't seem right to make the whole family suffer. So Diane Crosby tried to teach her son not to eat them, but she couldn't bear to keep the cupboards empty.*

We've already said that you can't be the family cop, but you can make it easier for the person with diabetes if the whole family eats healthy. And make no mistake: the "diabetic diet" is a healthy diet for all. So most families find that it's better for all concerned if the "forbidden fruits" are kept out of the house.

We don't minimize the difficulty of this switch to a household free of junk food. Many a child will yell and scream if he or she doesn't have junk food easily within reach. Many a mother tries to provide whatever the family likes best, and many a father "needs" those snacks.

But the healthy approach is especially important if you have a child with diabetes. Young people are bombarded with temptations to eat things they shouldn't, and they all succumb some of the time. While you can't always keep your child from indulging, you can help by setting a good example at home. When you eat right, you show your child that it *can* be done and that you care enough to eat as he or she eats.

Lesson 4: Don't Criticize When Your Loved One Succumbs to Temptation

> - *"Linda, I saw that! You thought I was sleeping, but I wasn't. You went right down to the kitchen, opened up the refrigerator, and had a piece of that birthday cake. We agreed you wouldn't do that anymore. Didn't your promise mean anything?"*

It's natural for you to feel frustrated when you catch your loved one giving in to temptation, but adding insult to injury is a surefire argument starter.

You probably have to say something sometime, but saying it on the spot, when you are boiling (and your loved one is probably feeling guilty and defensive) is almost certainly a mistake.

Count to 10, then start thinking about what to do. If your loved one is generally pretty good about sticking to her diet, keep the current indiscretion in perspective. Remind yourself that no one's perfect, and that keeping to the diabetes regimen is hard. An occasional slip is unlikely to cause serious long-term health problems.

If your loved one succumbs to temptation on a regular basis, there are still things you can do that might help, some of which we have already mentioned. You might look into the possibility of joining a support group with your family member, or participating in a diabetes education program together. In these settings, you might both learn some helpful facts and approaches to the problem.

Lesson 5: Don't Talk in Public about Your Loved One's Diabetes Unless He or She Is Comfortable with Such Talk

Jeanette struggled at home every day, all day, with her husband Frank's diabetes. Being a naturally open, talkative person, Jeanette had a habit of mentioning it to others. She made benign little comments to waiters ("Frank can't have any dessert because he has diabetes") or to friends ("Frank's diabetes is acting up today, so I hope you don't mind if we leave early"). Their friends all knew Frank had diabetes, and it just seemed natural to Jeanette to refer to it. But one night, maybe during a low, Frank blew his stack and roared, "I don't want you ever mentioning my diabetes to anyone, ever again. It's my diabetes, I take care of it, and that's it!" Jeanette was stunned and hurt.

Public comments tend to be taken as criticism. They also highlight the "difference" of the person with diabetes. What seems natural to one person may be taken entirely differently by the other. Try discussing the question with your loved one: "Do you mind if I mention the diabetes every now and then, or does it bother you?" It may be an adjustment for you not to mention something that is so much a part of your life together, but the adjustment may be necessary. Be sure your loved one is comfortable about having you talk before you do so.

Lesson 6: Offer Support and Comfort, Especially When Things Aren't Going Well with the Diabetes

> *George knew his wife Sue's diabetes was getting to be more and more of a struggle. What used to be easy—taking one shot in the morning and not worrying about it—had intensified into a multidose daily insulin regimen that seemed to consume her time and energy. Then she went to the ophthalmologist and was told she had "a spot of diabetes in one eye." Sue was devastated.*

People with diabetes are especially sensitive when their blood sugars are bouncing around or when they get news they interpret as bad. In Sue's case, the "spot of diabetes" was in fact of very little importance, but to her it was devastating. A little extra thoughtfulness in word and deed can go a long way toward keeping things positive.

Much has been written about the tendency to want to *do something* instead of just offering support. It's much easier sometimes to react by saying, "Well, I'm going to make you an appointment with two other ophthalmologists to see if your doctor is really right, and then I'm going to the library to look up exactly what the diagnosis means and what to do about it." This is not always the most helpful response. What Sue needs is a good hug, maybe a cry, and the feeling that George will always be there. The skill required here is the ability to give one of the world's greatest gifts—genuine, loving support.

Speaking of gifts, everyone loves them, and maybe they should be tangible. What are the gifts your loved one most appreciates? Cards, unexpected phone calls, flowers, a special night out, a back rub? Gifts are great to cheer up someone who is down. Spontaneous thoughtfulness is especially nice. It's bound to help your loved one feel better about himself or herself, and that will undoubtedly provide extra motivation for diabetes care.

Another true story can drive home the importance of simply showing your unconditional love, letting it be known within the family.

> *When Stefan was 10 years old he went through a period when he tried to minimize the pain of his insulin injections by giving his shots as slowly as possible. He would sit with the needle poised, often for minutes at a time, while his dad exhorted him to get it over with, arguing that he was actually prolonging his agony. Needless to say, his father's approach didn't help matters. Finally one day his dad took a different tack. He said, "I know those shots must really hurt, and I wish I could take*

some of them for you. You're really brave and I love you." Stefan smiled at his dad and said, *"It's not that big a deal."* Then he pushed the needle right in.

Stefan needed that extra bit of loving support that goes a long way toward making life with diabetes more manageable. This support may even explain Stefan's attitude toward his diabetes. When he was 11 years old, his father told him that one of his greatest wishes in life was for Stefan to no longer have diabetes. To this Stefan responded, "I don't like having diabetes. In fact, there are times when I hate it. But it has forced me to learn how to take care of myself, and I wouldn't trade that for anything in the world."

We hope that everyone who has diabetes will find a way to grow stronger and closer to those who love them.

Lesson 7: Be Especially Patient When Your Loved One Has a Low Blood Sugar

This point is so obvious and so common that it doesn't even need an anecdote to illustrate it. As you know if you've lived with hypoglycemic reactions of a loved one, the trauma may be worse for those witnessing it than for the person with diabetes. You have to keep reminding yourself that when hypoglycemic, the person with diabetes just isn't the person you know and love. When they are hypoglycemic, people will say things they don't mean, be violent when it's not in their real nature, and act in all sorts of ways that seem calculated to make you miserable. What's more, when it is all over, they will not remember a thing!

When your family member is having a low, you have to keep your wits about you and your emotions under control. The behavior is really not controllable, but it will pass.

Lesson 8: Look for Opportunities to Help, Especially in Public Situations

After 30 years of living together, Fred knows his wife Frieda's diabetes routine, and he has learned many little things he can do, unobtrusively and almost without thinking, that make life easier for Frieda. He buys the glucose test strips, makes sure there's always a supply handy. He orders the food in the restaurant, keeping control of that roving eye that spots the most tempting dessert on the menu. And he makes a point of quietly calling the host well before they go to someone's home for dinner, talking over the fact that there are certain foods they'd rather avoid. This last action seemed awkward at first, but it has become so natural that Fred doesn't even think twice, and the friends who are inviting them are thankful to have the advice, since they otherwise wouldn't know what to serve.

Eating right, testing, and taking shots can be particularly stressful when you are away from home, so your loved one may be edgier at these times. Be alert for opportunities to make things a little easier. The key to success here is to do things your partner wants you to do and not to make a big deal of it. It's not something you're doing for praise or thanks, it's just part of your love and support.

Lesson 9: Figure Out the "Hot Button" Issues and Work on Fixing Them

There are certain things that always create friction in the Parks household. One is when Sam, who has diabetes, sees his wife Joan eating chocolate. Another is when Joan finds Sam's used syringes lying all over the bathroom. These behaviors may not seem all that outrageous on the face of it, but they sure do get the Parks family going!

In most families, certain diabetes-related situations seem to press the "hot button." In one family the issue might be dietary indiscretions, in another battles triggered by low blood sugar reactions. Everyone has hot buttons, so the best thing is to identify your family's issues and figure out how to avoid them. It's amazing how successful this simple approach can be for solving problems and avoiding fights.

Lesson 10: Try a Little Humor

Glynda told us about an experience with her husband Jeff. One night after they had been asleep for several hours, Jeff started thrashing around. Glynda woke up and realized he was in the throes of a severe hypoglycemic reaction. She got him to drink some orange juice, and Jeff slowly regained full consciousness. Finally, at about 3:30 A.M., he was back to normal. Glynda, exhausted and a little frustrated, tried to go back to sleep. But no, Jeff decided it was time to make love. This was the last thing on Glynda's mind, so thinking quickly, she said, "Honey, we already did that." Jeff gave her a puzzled look, started to laugh, and fell asleep.

Stefan (whom we have already mentioned) developed diabetes when he was seven years old. To confirm the diagnosis and to begin learning to live with diabetes, Ste-

fan and his mother and father went to the pediatrician's office. There they were given instructions about diet, insulin, exercise, and the countless other things they would need to know. All through this process, Stefan's father was feeling more and more discouraged, overwhelmed by the prospect of living with his son's disease. At some point the pediatrician suggested that Stefan's father pull down his pants and stick his leg with a syringe to show his son that it didn't hurt too much. Spontaneously, Stefan's father blurted out, "At least I'm wearing clean underwear." At this, everyone laughed, and the tension level came down a bit.

Along with clear communication and love, humor can go a long way toward making your family's life with diabetes easier. You've probably heard people describe some difficult situation they lived through and then add, "I don't know how I could have made it if I hadn't been able to laugh about it." And you surely know people who can make a whole room happy just by their own sense of humor. Identifying something humorous in an otherwise difficult diabetes-related situation helps restore the problem to manageable proportions. Our patients have offered us many examples of how this helps keep all members of the family working together. And you don't need to be a comedian to lighten your load through humor. Humor is everywhere, and the more trying your day, the more important it is that you find a light side.

It is essential to stay strong and close as a family when you are living with diabetes. The problems of living are hard enough, without adding unnecessary family friction. We find that very often the things that create friction in a family are trivial when they are considered in isolation. But they do usually form patterns: specific hot-button issues, as we have described them, specific actions and failures to act. We also find that in most cases they can be easily remedied. You don't need to be a professional family counselor to become aware of your own family's dynamics. Think over the 10 lessons described above and see what applies to your family. Then do something positive about it.

Chapter 17

Balancing Your Social Life, Your Work Life, and Diabetes

- *"I was at my future in-laws' for dinner. It was the first time I had met them and I got hypoglycemic just before we sat down to eat! I told them I had diabetes and ate a glucose tablet. But afterward they all treated me as if they felt sorry for me. I hated it."*

- *"When I go out to lunch with people from work, I have to be much more careful than they are about what I eat. Sometimes that's hard, and I envy them."*

- *"I used to keep my diabetes a secret as much as I possibly could. After a while I realized that it just took too much energy to hide it, so now I let a few friends in on 'the secret.' I still don't let colleagues at work know, but this is easier."*

When you have diabetes, feeling different is inevitable. That's why managing diabetes in social and work settings is a big issue for many people. In this chapter we will discuss some common problems of integrating diabetes into your life and some potential solutions to these difficulties.

The key to minimizing uncomfortable feelings is integration of your diabetes with other aspects of your life. You can't sacrifice everything else in an effort to stick perfectly to your diabetes regimen. If you do, you're likely to feel you have no life at all. Neither can you go all the way in the other direction and ignore your diabetes—skipping shots, not testing your blood, or eating whenever and whatever you want. You have to find a way to balance the need for self-care with the need for a life that's as normal as possible. Each person balances these needs a bit differently.

Privacy and the Case of "Closet Diabetes"

Judy worked with lots of other young single people. Quite often, her colleagues would suggest going out for dinner after work. Since Judy always carried her insulin with her, she was free to join them, and she usually did. The only question was, where to test her blood and take her shot? Judy didn't like testing herself and giving herself insulin at the table, so her only option was to go to the restroom. To avoid embarrassment, she generally went into a toilet stall and sat there balancing her meter, syringe, insulin, and other paraphernalia on her lap and on the toilet paper roller. After she was done, Judy was free to join her friends, most of whom were unaware that she had diabetes.

Most people feel comfortable with letting it be known that they have diabetes, but Judy felt a need to keep her diabetes care private. She even hid it from her friends and co-workers. She may have had some bad experiences in the past when people found out about her diabetes. Or she might just be a private person.

It is each person's choice whether to tell and how much to say about diabetes. There are some dangers, however, to keeping your diabetes a secret. You could have a diabetes-related emergency and no one would be able to help you. Your friends could present you with all sorts of temptations without even knowing what they are doing. Besides, you should always remember that there is absolutely nothing to be ashamed about in having diabetes. Diabetes is just something you have, like brown hair and dark eyes. Making a secret of diabetes can create much more stress than it's worth.

At least your closest contacts at home and at work (or at school) should know enough about your diabetes—especially about recognizing and treating hypoglycemia—to help if you are in trouble.

If you want to start being more open about your diabetes, think about what you want to say and to whom. Do you simply want to acknowledge this important fact of your life, or do you want to ask someone to be available to help you in an emergency? Then try to create an opportunity to talk. If you've picked the right person, the conversation should work out fine.

Can You Be Too Open?

We all know some people who just seem to feel easy about themselves. They don't mind "letting it all hang out" or "wearing it on their sleeves." These people don't feel much need for privacy when it comes to diabetes or most other things in their lives. They test, take shots, and do whatever else they need to do wherever they are, and they may want to tell anyone who is willing to listen all about their diabetes.

If you are one of these "let it all hang out" people, there is a risk that you will actually be *too* open about your diabetes, especially in talking about it. Even your closest friends may not want to hear all the details of your diabetes management. If you feel this might be true of you, you may have to stop and remind yourself, "Just because I have to worry about diabetes all the time, that doesn't mean my friends have to. Maybe I'm even turning them off by talking about it so much." Whether it's your diabetes or pictures of your family vacation, be aware when enough is enough and know when it's time to change the subject.

Eating in Public

Food-related situations are probably the most common source of stress and embarrassment for people with diabetes. How often has someone said to you, "Oh, go ahead and eat it. A little bit won't kill you." Or maybe you've found yourself at a dinner party where the host announces proudly, "I made this dessert especially for you. It has no sugar at all—only maple syrup." What do you do in such a case? You could, if you know the person well, explain the facts. You could ask for a very small piece or take just a couple of bites, noting that you already filled up on the delicious dinner. You might even say you are too full for the dessert right now but would like a piece to take home for later. (When you get home, someone else is sure to love it.) Of course, it's perfectly true that the sweet won't kill you. But on the other hand, you don't want to get in the habit of eating whatever's out there to eat. There are many ways to turn down food politely, and it's a good idea to plan your moves ahead of time, so that you're not at a loss for how to respond when an awkward situation arises, as it surely will.

Does Your Diabetes Stop the Action?

Anthony went canoeing with his friends, to an island in the middle of a lake, where they all planned to enjoy a midday picnic. The canoers got off to a late start, though, and all of a sudden it was 1 P.M. Anthony needed to eat, but the party hadn't even reached the island yet, much less set out the picnic. Luckily, Anthony had anticipated the possibility of a delay and brought some fast-acting sweets along. He just popped some candies and kept paddling.

The key here was that Anthony, like so many others with insulin-requiring diabetes, knew enough never to leave home without a ready source of sugar. You never know when a meal will be delayed. If he hadn't had the sugar on hand, think of the disruption. He might have had a hypoglycemic reaction out on the water, while a bevy of canoes circulated around and his companions panicked, having no notion of how to help. Anthony, at a minimum, would have felt awkward, frustrated, embarrassed, and guilty. So it makes sense to do everything you can to minimize how often your diabetes stops the action.

Taking care of your diabetes can be especially difficult when you are with friends or at work, but it can be done. And when you do find a way to balance your diabetes needs and your social and work needs, your whole life feels more balanced.

We have talked about balance as the key to living a normal, relaxed life with your friends and co-workers. The balance is between hiding your diabetes altogether, with all the risks and difficulties that entails, and letting the diabetes dominate not only your life but also the social situations you find yourself in. We hope you will find that balance so that your diabetes can be well cared for and your life as a whole can be as stress-free and normal as possible.

Chapter 18

Dealing with Psychological Problems

- *"With my diabetes it's just one thing after another. I'm really discouraged. What's next?"*
- *"Before diabetes, I was a person in control of my life. But for the past few years my diabetes has been controlling me. I come home from work exhausted, so I grab something unhealthy to eat, which pushes my blood sugars way up and makes me feel even more exhausted. The whole thing's getting to me."*

Sometimes the daily stresses of life with diabetes can take a terrible emotional toll, beyond what is normal for you or for most people. Emotional problems can and do result. Among the more common and serious problems for people with diabetes are depression, anxiety disorder, and eating disorders. Also, the consequences of an emotional problem are especially severe for a person who has diabetes. The episodes last longer, feel worse, and recur more often. In addition, they make diabetes management much more difficult. Putting it plainly, having both diabetes and a psychological problem is a bad combination.

How can you tell whether you have a significant psychological problem or are just down in the dumps? And if you do have a serious emotional problem, where can you turn for help? These are the issues we address in this chapter.

It isn't always easy to distinguish between garden-variety distress and true emotional disturbance, but we hope our description of each disorder will give you an idea of where you fall on the spectrum. If you aren't sure, it makes sense to seek professional help in evaluating the seriousness of your problem. A single meeting with a mental health specialist, especially if the person has experience treating people who have diabetes, may be enough to determine whether you need treatment. Of course, you don't need to be suffering from a diagnosable emotional disorder to benefit from a visit to a mental health professional. Counseling from such a person can help you cope with the normal stresses of life with diabetes.

Depression

When most people say they are depressed, they aren't using the term in the clinical sense. They just mean that they are sad and dragged out emotionally. Everyone feels down from time to time. But these normal downs come and go, usually in a couple of hours or a couple of days and usually in response to a fairly clear cause. Clinical depression is different. It takes you down further and keeps you there longer. Often, it has no particular precipitating event, or if there is such an event, the emotional response to it is extreme. *Clinical depression is diagnosed when a person has five or more of the following specific symptoms for a period of at least two weeks:*

1. Depressed mood (feeling sad or empty) most of the day, nearly every day
2. Significant weight loss when not dieting or weight gain (more than 5% of body weight in a month), or decrease or increase in appetite nearly every day
3. Trouble sleeping or sleeping too much nearly every day
4. Feeling either very agitated or physically sluggish nearly every day
5. Fatigue or loss of energy nearly every day
6. Markedly diminished interest or pleasure in all, or almost all, activities most of the day, nearly every day
7. Feeling worthless or excessively or inappropriately guilty nearly every day
8. Diminished ability to think or concentrate, or indecisiveness, nearly every day
9. Recurrent thoughts of death (not just fear of dying), recurrent thoughts of suicide, or a suicide attempt or a specific plan to commit suicide

As you can see, clinical depression is different from a case of the blues.

Diabetes and Depression

Does having diabetes increase your risk of depression? The answer is almost certainly yes. We say almost certainly because although the evidence is strong, there is no conclusive proof. One reason for the uncertainty is that many of the symptoms (specifically numbers 2–6 above) resemble the symptoms of hyperglycemia. It is difficult to say whether a person with diabetes who has these symptoms is depressed, hyperglycemic, or both. Recent research, however, suggests that even given this confusion, clinical depression is about three times more common in individuals with diabetes than in the general population. The reasons are unclear, but we do know that having several complications (three or more) increases the risk of depression. That makes sense: if you have multiple major complications, life gets harder, and normal sadness can easily spin out of control. Also, poorly controlled diabetes (as indicated by elevated hemoglobin A1c levels) is associated with an increased risk of depression.

Whatever the cause of the relationship between depression and hyperglycemia, it's clear that at some point a negative cycle begins in which each problem reinforces the other. As we noted, depression makes it very hard to perform good self-care. So how can the cycle be reversed? Just as hyperglycemia and depression reinforce each other, so do improved blood sugar control and relief from depression. You can interrupt the cycle at any point.

Treating Depression

We strongly recommend professional counseling if you are clinically depressed. But there are also self-care approaches you can take. It may be very hard to take positive steps on your own, but it's worth a try. To be manageable, the steps must be small ones, the easiest you can think of. For example:

—Get out of bed by 9 a.m. every day and shower.
—If you have gained or lost a lot of weight during your depression, buy a piece of new clothing that fits.
—Call a friend frequently.
—Take a walk outdoors each day.

Add positive thoughts to your list: "A little at a time, and the easiest first." "I won't be depressed forever. If what I'm trying doesn't help, I'll find something else that will." One of our patients kept her list with her at all times. Her parents also recognized the value of the list. When she seemed to be feeling particularly bad, they would say, "Pull out your list, Sal." And she did. She would pick an item on her list, she would do it, and it helped.

You can also do things to help improve your blood sugar control. Trying any harder when you are depressed might seem impossible. But keep in mind that lower blood sugars will probably contribute to relieving your depression. Every little bit helps.

When we work with people who are struggling to make changes, we introduce the idea of an experiment. Change one part of your self-management, no matter how small, and keep notes on how hard or easy it was to do, how different you feel for having done the experiment, how you feel about doing another experiment, and what experiment you might try next.

What self-care experiment are you willing to try? How about taking your insulin on time for the next three days? Or testing your blood sugar level more often for the same period? Or making that appointment with your doctor that you've been putting off for months? Or walking around the block three times in the next week? Each of these is a small but meaningful step. Each could help you begin to turn things around, if the information you get from the experiment takes you to a next step, and the information from that experiment takes you to the one after that. At this point the only thing that matters is to get moving; your momentum will carry you along once you get going.

Speaking of getting moving, physical activity of any sort can help improve your situation. Exercise is probably the last thing you want to do when you are depressed, but it offers several benefits. First, exercise can improve your blood sugar control quickly and dramatically. The results are often amazing. Second, exercise can activate the brain chemicals called endorphins, which produce a mellow feeling. Even if you don't do enough exercise to get much of an endorphin effect, any physical activity is likely to improve your self-esteem and self-confidence. It helps you begin to overcome the feelings of helplessness and hopelessness that are dragging you down, and it reminds you that *you can do it*. Finally, exercise can be relaxing; it can help you sleep, clear your mind, focus your thinking.

Using some of the suggestions we have made should help you begin to turn things around, with improved mood and blood sugar levels. But you may not be able to muster enough energy to reverse the cycle, or your depression may be so powerful that even your best efforts are not enough.

Getting Professional Help

Seeking professional help is a big step. When you're feeling pessimistic and hopeless, not only about yourself but also about the possibility that anyone or anything can help, it's not easy. Maybe you are also a private person and the idea of discussing your problems with a stranger doesn't appeal to you. Or you may not "believe in" mental health professionals. Many people don't.

You are the only one who can decide when you are ready to seek professional help, but we can tell you that help is available. It isn't really a question of whether you believe in therapy; it does work. But you have to make the first move, to decide to get help. And as we mentioned before, you don't need to have a major psychological disorder to benefit from professional help. If you are psychologically intact but emotionally exhausted by your efforts to manage diabetes and the rest of your life, you too can benefit from some solid professional support.

Choosing a counselor.   The most important consideration is that you feel comfortable with the counselor you choose. We don't mean comfortable in the way that you are with a friend or spouse, but you should feel comfortable saying what is on your mind, knowing that the therapist is listening to what you say, and recognizing that the therapist's comments reflect a basic understanding of what makes you tick and that he or she is helping you to understand yourself. Don't stick with a counselor if you don't have confidence in him or her, and certainly don't stay if the counselor (or any other health professional) acts in any way that you consider inappropriate or questionable. The key issue is getting the help you need, not worrying about a health professional's feelings.

Another crucial requirement is that the therapist have some basic understanding of diabetes in general and of your diabetes in particular. Unfortunately, very few counselors specialize in treating people with diabetes, so you may not find such a person. You can call your local affiliate of the American Diabetes Association or the American Association of Diabetes Educators for information. They may be able to provide you with the name of a certified diabetes educator (CDE) in your area who specializes in providing mental health services for people with diabetes.

Cognitive-behavioral therapy is especially effective in treating diabetes-related psychological problems, so we recommend that you try to find a therapist who specializes in this approach. Cognitive-behavioral psychotherapy is designed to break the cycle of negative thoughts leading to negative feelings leading to negative behavior. Studies show that this kind of therapy is at least as effective as medication for people who are depressed.

Length of treatment.   This is such an individual matter that it's difficult to make a general statement, but if your goals are to improve your skills in coping with diabetes or to relieve acute symptoms of depression, you should expect some results within 10–12 sessions. That's not to say that your problems will be all gone by this time, but you should experience some meaningful relief by then. If you have found a therapist who is right for you, you will notice one thing quickly—that you have confidence in him or her.

Medications. Antidepressant medications can be a big help in treating depression, but they are much more effective if they are used in combination with counseling. The more commonly used antidepressants fall into two classes: *tricyclic antidepressants* and *selective serotonin reuptake inhibitors.*

The tricyclic antidepressants include such drugs as Elavil (generic name amitriptyline), Tofranil (imipramine), Sinequan (doxepin), and Desyrel (trazodone). Until recently, they were by far the most commonly prescribed antidepressants, but that's less true today. Tricyclics may have side effects, including dry mouth, sedation, increased appetite and weight gain, or sexual dysfunction. Most people don't experience these side effects, but some of them can be especially troublesome for people with diabetes.

The antidepressants called selective serotonin reuptake inhibitors, or SSRIs, are a newer class of drugs. These include Prozac (fluoxetine), Paxil (paroxetine), Zoloft (sertraline), and Effexor (venlafaxine). These medications seem to be less sedating and contribute less to sexual dysfunction. In addition, they actually tend to decrease appetite and lead to weight loss in some people. This benign side-effect profile helps explain the dramatic recent increase in the prescription of this class of antidepressants. Serotonin reuptake inhibitors do cause gastrointestinal distress or overstimulation in some people.

If you begin taking an antidepressant medication, it's important to keep in mind that the drug usually takes a couple of weeks or longer to produce its full beneficial effect. Unfortunately, the side effects, if you are going to experience any, begin much earlier but become less troublesome over time. So there may be a period of days or weeks after you begin taking an antidepressant when the only real effect you get will be a negative one. Be sure to tell the physician who prescribed the medication about both benefits and side effects you are experiencing. And don't give up too soon.

You should also know that the effectiveness of all mood-altering drugs is an individual matter. Different medications, even those closely related chemically, seem to affect different people differently. So you may need to try more than one medication before you find one that is right for you.

Anxiety Disorder

Everyone who has diabetes worries about diabetes-related concerns. Worrying about your blood sugars or about the possibility of developing complications is as normal as worrying about your job, your marriage, and your children. A clinical anxiety disorder, like clinical depression, is different from this kind of normal worry. It makes the worrying so intense, so uncomfortable, and so long-lasting that you may hardly be able to function.

A *clinical anxiety disorder* would probably be diagnosed if you are uncontrollably anxious for at least six months and if you worry excessively about a number of events or activities (such as work or school performance or your diabetes management), *and* if during that period you had at least three of the following symptoms for more days than you did not:

1. Restlessness or feeling keyed up or on edge
2. Easily growing tired
3. Difficulty concentrating or mind going blank
4. Irritability
5. Muscle tension
6. Sleep disturbance (difficulty falling or staying asleep, or restless, unsatisfying sleep)

You probably noticed that some of these symptoms are identical to those of clinical depression. There is an overlap, because some psychological problems share similar symptoms and because some people suffer from more than one disorder. This again brings up an important point: if you have any signs of a clinical psychological disorder, get help. What particular disorder you may be suffering from matters less than the fact that you are suffering.

Very little is known about the rate of anxiety disorder among people with diabetes, but studies conducted at the Johns Hopkins Diabetes Center suggest that it is as common as depression among people with diabetes and that both anxiety disorder and depression occur at a much higher rate among people with diabetes than among those without diabetes.

Fortunately, there are things you can do to help yourself if you have an anxiety disorder, including some you can do on your own. First, identify the fears that are creating your disorder. Then see if you can do anything to relieve those fears. If fear of hypoglycemia is disturbing you, for example, read some of the suggestions in Chapter 5 and see if they provide any relief. If you are afraid you may develop complications, ask your health care provider for the facts about exactly where you stand and what you can do to minimize your risk. If you are anxious about the effect your diabetes may be having on your family life, refer to the discussion in Chapter 16 and try talking out these fears with your loved ones.

If these self-help efforts are not enough—and they may not be if your anxieties have a real hold on you—get professional help. All the guidelines for depression counseling we offered above apply here as well. There are also medications you can take which may help relieve your anxiety disorder. Commonly prescribed anti-anxiety drugs include Ativan (lorazepam), BuSpar (buspirone), Serax (oazepam), Tranxene (clorazepate), and Xanax (alprazolam).

Eating Disorders

If you take good care of your diabetes, you probably spend a good deal of time thinking about food and watching what you eat. Especially if you are a young woman, you are probably concerned about your weight as well. That's why many young women who have diabetes tend to be preoccupied with what they eat and how much they weigh. For some of these women, this preoccupation may lead to an eating disorder. Some young men with diabetes also suffer from eating disorders, but these problems are about ten times more common among women. This is probably a result of the far more intense pressure on young women in our society to be thin.

Eating disorders come in two forms, and each has disastrous consequences for a person with diabetes. The first type is *anorexia nervosa.* People who suffer from anorexia severely restrict the amount of food they eat, often to below 1,000 calories a day, and they frequently exercise at extreme levels as well. The other eating disorder is *bulimia nervosa.* People who suffer from bulimia binge by eating very large amounts of food in a short time and then try to get rid of what they have eaten by vomiting or by using laxatives or diuretic medications (water-loss pills). Having either anorexia or bulimia makes it impossible to take good care of your diabetes.

How can you tell if you have an eating disorder? It's commonplace to want to be thin and to be disappointed if you are not. It is also normal, of course, to exercise as an aid to weight management. And it is normal to eat more than you should on occasion and to wish afterward that you hadn't eaten so much. The following symptoms aren't normal, however, and you may have an eating disorder if you:

1. Weigh less than 85 percent of normal for your height, body frame, and age
2. Have an intense fear of gaining weight or becoming fat, even though you are underweight
3. See yourself as fat when others say you are too thin

4. Exercise far more than is necessary to stay fit
5. Are a woman of menstruation age and miss at least three consecutive menstrual cycles
6. Deny the seriousness of your low body weight
7. Binge (eat very large amounts of food at a single sitting) at least twice a week for three months
8. Feel you can't stop eating or control what or how much you are eating

Many people eat prunes or use other approaches to manage occasional constipation. They may use diuretics, when the doctor prescribes them, to treat fluid retention or high blood pressure. But using laxatives, diuretics, enemas, or other medications for the purpose of reducing weight is not normal. Forcing yourself to vomit the food you have just eaten in an effort to prevent weight gain, even if it works for that purpose, is a clear sign of bulimia.

Finally, adjusting insulin doses to improve blood sugar control is good, but purposely taking less insulin than you need in order to control your weight by "purging" some of the calories you have eaten as urine sugar is not good. In fact, this kind of insulin manipulation is a clear sign that you have an eating disorder. Unfortunately, this behavior is very common; by some estimates as many as half of all young diabetic women frequently manipulate insulin doses to control their weight.

Disordered eating behavior in any form—severe restriction, binges, purges, or insulin manipulation—leads to acute medical emergencies. Eating disorders also contribute to an increased risk for the chronic complications of diabetes, because the blood sugars of people with eating disorders are so often out of control.

If you have an eating disorder or suspect you might be suffering from one, get help. We make this recommendation in full awareness of how difficult it is to admit you have an eating disorder and to ask for help. If you are like most people suffering from these problems, controlling your eating this way feels crucially important and you feel terrified at the prospect of giving up control. In fact, you are probably even terrified at the prospect of anyone discovering that you have an eating disorder. Besides that, you are probably ashamed.

You may also believe that no one can understand your problems and that no one could possibly help you. But there are people who can help. Tell someone you can trust about your problem and ask for help. If you aren't comfortable talking to your parents or spouse, maybe there is a relative, teacher, religious adviser, or health care provider you could approach. What you need to do, with the help of someone you trust, is to see a mental health professional who treats people with eating disorders; you may find such a person who knows something about diabetes as well.

As hard as it is to admit you have any of the emotional problems we have discussed in this chapter, it's critically important to do just that and to ask for help. Your life is at stake, and that is precious. So get the help that could save your life. Many of our patients have discovered the relief of living with just one medical condition—diabetes—rather than two.

Chapter 19

Interacting with Health Care Professionals

- *"I just found out that I have diabetes. Should I see a specialist?"*

- *"I spend months keeping a detailed record of my blood sugars, diet, and activity, and then my doctor spends less than five minutes looking through it!"*

- *"Everyone says I need to lose weight to get the diabetes under control, but nobody tells me how to do it."*

- *"Now that I've learned how to manage the diabetes, my doctor and I can work together as a team."*

The relationship between you and your health care professional has tremendous potential for satisfaction—and for frustration. It is, after all, your comfort, your body, your very life at stake. You look to your health care professional to make you well. You have all sorts of reasonable expectations, and maybe some unreasonable ones too. The opportunities for disappointment and disillusionment are great.

Still, according to surveys, most people like their own doctor, regardless of what they think about doctors in general. This chapter will discuss what you can do to foster a good relationship with your doctor and with other health care providers. We begin by describing the members of the health care team. We will then suggest some keys to building and maintaining a good relationship between you and your health care providers.

The Health Care Team

The *health care team* is a model that has much to recommend it. It involves coordination and communication: multiple players all working together for your benefit. A reality test is occasionally needed for this dream-team concept, however. Sometimes the members of the health care team don't communicate all that well. In this, as in so many other aspects of diabetes management, you may have to take charge yourself.

> *A patient of ours is an extremely well-organized person who is accustomed to being in charge. He comes to office visits well prepared, with his data nicely summarized and his questions lined up. Last year, when he developed a serious orthopedic problem, he not only communicated with each of the people on his health care team but went so far as to arrange a conference call for the whole team—four doctors and a patient. It was an unusual step, but it was a good example of the patient making sure that all the members of his health care team communicated, and it was done in such a friendly and gracious manner that all the doctors enjoyed it.*

Even if you are not such a take-charge person as the patient we described, you can still manage your care very well if you make the best use of available resources and know whom to seek out when. To do this, you have to start with a list of the players who might belong on your diabetes health care team.

You

You are the central person on your health care team. You make the decisions: what to eat, when to eat, how to exercise, how to take medications, when to seek help, and so on. You may be the sort of person who wants everything spelled out for you, who just wants to follow directions, or you may be the kind of person who bridles at the thought of losing control of your own decisions, who wants always to do it your way. Wherever you are on that spectrum, you are the one who leads the life and experiences the consequences of your actions. Still, we haven't met the person who doesn't need some help at some point. This usually starts with a primary care provider.

The Primary Care Provider

The medical professional who takes responsibility for and coordinates your overall health care is the *primary care provider.* You should know who this person is; you should not have to wonder. You should have his or her name and telephone number posted near your home phone, on a card in your wallet, written out for your friends, and so on. This is the person to call first in an emergency. This is the person who knows you and cares for you on a regular basis.

In this day of shifting health care systems, primary health care providers might change with disturbing frequency. We suggest only that you be aware of any changes. Visit the "new doc" early, get to know him or her, and let the doctor get to know you.

The training and background of your primary care provider is less important than clear identification of the role. Most often, we recommend a general internist (a physician trained in internal medicine) or family practitioner. Less often, it will be a nurse practitioner or physician assistant. Primary care providers have varying levels of expertise in managing diabetes, but they can recognize the problems, provide advice about many parts of treatment, and coordinate whatever specialty care is needed.

Remember that a general physician or nurse practitioner probably won't be a specialist in diabetes, and this is not a bad thing. She or he will be able to deal with the variety of health care problems you have. Most important, when the need arises, the generalist should freely refer you to a specialist.

Endocrinologist or Diabetologist

An *endocrinologist* is a physician who took advanced, specialized training in the field of endocrinology (hormones and glands) after completing training in internal medicine or pediatrics. *Diabetologist* is less well defined as a specialty. A diabetologist is generally a physician, usually an endocrinologist, who has special expertise in the treatment of diabetes. Most often, a diabetologist is an endocrinologist who subspecializes in the treatment of diabetes. Health professionals who are not physicians and whose primary training is as a nutritionist, herbal specialist, or "holistic medicine" specialist would not be called diabetologists.

Do you need an endocrinologist or a diabetologist on your team? Our opinion is that not everyone with diabetes does, but that quite a few people do. A simple way to decide is to think about how you are doing with your current provider. Are your questions answered reasonably well? Are your examinations reasonably thorough? Most important, is your diabetes under good control? If not, then you should consider whether specialty input from an endocrinologist or diabetologist is needed.

Endocrinologists or diabetologists may be primary care providers, or they may work on a referral basis, in tandem with primary care providers, in treating persons with diabetes. Let's consider four different patients with different needs:

Edgar is a 72-year-old man with Type II diabetes who has several other health problems as well: high blood pressure, arthritis, and a prostate problem. He has a pri-

mary care provider who is a general internist, and he has also seen a diabetologist about every six months, or whenever the primary care provider would like to get the specialist's opinion on some aspect of Edgar's health.

The variety of Edgar's illnesses makes it important for him to have a generalist coordinating his care. The diabetes is only one of several problems, and the generalist is asking for help as needed.

Sandy is 27 years old, with a 14-year history of Type I diabetes. An endocrinologist is her primary care provider. Her blood sugars are unstable, she has some developing problems with her diabetes, and the endocrinologist is best suited to give her most of the care she needs. He refers Sandy to a gynecologist and an ophthalmologist on a regular basis.

In this case, Sandy's Type I diabetes is her most significant health problem, and it's a difficult problem to manage. It makes sense for her to have a specialist for on-going care.

Michael has signed up for a managed care option in his health insurance that turns out to be quite restrictive. He wants to perform self-monitoring of blood glucose but is told the company won't cover the cost of the strips. He is having significant insulin reactions and thinks his insulin regimen needs adjustment, but the generalist seems unfamiliar with mixing insulins. Worse, when Michael asks about the possibility of seeing an endocrinologist, the generalist makes a few phone calls and then tells him that it really isn't necessary. Translated, this means that Michael can consult whomever he wants, but he will have to pay for it out of pocket.

Often managed care organizations are perfectly willing to approve needed consultations or on-going primary care by a specialist. But apparently not in Michael's case. The roadblocks he hit, such as no coverage for strips and an unwillingness to refer despite clear indications that the regimen wasn't working, clearly suggest that Michael needs help. He should get it from his managed care organization, and he should not have to pay out of pocket.

Antoine is 30 years old and has had diabetes since the age of 5. His primary care provider is—well, in fact, Antoine's not quite sure who his care provider is, since his company changed health coverage plans a year ago. He liked his old endocrinologist and may return to her for care, but he will now have to pay out of pocket

since the new plan doesn't include her as a care provider. As a result of the confu-
sion, Antoine hasn't actually seen a doctor in 18 months.

Antoine has let inattention get the better of him. Maybe he's in denial about his diabetes. Whatever the cause, Antoine, like all people with diabetes, needs regular care by a good medical care team.

Diabetes Nurse Educator

A nurse educator may provide a variety of services for the person with diabetes. A primary role is teaching self-management skills. Just what this involves will vary from place to place and person to person. For example, a nurse educator may be associated either with a large hospital or diabetes center or with just one practitioner's office. After assessing your individual needs, the educator may decide to concentrate on certain facets of self-care, such as insulin durations of action and injection technique, foot care, or diet.

Just how much individual patient management a diabetes educator does varies as well. Some diabetes nurse educators may work with a physician in providing follow-up care. A physician may prescribe an initial insulin regimen, and the nurse educator then helps the person fine tune it over time, under the direction of the physician. Only doctors, nurse practitioners, and physician's assistants (with various state regulations applying to each profession) have the right to practice medicine independently, but a nurse educator can often help the patient a good deal in addition to helping him or her learn good self-management.

To find out if the educator you see has special expertise in diabetes, ask if he or she is a *certified diabetes educator,* or CDE. Any health professional can become a CDE, but earning the certification requires considerable experience in patient education and passing an examination.

Dietitian

A dietitian provides nutritional care, education, and counseling. A *registered dietitian,* or RD, has met standards of the American Dietetic Association. Dietitians with a CDE designation have specialized in the dietary aspects of treating diabetes.

It is hard to imagine treating diabetes effectively without having a dietitian involved. Contrary to popular belief, the principles of healthful eating for diabetes are *not* well known and certainly not the same as they were 20, 10, or even 5 years ago. Individualizing diets requires expert professional knowledge. Matching the requirements of a particular diet with the individual's personal preferences takes another level of skill. Don't try to learn diet by yourself. Talk with a dietitian.

Mental Health Professionals

The term *mental health professional* encompasses people with a variety of different backgrounds, degrees, and skills. Some are trained formally in psychology, some in social work with an emphasis on psychiatric social work, some in sociology and counseling, and some in another area. The level of education is signified by the degree obtained: a bachelor's degree (B.A. or B.S.) means that the person has graduated from college; a master's degree (M.S.) usually requires one to two years of postgraduate work; and a Ph.D. requires about four to six years of education after college. Psychiatrists are medical doctors (M.D.'s), with four years of education and training after college, plus three to four years' training in psychiatry. A psychologist is a Ph.D. Most counselors trained in social work have a master's degree.

In essence, the mental health professional can help you reduce the psychological, emotional response to stresses in life. This may involve helping you learn coping skills to deal with the additional demands of diabetes in an already busy life. It could mean providing counseling and training in coping skills as part of a larger treatment plan for diabetes or for a specific psychological problem. Only medical doctors can prescribe medications such as antidepressants, but other mental health professionals are able to recognize the need for psychiatric care or medications and can refer the patient to a psychiatrist or another M.D.

The most important point about mental health counseling, in our view, is for people to recognize the need and take advantage of what's available. Thinking of the person who gets counseling as somehow weak or inadequate is a very old-fashioned notion. Working with a counselor is really no different than an athlete working with a coach. Please take advantage of all the help that's available for all your needs.

Ophthalmologist

An *ophthalmologist* is a medical doctor (M.D.) with specialized training in diseases of the eye. Chapter 25 describes the work of ophthalmologists in more detail. But everyone with diabetes needs an expert eye exam on a regular basis. This examination should be arranged by your primary care provider.

Optometrist

Optometrists are not physicians but professionals who have been trained in specific aspects of eye care. Optometrists vary widely in their experience in examining eyes for evidence of the diabetes-related eye condition called diabetic retinopathy. Some are experienced at picking it up with a careful dilated-pupil eye examination, while others are not. How can you evaluate this? First of all, no eye exam for diabetic retinopathy is adequate if the pupils are not dilated. Beyond that, you have to look out for yourself by asking questions of the optometrist, asking friends and associates to recommend an optometrist they trust, and checking back with your primary care provider or diabetologist.

Physical Therapist

The *physical therapist* is a professional with special training in improving physical function. Usually they work with rehabilitation after injuries or strokes, but they also have a role to play in prevention, for example, avoiding foot injuries. Physical therapy services are often underutilized. Just as people don't automatically know how to prepare a diabetic diet, they are not born knowing how to build strength, endurance, and flexibility safely. The physical therapist does have this knowledge. He or she can get you started on a safe exercise program, especially if you have a physical problem, such as a bad back.

Podiatrist or Other Foot Care Specialist

Podiatrists, orthopedists, and even physical therapists may specialize in the foot care for people with diabetes. But the *podiatrist* is the person who deals with feet as the only focus of his or her professional activity. Podiatrists can provide a variety of services, from trimming the toenails to examining the foot for structural abnormalities that could develop into ulcers without proper treatment. Chapter 28 describes how to use the services of the foot care specialist.

Other Health Care Specialists

There are other health care specialists who are involved in caring for people with diabetes. A social worker or an eye care nurse may be important, for example. Other medical specialties, such as obstetrics, gastroenterology (for stomach or intestinal problems), dermatology (skin), nephrology (kidney), and urology (bladder and sexual function), offer their own special focus. Your care team has to be customized to your needs as well as to the resources available where you live. Once you've assembled your team, you have to know how to get along with its members.

Working with Health Care Professionals

How can you best establish a good relationship with your health care professional? First, you need to understand your own expectations, the expectations that the health care professional may have, and how to meld the two.

Your Reasonable Expectations

As the person with diabetes, you quite naturally think of your own needs first, especially when it comes to health care. You have a right to expect communication, honesty, competence, professional standards, and quality care from your health care professional. You can also expect clear communication between members of your health care team. You have a right to switch doctors (although, as we will discuss, your health plan may have strict regulations about whom you can see under what circumstances). In Chapter 20 you will find a "patient's bill of rights," and we urge you to check it out. It is what you deserve.

But it makes sense every now and then to step back and consider the viewpoint of the health care professional. What is he or she dealing with and thinking about—and what is he or she thinking of *you*? Are any of your expectations unreasonable?

The View of the Treating Professional

It's certainly fair to assume that the treating professional wants what is best for you, that his or her motives are good ones. If you have any doubt about that, you should definitely move on to someone else. But all health care professionals operate within certain constraints and restrictions. First, the care provider must know what's medically *possible* and what is not. As much as you may want a cure for the circulatory problem in your leg, for instance, an experienced vascular surgeon may know that it is not possible.

The time element. There is always a time limit. These days very few professionals can spend as much time as they might like talking with each patient. To be sure, you deserve whatever time is necessary, and you shouldn't feel pushed out the door. But reality may fall somewhat short of the ideal in this modern world of time management. It's better to expect a specific amount of time, say 15 or 30 minutes, and use it well than to have unlimited expectations and be disappointed.

Specialist or generalist?   If you find the doctor who knows everything, please call us right away—that would really be a find! More likely, the specialist will know a good deal about diabetes, insulins, pills, complications, and so on. The generalist will know something about the general aspects of diabetes and a lot about all aspects of health care for you. Neither one will know your particular diabetes as well as you do. If you've just read something in a diabetes magazine or on the World Wide Web, it's very possible that your treating professional won't know what you're talking about. A good professional is one who will admit, "I don't know." Then, if the issue is potentially important, the professional will find out or tell you how to find out. But good health care is not a quiz show where the smartest doctor or the smoothest talker wins.

The human being behind the white coat.   And then, dare we say it, there's the matter of being human. Is a health care professional allowed to feel frustration, disappointment, defensiveness, or even anger? To a degree, there is probably no avoiding it. The care provider must maintain a level of professionalism, but you can't expect, and probably wouldn't want, a person with absolutely no emotion.

Making a list, checking it twice.   One of the relatively simple steps you can take to improve your interaction with health care professionals is to make a list of your main points before you go into the office: what's bothering you, what questions you have, what your priorities are. Show your doctor the list early in the visit. If 15 minutes of a 20-minute visit are spent on unimportant chit-chat, the doctor isn't going to be excited about addressing a whole new set of serious issues just when he or she thought the visit was ending.

Try to have your records, your diaries, and your dates in good order. You may become nervous in the office, so if you have prepared everything neatly and legibly and organized it well, you will save a lot of time.

Turning on the charm.   Don't be afraid to use your own charm, your own tact, your own "bedside manner." You should recognize two different interaction styles:

- *"You said take 16 units of insulin in the morning. Dr. Jones said take 20 units. What's the deal, don't you two talk, and are you right or is Dr. Jones right?"*

- *"I saw Dr. Jones after seeing you, and she suggested that maybe 20 units of insulin would help. What do you think, does that sound like a good idea, or do you want to talk with her first?"*

The first style is brusque, even combative, and is not likely to help the relationship with your health care provider. The second style is not only more tactful but also more cooperative; it is more of a teamwork approach.

Don't take offense too easily. Some doctors may seem abrupt or even gruff: "You're too darn fat." Others say the same thing rather differently: "I believe you would benefit if you could lose a few pounds." Some seem to accuse you of "cheating" if the treatment isn't working perfectly, others don't. But in the end, the words they use may not be as important as the care they give. So if you are truly offended by a professional's approach, leave. But our advice is to try to ignore the superficial and concentrate on what really matters.

Communication between professionals.   Don't expect instant or perfect communication between professionals. They all have busy days, and even telephone or fax communication may take some time. Furthermore, some communications are simply more important than others. It probably doesn't matter much whether your ophthalmologist knows the exact status of your prostate, but it's important for your primary care doctor to know if you see a cardiologist who changes your medications.

Changing horses.   A final word about talking to doctors and changing doctors: try not to worry about speaking out and asking questions. See if you can make the relationship work so that you get what you need out of it. But if you can't, and if you want to change doctors, don't worry about that either. We are amazed at how far some people go to protect the feelings of a doctor. He or she will be okay. There will be other patients. If you feel you have to change, just do it. The important thing is for you to get your health care problems solved.

Problem Solving

So far in this discussion we have put the emphasis on personalities and interpersonal communications. But in the end the issue is not how closely your personalities match, it is whether you and your health care professional can get the job done. And the job, quite simply, is problem solving. There must be clear communication between the two of you concerning the nature of the problem, from both your point of view and the doctor's. Once you agree on the problem, you can put your heads together and work out a plan.

Jean comes in to her endocrinologist's office with three things on her mind: she has a sore ankle, which she sprained a few days ago playing tennis; her hair is full of split ends; and she has had some insulin reactions at night. Her doctor comes into the room with other concerns: Jean has not had an eye exam in two years, and her glycohemoglobin was considerably higher than the doctor would like. In the interview, Jean gets a little nervous and keeps coming back to the ankle. She mentions the split ends mostly as a joke. Her doctor gets irritable, not showing much interest in the ankle, and he doesn't even smile at the reference to split ends. Jean leaves with a sense, shared by the endocrinologist, that it wasn't a very useful visit.

In Jean's case, she and her doctor never got to the stage of problem solving. They didn't even begin to work on some changes that might help with three important features of Jean's case: her need for better average blood sugars (glycohemoglobin), her need to avoid nighttime hypoglycemia, and the need to revisit her ophthalmologist. The reason? Jean and the endocrinologist had different agendas. Her ankle was bothering her, and she thought she'd make a little joke about the split ends. The endocrinologist's agenda was to talk about blood sugar control, but he let himself get sidetracked by things he wasn't going to do anything about.

Let's run that scene over again, slightly rescripted:

Jean comes in to her endocrinologist's office with three things on her mind: she has a sore ankle, which she sprained a few days ago playing tennis; her hair is full of split ends; and she has had some insulin reactions at night. But she thinks, "Wait a minute, he's not going to deal with ankles or hair. He's a specialist. Let's talk diabetes." Her doctor comes into the room with some other concerns: Jean has not had an eye exam in two years, and her glycohemoglobin was considerably higher at the last visit than the doctor would like. He's sorry to see her limping on a sprained ankle, and says so. In the interview, they immediately agree on the problem: how do they improve the blood sugar average and still avoid the nighttime hypoglycemia? Together, they work on problem solving. Before Jean leaves, the doctor jots down his suggestions for changes in insulin and also reminds her, in writing, to have her eyes examined.

This version seems a lot more satisfactory, doesn't it? The key to a better outcome was Jean thinking over what she really wanted out of the visit and making that clear. Of course, the endocrinologist helped by being sympathetic about the ankle even if he wasn't doing anything about it. But getting to the problem solving was the important thing—plain and simple.

Sometimes too many suggestions are made, too many warnings are given, too much is said. Many people will feel overwhelmed as they walk out the door. Don't think that it will all be more clear once you leave the office: It is well known that as soon as people leave the doctor's office they *forget* most of what was said.

There are several ways to fend off the barrage of information and prevent information overload. Sometimes your doctor will write down the points he or she is making. You could also take notes yourself as the doctor is talking. It's a way to slow the doctor down and for you to see if you understand what he or she is saying.

Another approach to enhance communication and hold instructions down to a reasonable number is to draw up a contract. Your contract is an agreement between you and the health care professional as to what you will do as a result of the office visit. Any contract involves benefit to two parties, and in this case the patient gets improved health care, while the doctor gets the satisfaction of helping. By "contracting," you end up with a short list of instructions that you understand and agree to try to carry out.

Whatever the interpersonal chemistry and methods of communication between you and your health care professional, you want to leave that office with some problem-solving suggestions. Then you can work on them yourself, making use of available resources.

Other Resources

As you leave the health professional's office, especially if it has been a supportive and positive setting, you may well have a sudden sense of being alone. You're the one with the diabetes—and no one else out there knows what it feels like. Even if your doctor and nurse are caring people, they have only so much time to interact with you. You may find it helpful to seek out other people with diabetes.

One avenue is a diabetes support group. Affiliates of the American Diabetes Association usually sponsor such groups, as do some hospitals and universities. Joining the American Diabetes Association and the Juvenile Diabetes Foundation can bring a lot of information right to your door and provide opportunities to interact with others in educational or fund-raising activities.

One particularly useful service of these organizations is the magazines they publish. The American Diabetes Association has a monthly magazine called *Forecast* that features articles on people with diabetes, recipes, research updates, discussion of specific treatment measures in the management of diabetes, and product information. The magazine of the Juvenile Diabetes Foundation, called *Countdown,* focuses on research.

There are many other resources out there as well. If you have access to a computer, modem, and Internet service provider, you will be able to locate chat pages, bulletin boards, Web sites, and discussion groups about diabetes. A healthy dose of skepticism is useful when you listen to nonprofessionals discuss any topic, however. Remember that if someone makes a statement about *their* diabetes, their situation, their understanding, that doesn't make it true for you. We recently saw a woman in her late 70s who had just developed diabetes. Her well-intentioned granddaughter had collected all the information she could find on the Internet and sent a three-inch-high printout to her grandmother. Unfortunately, the material was haphazard and disorganized, and the older woman was overwhelmed. Information overload can be as dangerous as no information at all.

You and your health care professionals are a team working together to control your diabetes and help you lead a healthy life. Maybe your team is a small one, well versed in the intricacies of your diabetes management, or maybe it will involve many specialties. Maybe it's everything you want, maybe not. But in the end, the goal is the same: to figure out how the various team members need to come together to control your blood sugar and keep you feeling well. Whatever you can do to make this work, it's worth the effort.

Chapter 20

Interacting with the Health Care System

- *"My insurance covers some things, like pancreas transplantation, that seem so useless to me, but it doesn't cover blood glucose testing strips, which are obviously essential. It makes me get special prescriptions that are so complicated I can hardly understand the restrictions: only 30 days' worth, no refills, written as a generic, signed by the doctor. Why are they hassling me?"*

- *"I just don't understand all these plans offered by my employer. It's the old alphabet soup problem: HMO, PPO, IPA, MCO, PCP. Some are much cheaper than others, but are they as good?"*

- *"My daughter has diabetes. She just left school, and all of a sudden I realized that she is no longer covered by my insurance plan. Is this a problem?"*

Whatever else you think of the health care system in the United States, you probably recognize that it's not really an organized system at all. It's a complicated set of policies, plans, providers, and insurers that evolved with no apparent overall planning. You may believe that it is the best system in the world, that it is in serious need of reform, or both. But if you have diabetes in your family, your immediate problem is how to get along in the current system. In the United States, no more rational approach is likely to come along anytime soon.

This chapter provides an overview of the *system*. It doesn't look closely at your personal interactions with individual health care providers (a topic covered in Chapter 19). Instead, we are dealing here with aspects of health care that may be even more frustrating: the forms, the phone calls, the coverage, and so on. Although we can't discuss all the innumerable existing plans and options or unscramble all the acronyms, we will discuss your own rights and concerns, what's out there to help you, and ways to make the system work to your advantage. Your primary interest is your own good health.

We start with a brief description of your rights *as we see them* (we're not implying that all insurers see things as we do). We will then describe the various kinds of health coverage. Finally, we will summarize the most important considerations when choosing a plan or using a plan to your best advantage. No matter what the advertisements say, there is very little that is simple or obvious or even logical about health insurance. It takes some thought and a lot of persistence to come out on top.

A Patient's Bill of Rights

A bill of rights for patients is not an uncommon document these days. The American Diabetes Association, for example, spells out as a matter of policy what your rights are when it comes to quality diabetes care. Many hospitals, too, have a patients' bill of rights framed and prominently displayed. Unfortunately, the framers of the U.S. Constitution did not write health care, much less glucose monitoring strips, into the Constitution. On the contrary, to this day federal law is very nonspecific in regulating what must be provided and what need not be provided as part of health insurance. So you have to be careful in selecting a plan and assertive in claiming your "rights."

We believe that the right to quality diabetes care starts with your own responsibility to do what you can for yourself. No amount of technology, no team of specialists or education program will be adequate if your own self-management is poor. But assuming that *you* are acting responsibly, then what should the system provide? In short, what constitutes quality diabetes care? This is where the debate begins. Let's start by setting out the basic elements of quality diabetes care to which we believe everyone is entitled:

—An accurate diagnosis and on-going care
—Diabetes education
—Provision of necessary supplies and pharmaceuticals, both disposable and permanent
—Access to health care professionals, both for primary care and for any specialized needs

Accurate diagnosis.   A problem that we covered at the start of this book (see Chapter 1) is how often people are unclear about whether they have diabetes or not. You really should know. We recommend that you be tested if you are at high risk (overweight, strong family history, unexplained weight loss, or other typical symptoms) and, most important, that you ask for a straight answer from a health care professional.

Diabetes education.   Nothing is more important in managing your diabetes than understanding it. People are not born knowing about diabetes, and usually the information they pick up from general sources (Aunt Matilda's second cousin, the man down the street, a 30-second news clip) is incomplete at best and often totally inaccurate. It is up to you to learn about diabetes.

The settings for diabetes education vary widely. Some people will have several one-on-one visits with a diabetes educator, while others may get their diabetes education in a group, along with other people who have diabetes. Sometimes diabetes education consists of a single intensive class and sometimes it is extended over a longer period of time. It is rarely necessary for someone to be hospitalized for education.

These days the educator should be a certified diabetes educator (CDE), and the program should be well structured and comprehensive. Education does not consist of a few casual comments or a simple diet handout. In addition to sessions with a CDE, there is no substitute for having an individual consultation with a qualified dietitian.

It is sometimes difficult to get reimbursement for the cost of diabetes education, although some managed care programs provide regular diabetes education classes, and outpatient education is often a covered benefit. Some programs, such as ours at Johns Hopkins University, include a reimbursable visit with a physician each day during the education program.

Necessary supplies and pharmaceuticals.   The things people have to buy just to manage their diabetes, to fill their prescriptions, can be expensive. These include pills, insulin, syringes, glucose test strips, meters, pumps, and so on.

The supplies and pharmaceuticals that are recommended by your doctor ought to be covered by an insurance plan. Unfortunately, many of them are not. Medicare, for example, does not pay for medicines. You may not be in a position to insist on getting reimbursement for supplies and pharmaceuticals if they are specifically excluded from the coverage in your plan, but you should try.

Access to health care professionals.   People with diabetes want, deserve, and need to have continued care by competent professionals. In Chapter 19 we mentioned that although primary care physicians are usually not diabetes specialists, they may be excellent physicians who can care for you very well without knowing all the details about meters, new insulins, and other diabetes-related matters. Most people with diabetes can be well managed by a primary care physician. However, people with unusually unstable diabetes, complications, or other special problems need to have their diabetes managed by a specialist.

In addition to a primary care physician, many people need to have at least some contact with specialists. For example, all people with diabetes should be followed regularly by an ophthalmologist (specialist in eye diseases). Input from other specialists is often indicated, such as that provided by a nurse educator, psychologist, podiatrist, or dietitian. Whatever your health plan coverage, you are entitled to both primary care and necessary specialty care.

Types of Health Insurance Plans

A convenient way to consider health insurance options is to divide them into government entitlements, traditional insurance coverage plans, and managed care plans. (A glossary of insurance terms is provided in the appendix that follows this chapter. It defines some of the many terms used in defining insurance coverage and health plans.)

Government Entitlements

Government entitlement programs have fixed criteria for eligibility, which are written into law. The eligibility criteria may be complicated, and to interpret them many people need the assistance of a social worker or benefits manager. In most cases, such as Medicare and Medicaid, the programs represent a commitment by the state or federal government to pay bills; within the military and veterans' health care systems, however, the programs actually deliver the care. These federal entitlements are probably the largest health care delivery systems in the world.

Medicare, the health insurance program for the elderly and disabled, is the largest single expenditure of our federal budget after payment on the national debt. (We recently heard of a woman who complained, "I'm not going to let government get in the way of my Medicare"—a nonsensical comment.) Medicare is not a means-tested program, so age, rather than income, is generally the basic criterion for eligibility. Medicare has significant co-payments and limitations of coverage. For example, insulin is not covered, and very little coverage is available for long-term care. Many senior citizens are therefore wise to pay separately for so-called Medigap policies that specifically fill the gaps in Medicare coverage.

Medicaid is a combined federal and state program that pays for health care for the poor. Unlike Medicare, Medicaid is a means-tested program, meaning that eligibility depends on the income and net worth of the potential insured person. Income and size of family are the basic criteria for eligibility. Benefits vary considerably from state to state.

There is no doubt that if you qualify, the government entitlements are the most advantageous programs for you. They adhere to insurance principles in that they are supported by a very large base of people paying into the system (taxpayers), and they do not exclude people for preexisting conditions or high health risk. Increasingly, though, they are being scrutinized as budget items that should be limited. Many Medicaid and Medicare programs, for example, are entering into managed care plans rather than simply paying bills. This often means that people are either forced or induced (by the lure of lower out-of-pocket payments) to join specific health plans. Be aware of this trend when you see the ABC Health Plus Network offered in your Medicare package. There is talk among politicians about changing the entire face of Medicare not only by further limiting payments but also by making it a means-tested program. The fact that you are enrolled in a government entitlement program does not guarantee any particular level of coverage. Increasingly, benefits are being limited as part of the overall effort to lower government expenditures.

Traditional Insurance Coverage Plans

The idea behind *traditional (indemnity) insurance* is really very simple: every person in a large group of people pays premiums to an insurance company; then, when a person gets sick, the provider (doctor, hospital, pharmacy) generates a bill, and the insurance company pays it out of the pool of money it collected as premiums. Interestingly, insurance companies make most of their profits by investing the premiums before they are paid out to providers, rather than by paying out less than they collect. State insurance commissioners regulate how much the insurers are allowed to skim off as administrative expenses and profit. By calculating the likely amount of illness in a given group of insured people, the insurance company tries to anticipate what the payouts will be and to charge adequate premiums to cover these payouts plus expenses and profit. When faced with uncertainty, the traditional response of insurers is to increase premiums to cover potential loss.

Blue Cross and Blue Shield plans across the country are a slightly differ-ent type of insurance. They generally operate as nonprofit corporations and thus receive certain tax breaks. Increasingly, like the for-profit insurance companies, they are diversifying into managed health care and, in some states, taking on a for-profit status.

The theory of insurance dictates that the insurer collect a large pool of members (called *covered lives*) so that the risk of illness is spread widely and is therefore relatively predictable. Some members will get sick, but many will remain healthy. You can see that it makes quite a difference for insurers whether the population being covered is elderly or young.

Insurers prefer to cover large groups, assuming that they will spread the risk among the healthy and the sick. When individuals or very small groups (such as a mom-and-pop store) apply for coverage on their own, the insurer is much more skeptical: are any of these people already sick? Will they re-quire payouts from the insurance company right away, no questions asked? How much does the insurance company know about these people? What is the insurance company's risk and how can it be minimized? These questions lead to some obvious answers. Faced with a request for individual coverage, an insurer is very likely to require a careful physical exam; to increase the pre-miums significantly if the person (or small group) is found to have signifi-cant illness or a higher average age; and to try to refuse coverage for preex-isting illness. While these are logical reactions in the for-profit insurance business, they do not work to the benefit of individuals or small groups ap-plying for traditional insurance, especially if a person has diabetes.

Even when covering large groups with actuarially sound premiums and low profit margin, traditional insurance has a tendency to become more and more expensive. This is because these insurers pay all the legitimate bills that are submitted. They pay on a fee-for-service basis—the insurance equivalent of piecework. This means that if a doctor does 20 operations in a week, she earns twice as much as if she does 10 operations in a week. If a person goes to the doctor five times in a month, the insurer pays five times as much as if the person goes once in a month. While the insurance company will proba-bly try to raise premiums the next time around, the fact is that as long as the company has little control over the volume of service, costs will tend to es-calate. This feature of traditional insurance, as much as anything else, has led to the explosion of health care costs generally. It has also led to new devel-opments in health coverage, typified by the managed care approach, which is rapidly replacing traditional insurance as the most common way Ameri-cans pay for health care.

Managed Care Plans

In the broadest sense, *managed care* refers to the management of who goes where for what health care services, and who gets paid how much by whom. Patients are "managed," meaning that they are not entirely free to go wherever they want for whatever medical service they want. The providers are tightly managed as well: they too are restricted not only in what they may charge for a given service but also in how often the service can be delivered.

As with traditional insurance, managed care plans depend on relatively large groups of covered lives. Typically, the plan receives payment on a per-capita basis. A large group of people (say, a large company) contracts with the plan to *deliver* all the health care for group members (not just pay for it, as with traditional insurance). The managed care company takes a fixed annual amount (for the sake of this example, say $100 per employee per month, or $1,200 per employee per year) for each of the company's 1,000 employees. It guarantees to deliver health care with the $1,200,000 it has collected for the year.

How the managed care company chooses to spend the dollars delivering care is up to the directors of the company. They can hire their own doctors or negotiate deals with independent doctors, own hospitals or negotiate deals with hospitals, even own suppliers of pharmaceuticals or negotiate deals for pharmaceuticals. This diversity of options is what makes the alphabet soup of managed care plans so complicated. And, as the managed care companies know very well, whatever they do *not* pay out, they keep as profit. This makes the business profitable.

To an even greater extent than with traditional insurance, the amount of illness in a population is crucial to the managed care company's profits. A traditional insurance company can adjust premiums, at least to some extent, and reduce its risk. But managed care plans usually offer one basic capitated rate and make their profit by controlling what they pay out for delivery of care. If the population is relatively healthy, the number of visits and expenses incurred can easily be controlled by using a gatekeeper. But every sick person who joins the plan eats directly into their profits.

Because there is so much profit to be made in collecting generous fees for the care of healthy people, managed care plans have long been accused of "cherry picking," or choosing a healthier-than-average population to enroll. Regulations have been made in an attempt to counteract this tendency of managed care plans, but if the regulations are not successful—if plans collect average fees for healthier-than-average people—the whole concept of managed care is undermined.

There is a science—some call it an art—called risk adjustment that is designed to calculate just how much the care of a given population should cost and to pay the insurer accordingly. It is a complex subject, however, filled with such imponderables as how much care is enough, what constitutes quality care, and who deserves what level of care. Ultimately, though, risk adjustments will be necessary if managed care is to have a lasting incentive to deliver excellent care.

Specific Types of Managed Care Plans

All managed care plans control, or manage, the expenses of providing health care. Exactly how they do so varies enormously from plan to plan.

Health maintenance organization.   The classic *health maintenance organization* (HMO) may be "closed panel" or "open panel." The closed panel HMO hires its own doctors and nurses, owns their office space, pays them a salary, and closely regulates their practices (controlling, for example, how many patients the professionals see in a day, what drugs they prescribe, and how many consultations or lab tests they order).

The open panel HMO may hire some providers, but it also negotiates with many outside doctors to deliver care at a reduced rate. While an independent practitioner may normally charge $60 for a visit, for example, the HMO can approach the doctor and offer 500 visits at $40 per visit. The way physicians are hired and how they feel about the organization can have consequences that may affect you. Sometimes the doctors get more personal income if they order less testing and make fewer referrals to specialists, and there have been cases in which physicians were prohibited from revealing such arrangements to their patients. The turnover rate of physicians in a particular plan can give you an idea of how happy the physicians are, which may also be an indication of how free they are to practice as they think best.

Preferred provider organization.   A *preferred provider organization* (PPO) manages the delivery of care somewhat differently, extending the practice of negotiation with independent providers. The company does not hire a large number of providers, but instead sets up a long list of physicians who have agreed to accept the PPO rates of payment and to play by PPO rules. The providers, for example, may agree not to refer to specialists without prior approval, or they may agree to have all laboratory work done through a particular commercial laboratory with which the PPO has negotiated favorable rates. Under this system, any physician who turns out to be more "expensive" than anticipated (in other words, one who makes too many referrals or orders too many tests) may be taken off the list. This would mean that you could no longer receive your care from that doctor.

Point of service plans.   The *point of service plans* allow members to see whichever doctor they want, but at a price. How much the members pay out of pocket depends on where they see the doctor: visits at the plan's regular office may involve no fee, an approved urgent care center may require the patient to pay 10% of the cost of the visit, a visit to an emergency room may cost the patient 15% of the bill, and a visit to an unapproved specialist may cost the patient 20% of the bill.

Hospitalization and Managed Care Plans

Hospitalization is a major expense and therefore a prime target of all managed care plans. Most managed care programs, and even traditional health insurers, now require preauthorization before hospitalization. This means that the physician has to call a special phone number, where someone (it is often not clear who this person is or what medical credentials this person has) takes the information provided and decides whether hospitalization is necessary and, if so, for how many days. Once the patient has been hospitalized, record reviews are a routine procedure; the reviewers decide when the patient should be discharged. This process, called *utilization review,* has resulted in much less hospitalization and the closing of many hospital beds and even whole hospitals.

We have tried to avoid the temptation to label different insurance plans as good or bad. Naturally, our opinions, like yours, are often based on our own personal experiences. But experiences will vary tremendously; a plan that one person has found to meet her needs perfectly may be terrible for someone else. There is no doubt, though, that systems of payment for health care are changing dramatically. New plans and companies are formed almost daily. Rather than bemoaning this (or wishing for the old days when the friendly local doctor pulled up to your door in his buggy and cared for your sick child in exchange for a plucked chicken), we recommend that you accept this new world and work on bending it to your own needs.

How Do I Get the Best Health Care Coverage for Myself?

There are two times to consider the question of how to get the best health care coverage for yourself: when you are choosing a plan and when you are in one. In either case, remember that if you have diabetes, you need to disclose and discuss that fact. Keeping a known health condition secret is a prescription for losing coverage altogether, and you should use every means available to you not to be without insurance. If diabetes is a fact of your health care life, it should be dealt with. There are predictable medical costs in sight, and the last thing you want is to have needed health care unaffordable due to lack of an insurance plan.

Qualifying for an Entitlement Program

As we mentioned above, government entitlements are often the best type of health care program. If you think you might be eligible, you should contact the relevant office of the federal or state government and find out whether you qualify.

Choosing a Traditional Insurance Plan through a Large Group

Earlier, when we described what goes on in the traditional insurance sphere, we explained that it is advantageous for people to enroll in large group plans rather than seeking insurance on an individual or small group basis. This is particularly true if the person has an illness, such as diabetes. Large group plans are most often offered by established, large employers. As few as 20 people may qualify as a group. Unions are another good source, since many unions have negotiated very favorable health plans over the years. But there are other ways to get into a large group. Consider associations, fraternal organizations, and clubs. Simply by bringing together groups of people, they may have developed plans that will allow you to join, despite having diabetes. A spouse's policy may be able to cover you. When you are choosing employment, be sure to consider whether the employer offers a group health insurance plan. It may well be worth sacrificing other elements of a job, such as a higher salary, to accept a job with good insurance coverage.

Some states have pooled risk plans, in which so-called uninsurable risks are allowed into a state-run plan. Where available, these plans can provide insurance at a reasonable rate even when you have serious expenses coming up.

Choosing a Managed Care Plan

You may very well find that managed care plans of one kind or another are increasingly favorably priced. This can be the deciding factor in choice of a plan, and there is certainly nothing intrinsically wrong with choosing a plan with a good price as well as good care. But you need to make the effort to understand what you are getting into. Here are some questions to ask about managed care plans. Be sure that you have the answers to these questions *in writing* from someone with the authority to be held responsible for the answers.

—To what extent can I choose my doctor?
—Is my regular doctor able to continue caring for me?
—As a person with diabetes, will I be seeing a board-certified internist? family practitioner? endocrinologist? Can I see a specialist if my care is not going well?
—Are retinal exams, glycohemoglobin tests, and other diabetes-related tests that I may need routinely covered?
—Are glucose meters and strips covered?

Our advice is to find out about the plan before you join. Use whatever sources of information are available: your employer's human resources department, people already enrolled in the plan, company brochures or lists of covered services, plan salespeople. No one likes having major coverage surprises.

Working within a Plan

Here are three suggestions to help you "work the system" once you have enrolled in a health insurance plan.

1. *Learn the rules for getting coverage and getting visits, and play by them.* Sometimes the rules seem almost cruelly complicated, and sometimes you will get the impression that they are nothing but barriers put up to confuse and discourage you. But if you learn the rules, you can profit by your knowledge. If the plan requires four identical prescriptions, each saying a certain thing, get them. If you have to have written preauthorization, get it. Whether or not the health plan has good reasons for establishing a set of complex regulations, chances are you will not be successful in going around them, so you may as well go through them.
2. *Be persistent.* If you think you deserve a certain coverage, keep asking. Make it a game, a personal challenge. Write back, call back, talk with a supervisor. Write down the date and time of every phone call you make, and write down the name of the person you talked to and what was said. You would be amazed at how many people end up getting positive responses just by coming back at insurers over and over again.

3. *Apply pressure when needed.* If some needed service is not covered, there is always the last resort of trying to force a change in coverage policy. Maybe a letter to the president of the company will work. Perhaps your union or association, the insurance commissioner, or a politician can help. There are certain necessary elements of diabetes care that you probably know better than most. Don't be afraid to speak up.

We think that health insurance coverage for quality diabetes care is your right. How such a statement actually plays out will vary, but it is worth making anyway. We have to assume that very few traditional insurance plans or managed care plans are oblivious to their responsibility to provide quality health care. We believe that by being smart and aggressive, we can all work our way through the maze that is the U.S. health care system and come out reasonably successful.

APPENDIX: GLOSSARY OF INSURANCE TERMS

ACTUARY   The person who tries to calculate exactly what the amount of illness will be in a given group of people and therefore what the payouts will be for an insurance plan.

ADVERSE SELECTION   The situation when a plan gets more than its share of sick people (the opposite of *cherry picking*).

CAPITATED PAYMENTS   Payments based on the number of people in a plan, providing the same payment per person. If a provider such as a doctor's office takes on the care of 100 people at a capitated rate of $50 per person, the provider receives $5,000 for delivering that care, regardless of what the care actually costs.

CATASTROPHIC COVERAGE   Insurance coverage that starts only when expenses are very high. It is a policy of last resort, not paying for small or even average expenses but only for the very high (catastrophic) ones. Because these catastrophes are relatively rare, catastrophic insurance is relatively cheap.

CHERRY PICKING   The practice of picking the predictably most healthy people to join a plan. This can be done subtly by steering advertising campaigns toward healthy people or overtly by excluding people with known illnesses.

CO-PAY   What a patient pays out of pocket for a partially covered service. If the insurance plan pays 80% of a given bill, the patient's co-pay is 20%.

COVERED BENEFIT   A material or service that is paid for. For example, glucose meters, insulin, or routine outpatient visits may or may not be covered benefits in a given plan.

DEDUCTIBLE   Amount that must be paid by the covered individual every year before any insurance coverage kicks in. If you have a $200 deductible, then you pay the first $200 of all expenses each year before your insurance policy pays for anything.

DISPOSABLE SUPPLIES   Supplies that are used and thrown away, such as syringes, glucose test strips, and alcohol wipes.

DURABLE MEDICAL EQUIPMENT   Supplies that last, rather than being thrown away on a regular basis. Blood glucose meters and insulin pumps are examples.

ENTITLEMENT   A program such as insurance coverage that a person is entitled to by virtue of situation in life. The term usually refers to government programs. Medicare, for example, is an entitlement for which one qualifies by being 65 years of age or older. Medicaid is usually based on low income, veterans' benefits on having served in the active military service, and so on.

GATEKEEPER   A person (or system) that directs the flow of people to particular providers. For example, if you have a cold, the gatekeeper (perhaps a nurse practitioner or a family practitioner) may decide that he or she can treat you and that you do not need to see a specialist. If you come with a broken bone, the gatekeeper may decide that you need to see an orthopedist. The gatekeeper is your entrance into the system; you cannot decide for yourself which specialists you see.

HEALTH MAINTENANCE ORGANIZATION (HMO)   An organization (usually a for-profit company) that essentially collects a premium from insured people or their employers and hires a staff to provide all health care.

INDEPENDENT PRACTICE ASSOCIATION (IPA)   A group of professionals linked in a group to provide service at a reduced fee to large numbers of patients (similar to a *preferred provider organization*).

MEANS-TESTED PROGRAM   A program in which eligibility depends on income and net worth. Medicaid is the classic means-tested program, meant to support health care for the disadvantaged. Medicare and the health insurance plans of the Department of Veterans Affairs are not at present means-tested programs.

MEDIGAP   Insurance policies that are designed to fill in the gaps of Medicare. Ideally, for a reasonable cost these policies will cover only what is left uncovered by Medicare. The buyer has to be wary, though, that coverage is not overlapped or duplicated.

OPEN SEASON   A period of time in which there is open enrollment to a plan. For a month or so, people can sign up for the plan (sometimes still subject to certain limitations). Between open seasons, a plan can decide whether or not to let you in.

POINT OF SERVICE PLAN   A plan that provides different levels of coverage depending on where the patient receives the service. For example, you may be covered 100% if you go to one of the doctors in the plan, but if you choose to go to an outside specialist, have surgery at a hospital other than the recommended one, and so on, you may have to pay 50% or more of the bill out of pocket.

POOLED RISK   Plans, usually run by a state government, that insure people who are otherwise too ill or too much at risk of illness to be eligible for usual coverage. The pooled risk plan may use government funds to pay some of the high premiums charged by insurers to take on high-risk individuals.

PREAUTHORIZATION   The requirement to get approval before any test, procedure, or hospitalization is done. Typically, criteria are set up at a central computer, so when a physician calls for preauthorization the information provided is put into the computer and the request is then approved or denied. If your plan requires preauthorization and you do not obtain it, you may end up paying the entire bill out of pocket.

PREEXISTING CONDITION   A medical condition (such as diabetes) that exists before a person signs up for a given health plan. Many plans state that they will not cover preexisting conditions or will cover them only after a certain period of time. There are laws being passed in some states and possibly at the federal level that prohibit exclusion on the basis of preexisting conditions.

PREFERRED PROVIDER ORGANIZATION (PPO)   A network of physicians and other professionals who have agreed to accept patients from a specific managed care plan, usually receiving a reduced fee per visit, in order to be sure that they have a flow of patients.

PROVIDER   Whoever delivers a health care service. A provider may be a doctor, a group practice, a nurse, a nutritionist, a hospital, or an entire health care system.

RISK ADJUSTMENT   The science of deciding how much risk for illness there is in a given group of people and adjusting the payments accordingly. For example, the risk is much higher if the average age of a population is 60 than if it is 30; a fair adjustment would be to have greater financial resources within the plan covering the 60-year-olds.

UTILIZATION REVIEW   The process of reviewing expenses in progress, usually applied to hospitalization, where teams of chart reviewers check the charts of patients daily to decide whether continued hospitalization is necessary. Utilization is now also being applied to outpatient care.

Chapter 21

Employment and Diabetes

- *"I want to be a police officer. Is there anything wrong with that? Why can't I be a police officer, if I want to?"*

- *"At the job interview today, they asked me if I have diabetes. I said yes, and the tone of the interview changed on the spot. I think I blew it."*

- *"I have a job in health care, where if I have a bad insulin reaction, it could really hurt someone. Should I get out of the field of health care altogether?"*

- *"What can I do to show my employer that I can be an excellent employee with diabetes?"*

Throughout this book, we encourage you to take control of your diabetes, and we provide tools to help you do so. But if diabetes keeps you from getting or keeping a job, it is controlling you, regardless of how well you manage your blood sugar. In this chapter, we talk about how to hold your job regardless of diabetes. We describe, first, responsibilities and rights—yours and your employer's. We discuss employment discrimination, how to make it through job interviews, and what to consider in various kinds of employment. Finally, we offer some real-life scenarios and practical advice about accommodating successfully in the workplace—how to keep diabetes from dominating the situation.

Ideally, every job should be available to every qualified person, every employer should have an enlightened and intelligent approach to diabetes, and every employee should be successful at managing diabetes without any interruption of work. But this is not a perfect world. Since every person and every workplace have unique features, employment problems can arise. Just remember: having diabetes is only one of your individual characteristics. You can work with it.

On the Job

Your Responsibilities

You have a responsibility both to yourself and to your employer. You need to take good care of yourself for the long run. If work is interfering with good self-care, you have to modify your regimen, modify the job, or seriously consider changing jobs. You will call unfavorable attention to yourself if you take too many sick days, make too many demands, or, in the worst scenario, have a severe insulin reaction on the job that causes injury to yourself or others. We have heard of a case that came to court for just this reason: the employee, a police officer, had one severe insulin reaction, in which he put people in serious danger by crashing his patrol car. The county wanted to fire him from the force without a second chance. This was a case of "one strike and you're out." It was a situation you never want to be in.

You have a responsibility to your employer to perform your job reliably and well. This means, among other things, not taking unnecessary risks that could interfere with your job performance.

It is a good bet that your employer will know little about diabetes—a lot less than you do—and it's also likely that he or she won't be all that interested. So the best option is to make your diabetes self-care compatible with good job performance. If push comes to shove, though, it doesn't hurt to have a working understanding of what constitutes employment discrimination.

The Employer's Responsibility

The Americans with Disabilities Act and Title V of the Federal Rehabilitation Act form the basis of your legal rights as they relate to employment and diabetes. The law states that employers cannot discriminate against a person because of handicaps, if that person can perform the job with reasonable accommodations made by the employer. Diabetes fits within the definition of handicaps covered by this law. When you are holding a job and have diabetes, it is not legal for an employer to use your diabetes against you unfairly. It cannot be a factor in your advancement or your continued employment, unless it keeps you from doing your job. In most cases, you cannot be fired simply because of diabetes; the employer must give a valid reason for firing you—one that would stand up in court.

There may be more subtle, but also damaging and illegal, limits put on you. For example, restrictions on your areas of work must be based on a realistic assessment of your capabilities and any potential dangers. In one case a worker was not fired, but his activities were so restricted that there was no chance of advancement. The employer must be able to justify such restrictions.

You are also legally entitled to reasonable accommodation for your condition. Just what is "reasonable," of course, can be a matter of serious contention. You may feel that you need regular work breaks, regular hours, no night work, and the right to have food with you at all times. That would be nice, but the employer may be unable to make these accommodations. From the employer's viewpoint, if your diabetes interferes with your job performance, or if the accommodations you need cannot reasonably be made, then all bets are off. Such disputes sometimes end up being settled in court. So think carefully about your responsibilities as a good employee.

Finally, one reason that employers worry about hiring people with disabilities is their concern that the company's health insurance premiums will climb if an employee becomes sick and makes more health care claims, or even if the health plan just finds out that an employee has diabetes. The employer may not be happy about keeping a person with diabetes for this reason, but it is illegal to let an employee go just because the employee's health may affect insurance premiums.

Looking for a Job

In our transient society, where people frequently change jobs and even locations, at any given moment many people will be in the process of seeking employment. The issue of employment discrimination often comes up at the time of a job interview. A potential employer is permitted to ask you if you have any health problem that would interfere with your ability to do the work. But he or she *cannot* ask you specifically whether or not you have diabetes, unless diabetes would affect your ability to do the job. Under no circumstances is the potential employer permitted to list a series of diseases and ask if you have any of them—even, as noted, if the reason is a wish to avoid increases in health insurance premiums.

What do you say, then, when the interviewer begins questioning you about your health status? This is a tough one. We don't recommend lying, but we do suggest that you try to answer only what the potential employer has a right to ask:

Employer. "Well, Ms. Perkins, I like you very much, and I think you'll be a valued employee with Acme, Inc. But I just want to be sure you'll always come to work and won't get sick on us—you know, raise our insurance rates or anything like that. You don't have any health problems I should know about, do you?"

Job Applicant. "Why, no, Mr. Dunning, I am sure I could do the job just fine. I've always been a very reliable worker with a good attendance record, as my recommendations attest." [*True.* And Mr. Dunning does not, in fact, have a right at this point to know that Ms. Perkins has diabetes.]

Employer. "Well, Ms. Perkins, I'm sure that's right. But I mean, you don't have any horrible *disease* or addiction or anything like that, do you?"

Applicant. "Why, no, Mr. Dunning. I take care of myself very well. I'm sure there's nothing horrible about me, Mr. Dunning." [*True.* And this is not the moment to educate Mr. Dunning about diabetes.]

We know that it's hard to sit in a hot seat and come up with the right answers, without antagonizing your interviewer or backing yourself into lies. There's no perfect solution. You don't want to be in a position of losing the job or filing suit. So we suggest that if you are interviewing for a job, you do not volunteer information about your diabetes.

There is usually a point in the preemployment process where the diabetes becomes known. Most often, an offer is contingent upon passing a physical exam. At this point, the fact that you have diabetes will inevitably come out, so it is important to understand your rights. *Diabetes is not a disqualifier. The issue is, can you do the job?*

Where Diabetes May Be a Problem

There are some specific jobs in which diabetes is a particular problem because of legal decisions against hiring people with diabetes. The Federal Bureau of Investigation is one such employer. We know at least one very successful special agent in the FBI who has Type I diabetes, but, the FBI's formal policy is not to allow people taking insulin to become special agents. The active duty military is another such employer. People with diabetes are not usually allowed to enlist, and people who develop diabetes while in the service, depending on which branch of the military they are in, may have difficulty holding their job whether or not the diabetes interferes with their work. A third problem area of employment is interstate trucking. Federal regulations state that people taking insulin cannot drive commercial vehicles across state lines, and many states extend the policy to intrastate driving as well, particularly to bus driving. The list goes on. People with diabetes who take insulin are usually excluded from being pilots, commercial divers, and often heavy machinery operators; police force hiring rules vary greatly.

What does this mean? Are these major employers breaking the law? Is it hopeless for a person taking insulin to try for employment in these types of jobs? The fact is that the FBI, for example, rightly or wrongly believes that the job of a special agent by its very nature is incompatible with taking insulin. Furthermore, the FBI has convinced the courts of this viewpoint. Likewise the military, the trucking industry, and many police forces have successfully defended blanket policies against employing people with insulin-requiring diabetes. So they are not breaking the law. This sort of legal ruling can change, and anyone is entitled to rechallenge such blanket exclusions in court. But if you choose to do so, do it with your eyes open, and expect a fight.

The Realities of Working with Diabetes

Having discussed some of the legalities, are there in fact certain kinds of work that are particularly hard to do if you have diabetes? The answer depends on your own personality and your own condition. Examples abound of people with diabetes succeeding in virtually every kind of work, from the National Football League and National Hockey League to politics, television, jazz, and scuba diving. But your situation is unique. If you can't control your diabetes during vigorous exercise (or if you don't have much athletic ability), then you should forgo professional athletics. If you have long-term complications, these also have to be put into the equation. If you don't have complications, we suggest that you not worry about whether you might develop them at some future date.

We are often asked whether stress on the job makes diabetes worse, and our answer is that there is no set answer. Any adrenalin rush does tend to raise blood sugar, but you can take extra insulin, tighten your diet, or fit in some regular exercise. On the other hand, if your response to high-stress situations is to forget about your diabetes self-care, then you'd better find employment with a low level of stress.

The issues become more subtle when you consider job demands that go beyond concerns of physical condition or stress. People worry about whether their diabetes is compatible with long hours, shift work, irregular hours, and unpredictable exercise. They worry especially about jobs that require a high level of intellectual function on which much depends. Can you climb to the top of your organization, with all that entails, even though you have diabetes? Absolutely! But again, you have to consider your own personality. If you love the challenge and can work variety into your diabetic self-care, go for it. There is certainly no ceiling on the amount of personal responsibility or intellectual demand a person with diabetes can manage.

Real-Life Scenarios

Kurt has Type I diabetes, which is quite unstable, with sugars that fluctuate widely if he is not very careful, and sometimes even when he is. He is assigned to the graveyard shift at an automobile plant, working nights five days a week, sleeping from 9 A.M. to 4 P.M. On Saturdays and Sundays, he lives "normal" hours, to see the family. Kurt's blood sugars go haywire because he can't get his insulin doses timed properly with these shifting hours.

Shift work, with changing hours of sleep, often causes a problem for people with diabetes. One solution, the most intensive, is to be on either an external insulin pump or a regimen consisting of twice-daily Ultralente (long-acting) insulin and a dose of Regular before each meal. This way, you can maintain a day-and-night low level of insulin (basal rate pump or Ultralente) while covering each meal, whenever it is eaten, with Regular. If you are not up to maintaining such an intensive schedule, you can at least try to mimic the principles involved: take two shots of longer acting insulin a day, and mix in your biggest doses of Regular before the largest meals of the day.

Marcia is a law enforcement officer who carries a gun in her daily work. Admittedly, she has never used it in action over a long career in police work. But she is concerned that if an insulin reaction were to occur at the wrong time, someone could get hurt.

It is a realistic worry that almost anyone taking insulin has at one time or another: concern that they will have a reaction when they are driving a bus, arguing a case in court, doing brain surgery, or driving their kids to school. An easy answer is to say that no one's risk is ever zero, and that no one ever knows when any type of health emergency might occur—a heart attack, epileptic seizure, or whatever. But that's not a good answer, because it is true that taking insulin does increase the risk of hypoglycemia. There are many practical steps you can take to avoid catastrophic insulin reactions. We go into much more detail about this in Chapter 5, but here are a few re-minders to carry with you into the workplace:

—*Know if you are at risk.* What treatment are you on? (Insulin is always more likely to cause hypoglycemia than pills, for instance.) Are you always aware when your blood sugar goes low, or does it sometimes sneak up on you without warning? Have you ever become confused and required the help of another person to treat your reaction? If you answer yes to the last question, then you are at special risk; if your answer is no, then the risk is much less.

—*Know when your most vulnerable times are.* Do you tend to be on the low side before lunch or late in the afternoon? Even if you are not frankly low at these times (for example, not in the 50s but in the 70s), recognize that you are cutting it close, and one day you may be very low at that same time.

—*Keep a source of concentrated sugar with you at all times.* This is just common sense, but it is absolutely essential if you take insulin.

—*Be sure that your co-workers know what an insulin reaction is and how to treat it.* By talking it over with them, you make it possible for them to be able to help (by giving you some sugar) if you have a reaction. If they have no idea what is going on, your reaction could be more traumatic for them than it is for you!

—*Anticipate the times when you want to be sure your sugar is okay.* Check it just before you drive the kids to school, kick off a key sales meeting, or prepare to do brain surgery.

Theresa is skating on thin ice at her job. She developed Type II diabetes a few years ago, a year after starting this job. Her attendance record, never that good, got worse. Between visits to doctors and a liberal assortment of days off for colds, al-lergies, and cramps, Theresa is nervous that her supervisor is just about fed up with her frequent absences.

In Theresa's case, we see the supervisor's point. Having diabetes entitles you to exactly the same number of sick days as any other employee. You may need to do some schedule juggling, stacking up several doctors' appoint-ments into one morning, or taking just an hour off at the end of the day. Hav-ing diabetes may mean coming to work when you are not feeling 100% per-fect. In the worst case, if complications really preclude full-time work, you'll need to consider working part time. A person hopes for understanding, but employers are not required to keep a worker who can't get the job done.

> *Tom sees that his co-workers are sloppier than he is, that they don't do their work as neatly or completely, show up and leave work at will, and are generally undisciplined. But he is the one with diabetes, and his supervisor is always bugging him about whether he is able to do his work.*

Chances are that Tom's supervisor is almost completely ignorant about diabetes and may well be prejudiced against it. Tom's challenge is to convince the employer that he is doing the job well—better than average, in fact. There may be a point at which the supervisor can actually learn something about diabetes. But if the supervisor isn't interested, then Tom should just concentrate on showing her that diabetes is not a factor in his job performance.

Having diabetes is readily compatible with the vast majority of work settings and potentially compatible with anything. But we know this is the rosy view. We know that you have to think about many things that your colleagues at work ignore: timing of your meals, work schedules, extra doctors' appointments, and so on. You can do it, but you will have to work that much harder to succeed.

If you are looking for a job or considering a change, be aware of which areas of employment are most compatible with you and with your diabetes. You can anticipate special problems in the military and interstate trucking, for example. While diabetes will inevitably play a role in your employment decisions, we hope it will not dominate them.

There are many things you can do to ensure that you do your work safely and competently. For example, make sure that some of your co-workers are aware of your condition so they can help in a pinch. If, despite your best efforts, you encounter illegal job discrimination, you will be faced with a personal choice between confronting it and sidestepping it. Either course of action is honorable.

Whatever your employer or your co-workers think, you should know in your heart that diabetes is just one of your personal characteristics. It shouldn't define you in the workplace anymore than it should define you throughout life. And there is even a positive side to diabetes in the workplace, especially from the employer's point of view.

Did you ever stop to think about who is more likely to be disciplined, a person with diabetes or a person without it? Who is generally eating a healthier diet? Who is generally more consistent, regular, and reliable? These traits are enormous strengths in the work environment. They are exactly what employment offices yearn for. And, in fact, they are very common traits among people with diabetes. So it is really no surprise that people with diabetes are usually excellent employees. As you know, the world is studded with outstanding, successful people who have diabetes, from Mary Tyler Moore to Catfish Hunter and hundreds or thousands more. Self-discipline is a key to success, and people with diabetes usually have it. On the whole, they make excellent employees. The world should know that.

Part IV

Complications

The complications of diabetes, both in the short run and the long run, are what make it such a frightening disease. If there were no complications, the high blood sugar would just be an abnormal laboratory test. But of course we all know that diabetes can cause serious complications. What many people with diabetes *don't* understand is that the complications are far from inevitable and can be very successfully managed. The horror stories you may have heard probably happened before the modern era of diabetes care, or they happened to people who did not take advantage of what is available.

Part IV describes the various complications that can occur. There are two broad categories of complications: immediate (or acute) and long-term. Acute complications are directly and immediately due to high blood sugar. They come on in a matter of minutes or hours when the sugar goes up and disappear as the sugar comes back down. Most commonly, they include thirst, frequent urination, blurred vision, fatigue, weight loss, and, in women, vaginal yeast infections. In the extreme, they lead to ketoacidosis or hyperosmolar coma.

The long-term complications occur only over many years or decades of diabetes and are not so easily cured. They can affect the blood vessels, eyes, kidneys, nerves, legs, and feet. For good reason, the long-term complications of diabetes are feared. But a great deal of misinformation is spread about them. We want to clear this up and tell the facts as they are.

Throughout most of the twentieth century, the long-term

complications were so common that doctors and patients alike began to consider them almost inevitable. Looking back, though, we can see that people who took extremely good care of themselves, even with the primitive tools available, did best in avoiding the complications.

Today, we know for sure that you can you can stack the deck in your favor. Good control of blood sugar over the years matters. You *don't* have to share the grim prognosis of previous generations with diabetes.

Even when a particular complication (such as nerve damage or eye disease) is detected, good management can keep it from becoming a serious problem. If you do develop complications, then there is much that can be done to limit the damage, reducing the chance that the complications will become disabling. Together with you, we are in the business of eliminating the complications of diabetes.

Chapter 22

Systemic Symptoms

- *"I'm tired all day, and then at night I don't get any rest because I'm up to go to the bathroom three or four times."*
- *"Blurry vision, feet tingling—I'm a wreck just worrying about what it all means."*
- *"I'm motivated to keep my sugars in control now, because I just don't like the way I feel when they're high."*

Too high blood sugar makes you feel bad. Some of the feelings, such as fatigue, may be so subtle you don't notice them. Others, such as a cottony dry mouth and painful feet, are uncomfortable, making it difficult for you to go about your daily activities. In this chapter we'll discuss the *systemic symptoms* of uncontrolled diabetes, meaning those symptoms due to high blood sugar that affect the body as a whole and go away as soon as the sugars are improved. After reading this chapter you may realize that you're bothered by these symptoms more often than you thought. Believe it or not, that's actually good news, because by learning how you feel when you're high, you can set yourself on a course to feeling better fast.

We will also discuss the dangers of becoming overly focused on high blood sugar as the cause of all your symptoms. You may forget that there are plenty of other reasons why you, or anyone else, might feel sick. Finally, we'll describe instances where you actually need to turn down the anxiety meter and realize that the episode is transient and you're doing what you can.

First, a definition: Symptoms are what a person feels. It's always helpful to think clearly and specifically about your symptoms. Saying "I feel just terrible" isn't nearly as helpful as pinpointing *in what way* you feel terrible: "I feel just terrible because I'm so thirsty" (or so feverish, or have such a headache, or whatever). Thinking clearly about your symptoms will help you and your health care professional identify what's causing them.

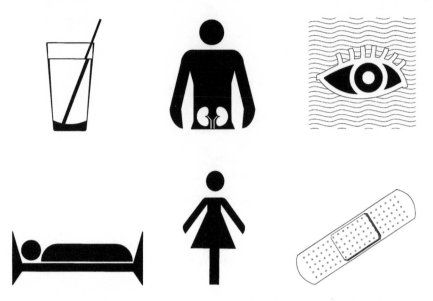

Figure 21. High blood sugars can make you feel miserable. The symptoms are thirst, frequent urination, blurry vision, fatigue, vaginal infections, and sores that don't heal.

Thirst and Frequent Urination

The blood thickens when the sugar is up. Think of a high concentration of glucose as making the blood more like syrup. The brain registers this thick blood as a sign of dehydration and sends you the message to drink fluids in order to dilute your blood back to normal. When you drink gallons of water, you can't just keep swelling up, so your kidneys get rid of the water by making large quantities of urine.

Thirst and frequent urination (*polyuria* and *polydipsia*) can be severe. We have known people to urinate as often as every half-hour and drink one glass of water after another. (This situation is made much worse, of course, if the person is drinking a liquid that contains sugar, such as soda or orange juice.) Being thirsty can make a person very uncomfortable. One woman was so desperate to quench her thirst that she had cupped water in her hand from the faucet and continuously brought it to her mouth. By the time she came to our clinic, her lips were chapped and raw.

Symptoms of thirst and frequent urination aren't always that obvious. Your diabetes may be well controlled much of the time. But even with well-controlled diabetes, mild symptoms can be present with a temporary rise in blood sugar after a particularly large meal or too little insulin. A slightly dry mouth or greater than normal thirst may be your only clue that this is a time of day when your sugar is creeping up. Check and see. Sugar usually has to be well over 200 mg/dl (and more often over 250 mg/dl) to cause thirst.

We should note here that not all frequent urination is due to high blood sugar. Try to determine whether you are actually urinating large volumes or just urinating frequently. Frequent trips to the bathroom to void small amounts of urine, especially if there is pain, blood in the urine, or (in men) difficulty starting the stream, are more likely due to a urinary tract infection or prostate problem than to diabetes.

Blurred Vision

Blurred vision can be scary. You know that diabetes can cause visual impairment, and you may begin thinking that your time has come (even if you've only had diabetes a few years, when serious diabetic eye disease rarely occurs). Actually, damage to the retina caused by diabetes (called diabetic retinopathy; see Chapter 25) occurs as a result of *longstanding* high blood sugar; it is a long-term complication, not an acute complication. By contrast, blurred vision regularly occurs as an immediate, and quickly reversible, effect of high blood sugar.

Here's how it happens: the lens is a clear little focusing device (like the lens in a camera) located toward the front of your eye. It focuses your vision, automatically changing shape when you move your gaze from near to far. When you look out at a distance, the lens flattens out. When you look at something close up, it becomes rounder. If your blood sugar is high for several days or more, the lens swells up and can't change shape as easily. Then, whether you're looking near or far, it's as if you're wearing the wrong pair of glasses. Things are out of focus, blurred. In the extreme, vision can be severely limited. Fortunately, the lens regains its elasticity fairly quickly with stabilized blood sugar control. Most people will see an improvement in vision within a few days, although it can take up to six weeks for the lens to return completely to normal. An important point comes up here: if your vision is blurry because of varying blood sugar control, this is definitely not the time to go have your glasses changed. If you do, chances are you'll just have to have them changed again in a week or so. Wait until your blood sugars are more stable.

Blurred vision is often the symptom that leads a person with diabetes to seek medical care in the first place. It may also get your attention following a few days of high blood sugar as a result of an illness. But almost always, blurred vision in someone without definite, established retinopathy is a temporary problem that will respond to blood sugar control.

Fatigue

One of the most annoying symptoms of high blood sugar is fatigue. It is generally caused by a lack of insulin or insulin function. Remember that without insulin carbohydrates are not converted to energy normally by the cells of the body; this causes the sugar to stay in the bloodstream and build up to a high level. The result is the sensation of running out of gas. You may be eating, but if sugar is not getting into the cells, then eating isn't doing you any good.

Fatigue from high blood sugar can be mild or severe. When it is mild, it is often ignored or attributed to age, overwork, or stress. In the extreme, some people become so fatigued that they literally fall asleep during a conversation. Insulin users often notice some transient fatigue after a meal, particularly if it is large, until the insulin "catches up" with the food and moves the sugar into the cells.

It shouldn't be hard to tell the difference between the fatigue of high blood sugar (hyperglycemia) and the fatigue that occurs due to low blood sugar (hypoglycemia.) Low blood sugar occurs when you haven't eaten in a while or when you are just starting to eat (before the food has been absorbed from the stomach.) In addition to fatigue, it usually causes other symptoms, like sweatiness, shakiness, palpitations, or trouble thinking straight. High blood sugar, on the other hand, is more likely to worsen in the few hours *after* a meal or when you are sick. The fatigue due to high blood sugar creeps up on you; it doesn't come on in a matter of a few minutes.

The best way to determine if you are high or low is always to test your sugar. But if you have a significant doubt, you may just have to eat something sweet and see if the symptoms go away (in which case, they were due to hypoglycemia.) As a person with diabetes who is knowledgeable about diabetes, you will learn to tell your highs from your lows.

Weight Loss and Hunger

Weight loss and hunger occur for the same reason as fatigue—lack of insulin or insulin function. As the sugar level rises in the blood, it spills into the urine. It may come as a surprise to you, but sugar in the urine actually amounts to a significant drain of calories. If you need 1,800 calories a day to maintain your body weight, and you eat 1,800 calories but lose 300 of them in the urine, that's like eating only 1,500 calories. You will lose weight. Eating doesn't do any good if the calories you take in just pass out of the body through the urine.

Weight loss out of proportion to dieting, then, is not a good sign. This may be a tricky point to recognize. Does the weight just seem to melt away now, even though in previous years you could never lose a pound? Are you not really following a diet but getting terrific weight loss results? If so, check your sugar. It may be high (200s, 300s, 400s). If it is allowed to continue, this situation will surely get worse, not better. High blood sugars are definitely not the recommended way to lose weight.

Excessive hunger, called *polyphagia,* is the third symptom of the triad that also includes polydipsia (thirst) and polyuria (excess urination). Hunger may be the hardest symptom to pin on high blood sugar. First of all, it is much less common than thirst and excess urination. Second, hunger is more psychological than physical: most people feel hungry if they see some food that looks or smells appetizing, no matter what their blood sugar is. Third, like fatigue, hunger is a common feeling when your blood sugar is low, not high. So, again, test your sugar when in doubt or until you have learned to recognize your symptoms accurately. Reacting to every "pang of hunger" may be exactly the *wrong* response.

Infections

High blood sugar increases the risk of infections for two reasons. First, the fungus and bacteria that cause infection thrive in a high-sugar environment. Second, the immune system, which fights off infections, doesn't work as well in the presence of high blood sugar.

The most common infection seen in out-of-control diabetes is a fungus (yeast) called candida or monilia. It is the organism that causes the infection all too familiar to many women—vaginal yeast. Men can also get yeast infections in the groin or other areas of skin. Yeast infections are effectively treated with creams, ointments, and suppositories, but they will keep coming back unless there is an improvement in blood sugar control.

Other common infections associated with high blood sugar include urinary tract infections (especially in women), gum infections, infections of wounds, and infections of the extremities, especially the feet. Foot infections have the potential to become serious. People with diabetes are also more likely to get a secondary bacterial infection (such as bronchitis) complicating a viral respiratory infection such as the flu. That's why we recommend flu shots for our patients with diabetes.

We are often asked whether having high blood sugars in the hospital after a surgical operation will keep a person from healing or even cause an infection. It is true that having very high sugars (for instance, over 300 mg/dl) continuously for days at a time can slow down healing. But this fact has to be balanced with the more immediate danger of severe hypoglycemia during the hospitalization, when you may not be eating well. We don't expect perfect control from people who are recovering from surgery; in fact, we tend to relax control a bit in the postoperative period.

Cloudy Thinking

Many people notice a change in their thinking with high blood sugar. Some people describe it as "being full of cobwebs" or "not being in touch with the immediate surroundings." Others describe a moodiness, especially feeling disinterested or depressed. High blood sugar makes work and study difficult. One woman said that she became aware of how much high blood sugar was affecting her thinking only after her control improved with an insulin pump. Her grades at college jumped from a low B average to mostly As (but we can't guarantee that good control will make you a brilliant student!). Moodiness and irritability are definitely associated with high blood sugars. When control is improved, family members often notice the difference: "Fred is back to his old self again. He's interested in doing things!"

Increase in Nerve Pain

Many people with diabetes feel the effect of high blood sugar on their nerve fibers. There may have been a tingling sensation in their feet even before the actual diagnosis of diabetes was made, or pain from their established neuropathy (nerve damage) may worsen when the blood sugars are high. While the sensations are more common in the lower extremities, some people experience distress in their hands as well.

Neuropathic pain (nerve pain) usually improves with improvement in blood sugar control, but if neuropathy is established, it won't resolve completely. Think of painful nerves as being like static on a radio: you can improve the sound quite a bit just by tuning into the station (like tuning up your blood sugars), but if the radio is old and dusty (like your nerves when damage over the years has caused neuropathy), reception won't come back completely to normal even with fine tuning. Chapter 27 describes the medications used to relieve nerve pain if it is interfering with daily functioning.

The Differential Diagnosis

One mistake that people sometimes make is seeing everything as related to blood sugar control. Although it's a good idea for people with diabetes to pay attention to their sugars and to explore options for control, it's not so good if they ignore other illnesses, always assuming that "it's just my diabetes." Professionals may fall into this trap, too. Our treatment of Stanley is a case in point.

> *We were sure that Stanley, a retiree, had high blood sugar when he described his frequent urination, which interrupted his woodworking activities and awakened him four times at night. He said he was tired all the time (who wouldn't be, waking up every other hour all night?), and we focused entirely on his blood sugar control. Imagine our surprise when his hemoglobin A1c came back excellent and his blood glucose monitoring confirmed that his sugars were mostly just fine.*

It turned out that Stanley's symptoms were caused by an enlarged prostate and some nerve damage to his bladder. He was urinating frequently because he couldn't empty his bladder completely. Only when he was treated for the prostate problem was the symptom relieved.

How can you tell if it's your diabetes or something else that's causing a particular symptom? Think about the *differential diagnosis:* what are the different possibilities? Just about every symptom can have more than one cause, and the list of possible causes is called the differential diagnosis. You may not know all the possible causes of a particular symptom, but there's one easy way to tell if the symptom is due to high blood sugars: check your sugar. And confirm your impressions with your health care provider. Don't wait until you are at your wit's end. Too many people put themselves through needless worry over something like blurred vision, which turns out to be easily reversed and managed.

How Serious Is It?

If you have diabetes, you will have high blood sugars at least once in a while. Diabetes cannot be controlled perfectly. But how serious is a particular episode of high blood sugar? Generally, it is serious if it is longstanding or if it produces severe symptoms. Checking the hemoglobin A1c is an easy way to determine if the high blood sugar has been persistent. If the hemoglobin A1c is above your target, investigate further by doing more intense self-monitoring of blood glucose and by keeping scrupulous records. You may find a pattern for your high blood sugars. Maybe you've gone overboard with afternoon snacking, or maybe you go high regularly after supper. But if there is no obvious pattern, or if you are having trouble getting your blood sugar levels back on track, get in touch with your health care professional to collaborate on some new self-care strategies.

Even if your A1c is within your target range, an acute episode of high blood sugar with severe symptoms should not be ignored. Infection, severe stress, or a bottle of bad insulin all can cause a rapid deterioration in blood sugar control. Get the blood sugar down! If you are unable to get it down quickly, if you have ketones, or if symptoms progress, then get in touch with your health care professional or go to the emergency room immediately.

In the end, there will be some sugar levels that you cannot explain. Focusing excessively on the odd bounces will only lead to frustration. We always ask our patients to look for *patterns* and not to fret about every single value.

Listen to what your body tells you about your sugar. In the process, you may discover why you have that thirst in the evening that leads you to drink several diet drinks when no one else seems thirsty. You may find out why on some days you just don't have any energy or any patience. You may learn why you are losing weight so easily. Listening will let you hear an early alarm that something is wrong and needs your immediate attention.

Chapter 23

Diabetic Ketoacidosis and Hyperosmolar Coma

- *"I was in the hospital once for diabetes, but I don't have a clue whether it was diabetic ketoacidosis."*

- *"I used to check my ketones all the time, and sometimes they were a little bit positive. I really don't understand what that all means. What's more, I don't know if it matters."*

- *"How high can the blood sugar go, and what happens when it gets there?"*

Diabetic ketoacidosis and hyperosmolar coma may seem like the sort of long scientific terms that you never really wanted to understand. But they can definitely be dangerous and are completely preventable. So let's try to make sense of them.

Diabetic Ketoacidosis

Doctors generally refer to *diabetic ketoacidosis* as *DKA*. It's also sometimes called "diabetic coma," but that is confusing, since coma in diabetes is far more often caused by hypoglycemia than by DKA. (Calling DKA "diabetic coma" really goes back to the preinsulin era before 1921, when children went into coma before dying of DKA.) We think it is important for you to understand what DKA means, why it happens, what to do about it, and how to prevent it.

What Is Diabetic Ketoacidosis?

As the name implies, diabetic ketoacidosis involves *ketones*. Ketones are the chemical by-products of fat breakdown, just as ashes are the by-product of burned wood. There is always some amount of fat breakdown taking place in the human body and always some normal amount of ketones in the blood. Ketones build up in the blood only when fat breakdown is increased, for example, when you don't eat for 12 or 18 hours. When high levels are in the blood, the ketones spill into the urine, just as sugar does. A small amount of ketones in the urine (called *ketonuria*) is not unusual. But it is important to understand the central role that insulin plays in the control of ketone production and disposal, because too high a level of ketones in the blood does cause ketoacidosis.

As we've said, insulin is needed to allow the body's cells to burn sugar. With the right amount of insulin (in a nondiabetic person), as soon as the blood sugar rises, as it does after a carbohydrate-containing meal, the body uses that sugar as fuel and stores away fat for later when there's no new carbohydrate fuel eaten. So sugar (carbohydrate) is the preferred fuel for the moment, and when it is available, it's used. Fat is backup, the storage form of energy. In this normal situation, if no carbohydrate is eaten, there's relatively little sugar in the blood, insulin goes down, and the body turns to fat for energy. Ketones increase a bit in the blood from the fat breakdown and may spill over into the urine.

The problem develops if your pancreas isn't making nearly enough insulin (as in untreated Type I diabetes) and you don't get enough insulin by injection. The sugar builds up in the bloodstream but is not used for fuel (since it lacks insulin to help it enter the cells). So the body must turn to its fat stores for energy, increasing ketones in the blood.

When ketones rise to a high level, not only do they spill over into the urine but also they can cause your whole body to become too acid: in other words, you have *acidosis*. That's because the ketones are actually acids. If the doctor thinks you may have DKA, he or she will look for the presence of too high a level of ketones in your blood and urine, and the presence of acidosis.

What Are the Common Causes of DKA?

In a person with Type I diabetes, DKA is caused by having far too little insulin in the blood. This could be due to neglect or to a particularly extreme case of denial or anger. It could be because the insulin went bad. Rarely, people run out of insulin in places so remote that they cannot get a new supply. Whatever the cause of not getting nearly enough insulin when it's needed, anywhere from a day to a few days later, the person with Type I diabetes will develop DKA.

If you have not stopped taking your insulin, the other major cause of

DKA is that you need much more insulin than you did take. There are many temporary conditions that increase your need for insulin. The most common are illnesses like colds, upset stomach, or flu. (By the way, it's not likely that stress alone would increase your insulin requirement enough to cause DKA, unless you forgot doses of insulin.) More severe problems, such as pneumonia or a heart attack, can certainly tip a person with diabetes over into DKA.

Unfortunately, a common cause of DKA is the mistaken impression that when you are sick and not eating well, you should not take insulin. The opposite is often closer to the truth: illness *increases* your need for insulin, and omitting insulin during the stress of an illness can very easily lead to DKA.

What Are the Symptoms of DKA?

DKA can make you very sick and can even be fatal. What clues should you look for that suggest you may have DKA? First, the blood sugar will be high. You will in all likelihood feel the symptoms of thirst, frequent urination, and fatigue. Second, ketones make you feel nauseous and usually cause vomiting. Finally, DKA can progress to the point that you are virtually bedridden with fatigue, dehydration, and all-over illness.

A more specific sign of DKA is called air hunger (or Kussmaul respiration). Breathing hard (as you would after strenuous exercise) is the body's way of getting rid of excess acid. The person with DKA, then, will tend to breathe deeply and rapidly, just as if he or she had been exercising.

DKA can sneak up you. It can be mistaken for the flu, or it can be a complication of the flu or other illness. Especially if you have Type I diabetes, when you are feeling sick for whatever reason, check your blood sugar and test your urine ketones regularly—it could be DKA. A person with Type II diabetes should only get diabetic ketoacidosis under severe stress. But rather than thinking of DKA as only occurring in Type I diabetes, it is better to think of it as very badly undertreated diabetes of either type. If your blood sugar is up, you're not feeling well, and you're spilling ketones in your urine, be sure to take your insulin, consider adding some extra Regular, and contact your health care professional if things do not improve soon.

How Is DKA Treated?

DKA is treated under medical supervision, usually in a hospital. The basic elements of treatment are simple enough: provide insulin, replace fluids, and check that the electrolytes (especially potassium) do not fall too low. The doctor will probably want to start an intravenous feeding line, because each of these parts of treatment has to be carefully monitored.

With proper medical attention, DKA is almost always successfully treated (the death rate is well below 5%). But without treatment, or if treatment is delayed much too long, it can be fatal.

Can DKA Be Prevented?

DKA can definitely be prevented. In fact, we consider DKA to be the result of a major breakdown in routine diabetes care. At least in theory, there is no reason for anyone to develop DKA, although there are some people with unusual insulin resistance or unusual lability who, regardless of everyone's best efforts, develop DKA.

Simply put, good self-care is the key to prevention. Check blood sugar regularly, more often when you are sick. Take insulin regularly, even when you are sick. Have the sticks available to check urine ketones, especially when you are sick. And act on the results: when the sugar is up, if you take insulin, you will need more. Take extra Regular insulin or lispro insulin, which will be the fastest acting, and test again in one to two hours. How much insulin to take depends on your own situation, but it is a reasonable estimate to take as much as 10% of your usual daily requirement every two hours until your blood sugars start to come back down.

If you do have an episode of DKA, it would be worthwhile to think over how it happened so you can avoid it the next time. Did something happen that caused you to take no insulin for a period of time? Did you not realize until too late that you had a bad bottle of insulin? Did you not increase your insulin enough when you had another stress, such as the flu? Asking yourself these hard questions will help you prevent DKA from happening again.

Hyperosmolar Coma

Hyperosmolar coma means "coma due to too thick blood." You can see for yourself what this means by pouring syrup into a glass of water until the water visibly thickens. This is what happens in hyperosmolar coma: the blood sugar goes up so much that the blood is actually thicker, or hyperosmolar.

How high do blood sugars go? In hyperosmolar coma, the sugar level is almost always over 1,000 mg/dl and can actually reach 1,500 or 2,000 mg/dl. As the blood sugar goes up, the person urinates frequently and becomes dehydrated. A vicious cycle is set up in which the blood sugar goes up, dehydration follows, and that increases the blood sugar still more. In fact, many conditions, such as fever, severe burns, or too many diuretic pills, can contribute to hyperosmolar coma.

Who is at risk for hyperosmolar coma? Hyperosmolar coma most often occurs in people who have Type II diabetes. In Type I diabetes, DKA develops well before blood glucose rises to that astronomical level of over 1,000 mg/dl.

Hyperosmolar coma is a medical emergency, fatal if not promptly treated in a hospital. Because dehydration is such a central part of the problem, large amounts intravenous fluids have to be given along with insulin.

Prevention of hyperosmolar coma depends on catching it before it becomes severe. Taking even basic measures, such as increasing water intake and treating a rising blood sugar with insulin, is usually enough.

Chapter 24

Hardening of the Arteries

- *"I had a heart attack at a pretty young age—I was just 55. My doctor said it was due to diabetes. But I thought that was something that happens to much older men."*

- *"My teenager has diabetes, and everyone keeps talking about foot care and cholesterol in the arteries. I don't understand whether this is really a problem for him or when it will happen."*

Hardening of the arteries (*arteriosclerosis,* also called *atherosclerosis*) results when fat deposits, or plaques of cholesterol, develop within the walls of arteries. The best analogy for arteriosclerosis is rust building up inside a pipe. Like rust in a pipe, hardening of the arteries is commonly associated with aging and can cause blockage, with all sorts of consequences. If the artery is partially blocked, the blood flow getting through may be marginal; if it is blocked entirely, then no blood gets through. In this chapter, we will talk about what causes hardening of the arteries and how best to prevent it. We will discuss which parts of the body are most often affected, the symptoms, and the effect. Finally, we will describe what can be done about arteriosclerosis when it does occur.

Risk Factors for Arteriosclerosis

It is becoming increasingly clear that the causes of hardening of the arteries are more complicated than just the amount of cholesterol in blood. Taken together, the things that increase your chance of having hardening of the arteries are called risk factors. Having a risk factor for a problem doesn't mean that you will get the problem, but it does mean that you have an increased *chance* of getting it.

There are five major risk factors for arteriosclerosis, most of which you probably know about: high LDL cholesterol (or low HDL cholesterol and high triglyceride) levels, untreated high blood pressure, smoking, poorly treated diabetes, and a family history of heart disease (coronary artery disease) at a young age. Aging and menopause also increase the risk. The risk factors are additive, meaning that the more of these risk factors you have, the more likely you are to develop arteriosclerosis at a young age, and the fewer you have, the less likely you are to have the problem.

High LDL Cholesterol (Hypercholesterolemia or Hyperlipidemia)

It's easy for a doctor to check the levels of blood cholesterol and other blood lipids (fats). The results can be confusing, however. Total cholesterol is the total amount of cholesterol in your blood. It can be subdivided (broken down or fractionated) in a lipid profile into LDL cholesterol, and HDL cholesterol. The LDL cholesterol is called "bad cholesterol," since it is the fraction of total cholesterol that when elevated (for example over 160 mg/dl) increases the risk of arteriosclerosis. HDL cholesterol, or "good cholesterol," on the other hand, actually protects you from hardening of the arteries. High levels of this kind of cholesterol (over 60 mg/dl) decrease your chances of developing heart disease, foot problems, and stroke; low levels of HDL cholesterol (under 32 mg/dl) increase your risk.

Finally, there's the triglyceride part of the lipid profile. There is still some debate about how important high triglyceride levels are, but most experts think that high levels do increase the risk of heart disease in diabetes. Furthermore, very high levels can increase the risk of pancreatitis. People with high triglyceride also often have low HDL cholesterol.

A national panel published recommendations for each of the blood lipid levels (Table 15). As you see, the recommended level depends on how many other risk factors you have.

The total cholesterol can be accurately measured whether or not you have eaten before the test, although lipid fractionation must be done after fasting for at least 12 hours. The first step in treating abnormal lipids is always a good cholesterol-lowering diet, such as the Step Two diet recommended by the American Heart Association. If this doesn't work, effective pills are available.

Untreated High Blood Pressure (Hypertension)

Blood pressure, like blood sugar, is one of those measurements that changes from minute to minute. Also like blood sugar, it is hard to measure blood

Table 15. Coronary Artery Disease: Evaluating Your Risk and Choosing Your Treatment

Evaluating your risk:

You are at *very high risk* if you have *already been diagnosed* with coronary artery disease (heart attack or agina), stroke or TIA, or poor circulation to the feet (peripheral vascular disease).

You are at *high risk* if you have diabetes and *one* or more of the following risk factors:
    You are a man over 45 years old
    You are a woman over 55 years old
    You smoke cigarettes
    You have, or have been treated for, high blood pressure
    Your HDL cholesterol is lower than 35 mg/dl
    Your father or a brother had a heart attack before the age of 55
    Your mother or a sister had a heart attack before the age of 65

You are *low risk* if you have *none* of the above risk factors in addition to having diabetes. If your HDL cholesterol is over 60, you are at *low risk* unless *two* of the above risk factors are present in addition to diabetes.

Choosing your treatment:

Based on your LDL cholesterol values and whether you are at low, high, or very high risk, you and your doctor should consider treatment according to the following guidelines:

If your risk is:	Consider *dietary treatment* when LDL cholesterol is greater than:	Consider *pharmacologic* (pill) treatment when, after dieting, LDL cholesterol is greater than:
Low	160	190–220
High	130	160
Very High	100	100

NOTE: To complete this evaluation, you need to know your blood lipid levels of LDL cholesterol and HDL cholesterol.
SOURCE: Recommendations of the National Cholesterol Education Program, published in *JAMA* 269 (1993): 3015.

pressure continuously. So when you go to your doctor's office, a single high reading may be due only to your momentary stress from being in the doctor's examining room (white coat hypertension). But a high reading should be rechecked so that persistent high blood pressure is not missed or minimized.

Hypertension is a very strong risk factor for hardening of the arteries, eye disease, and kidney damage.

As with high cholesterol, diet is the first step in treatment of hypertension. The mainstay of dietary treatment for high blood pressure is to cut down on salt intake. Weight control and exercise are also very effective. If these measures do not work, then oral medications may be indicated. A number of classes of pills are available. The thiazide pills (for example, Hydrodiuril) are often used, but they can worsen your diabetic control. Likewise, the beta blockers may slow your pancreas from putting out insulin and may decrease your awareness of insulin reactions.

A recent study found that the so-called ACE inhibitors are effective not only in controlling blood pressure but also in slowing the progression of kidney disease. The ACE inhibitors are generally recommended now to control high blood pressure in diabetes, especially for people who have some evidence of kidney disease, such as protein in the urine. Sometimes a dry cough is a disturbing side effect.

Smoking

Long known to cause lung cancer, cigarette smoking is now known to increase the risk of heart disease. Obviously, the best approach is to avoid smoking in the first place. Quitting is difficult, to say the least. Also, people have a strong tendency to gain weight when they first quit. But even in people with Type II diabetes, who often have a weight problem, the health benefits of stopping smoking far outweigh the effects of weight gain. The effect of smoking on risk of heart disease disappears within a few years of quitting. So put "quit smoking" high on your "to do" list if you have diabetes.

Diabetes

High blood sugar definitely increases the risk of arteriosclerosis. Poorly controlled diabetes also increases the chance that your lipid levels will be abnormal. There is as yet no definite proof that good diabetic control itself lessens your chance of developing early hardening of the arteries, but the evidence that does exist all points in that direction. Certainly, if you practice diabetes self-care in the broadest sense—improving your diet, exercising, and watching for other risk factors—you will considerably reduce your chances of developing early or accelerated arteriosclerosis.

Family History

This is the one risk factor that is out of your control—you cannot pick your parents. But you should be especially mindful of the need to reduce your other risk factors if your father or brother has had significant hardening of the arteries before the age of 55 or your mother or sister before age 65.

Heart Disease, Peripheral Vascular Disease, and Cerebrovascular Disease

The three major areas most often affected by hardening of the arteries are the blood vessels supplying the heart, the legs, and the brain. Heart disease—angina pectoris and heart attacks—is the most common of these problems.

Heart Disease

To understand heart disease, you have to understand something about the heart. It is a large muscle that pumps the blood around the body. Like all muscles, it has its own arteries that provide it with a blood supply. These arteries are called coronary arteries, and they are essential to the function of the heart as an effective pump. When a coronary artery is blocked, unless there is an alternate supply of blood for the part of the heart normally supplied by that artery, some heart tissue dies. And coronary arteries are often partially or completely blocked by arteriosclerosis (Figure 22).

Think of a rural county where a town depends on supplies trucked in on a single road. If a storm comes along and destroys that road, unless alternative supply lines can be opened up, the town goes without supplies. The amount of damage done would depend on how big the town is and how long it is left without supplies. But unless supplies are restored quickly, there would be pain and damage in the town.

When a coronary artery is partly blocked, enough blood may get through to keep the heart beating normally when the person is at rest. But when the heart has to pick up its speed—for example, during exercise—this partly blocked artery can't open up enough to let an adequate amount of blood through. The symptom produced by this marginal blood flow is chest pain on exercise, called *angina pectoris*. This pain is usually quite characteristic: when you walk quickly, carry groceries, or even become very emotional, a deep, tight pain develops in your chest, jaw, or left arm. It goes away as soon as you stop the exercise and calm down—in other words, when your heart rate returns to normal. There are many less typical forms of angina, so if chest

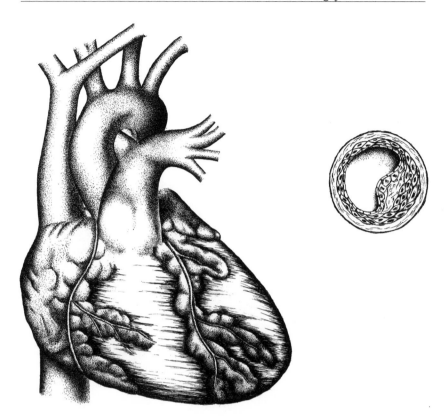

Figure 22. The heart is a big muscular pump that needs a supply of blood itself to remain healthy. The coronary arteries (circled) perform this function. If they become clogged (enlarged view), then they cannot perform this function as well. If the artery becomes completely occluded, then the heart muscle will be injured—a heart attack.

pain develops, you should definitely see a doctor to find out if it is cardiac pain or not.

If a coronary artery, large or small, becomes completely blocked (usually by a small blood clot on top of a plaque), it will cause some of the heart tissue to die. This is called a heart attack or *myocardial infarction.* The chief symptom is usually an angina-like pain that does not go away even with rest. If the area affected is big, the heart attack is severe; if a small artery is affected, the heart attack is mild.

Whether the heart attack is mild or severe, the outcome depends mainly on how quickly it is treated. Doctors these days are using drugs that break up blood clots and reduce the blockage, and they monitor patients carefully to see that any dangerous irregularity of the heart is promptly treated. These treatments are more successful if the person is seen by medical professionals within an hour after symptoms begin. Since early treatment significantly affects outcome, any persistent chest pain (pain lasting over about 15 minutes), especially if accompanied by sweating, faintness, or pain to the left arm, should be evaluated by a doctor *immediately*.

In addition to the immediate medical treatment of heart attacks, which is usually very successful, surgical procedures are often done. In one technique, called a *coronary angioplasty*, the inside of a blocked artery is essentially reamed out. More commonly, the blocked area can be bypassed by putting in some new vessels during coronary bypass surgery. One recent trial found that bypass surgery is more effective than angioplasty in people with diabetes. Given modern care, people can live long, productive lives after suffering a heart attack.

Hardening of the Arteries in the Legs (Peripheral Vascular Disease)

Just as arteriosclerosis can affect coronary arteries, it can also affect the long arteries going to the feet. The symptoms are somewhat similar. When the leg vessels are partially blocked, enough blood gets through except during increased exercise of the leg muscles. During such exercise as walking briskly, the muscles (usually of the calf or thighs) don't get enough blood, and they hurt. This is called *claudication*. As with angina, the pain (usually a cramping of the calf) stops soon after the person stops exercising.

Complete blockage of an artery in the leg can cause gangrene. In fact, this does not happen very often, partly because other arteries usually bypass the block. More often a foot gets into serious trouble when some degree of vessel blockage coexists with severe nerve damage and trauma to the foot causes a break in the skin, allowing infection to set in (see Chapter 28).

As with the coronary arteries, there are several surgical approaches to correcting severe blockage in a leg artery. The angioplasty procedure can be done, to ream out the middle of the artery, or an artificial artery can be put in place to bypass the blocked one.

Hardening of the Arteries to the Brain (Cerebrovascular Disease)

Essentially the same problem that takes place in the heart and the legs can happen to arteries supplying blood to the brain. Again, mild symptoms may appear with partial blockage, before any complete blockage occurs. In medical terms, the symptoms of partial blockage are called *transient ischemic attacks (TIAs)*.

The symptoms of partial blockage usually include temporary neurologic problems, such as a numb arm or loss of ability to speak clearly. They last only a matter of minutes, but they usually recur. Complete blockage of an artery to some part of the brain causes a stroke: a particular part of the brain is starved of blood and dies. (There are several other causes of strokes that are not specifically related to diabetes or to arteriosclerosis, such as hemorrhage into the brain or the blocking of an artery due to a blood clot traveling from the heart, called an *embolism*.)

A disturbing and essentially untreatable condition may develop when many arteries in the brain, large and small, are partially blocked by hardening of the arteries. This problem, called *diffuse cerebral arteriosclerosis,* can cause a gradual decline in mental function or even multiple small strokes without any one blockage being identified. It is one cause of senility or gradual falling off in ability to function.

A surgical endarterectomy can clear a partially blocked artery in the neck (the carotid artery) if a block located there is causing TIAs. It is not possible, however, to bypass arteries that are actually in the brain.

Hardening of the arteries, or arteriosclerosis, is a common feature of aging, occurring to some extent in everyone. Diabetes is one of the five major risk factors that increase the rate of progression of arteriosclerosis. To reduce your chances of developing accelerated or early hardening of the arteries, you should not only work to control your diabetes but also be very aware of your cholesterol level and your blood pressure. And you should definitely stop smoking.

If blockage of the arteries becomes severe, it can cause angina or a heart attack, claudication or gangrene in the feet, and TIAs or a stroke. But in each case there are preventive approaches that will significantly reduce your chance of developing these problems. There are also medical and surgical approaches that can often help correct the problem if it exists.

Chapter 25

Diabetic Eye Disease

- *"Ophthalmologists, lasers, surgery, hemorrhages, yellow dyes. I don't get it. I don't have problems with my vision, and I don't understand why I should keep seeing eye doctors unless I do have problems."*

- *"When my doctor said she saw some diabetes in my eyes, my heart just sank. The thing I dread most about diabetes is going blind. I just don't think I could stand that."*

Diabetic eye disease is among the most feared long-term complications of diabetes, and for good reason. Over the years it has been the most common cause of blindness in adults, and even today many people with diabetes require treatment for the effects of diabetes in the eye. But the subject also suffers from far too much misinformation.

To begin with, visual impairment is *not* inevitable. Diabetic eye disease is *not* untreatable. Found early and treated properly, most diabetic retinopathy never causes impairment of vision.

Understanding how diabetes affects the eyes and what to do about it is not that complicated (unless you get to the level of basic cause, which remains obscure even to researchers). A little knowledge can put you on the right track to avoid visual impairment in your lifetime of diabetes.

How the Eye Works

The eye is a wonderful little organ that works in amazing ways. Figure 23 shows the anatomy of the eye. The basic idea is to focus an image of something you're looking at (say, an eye chart) on one spot on the back of the eye. The "photographic plate" that picks up the image and transmits it to the brain is called the *retina*.

To get an image focused properly on the retina, the image passes first through the outermost clear cover (called the *cornea*) over the pupil. It then

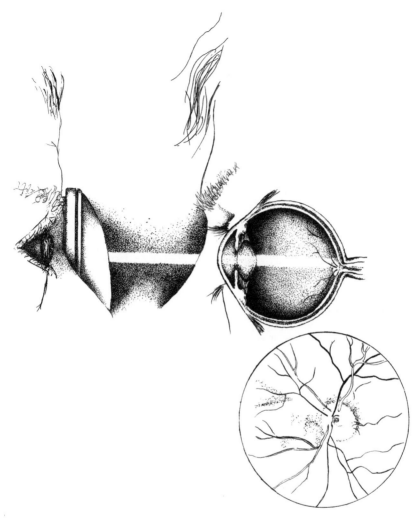

Figure 23. You can't see retinopathy on the outside of the eye, so the ophthalmologist must look through the dilated pupil to the back of the eye to get a look. There, he or she carefully examines the tiny veins and arteries for hemorrhages, outpouchings, or other abnormalities.

goes through the *pupil* (the black spot in the middle of the eye that is really a hole in the *iris*, which is the colored part of the eye). Inside the eye, the image is focused by the *lens*. The lens is a common spot for problems to occur, though not usually due to diabetes. If the lens is not strong enough to focus the image all the way to the back of the eye, it may need help in the form of a contact lens or glasses. If the lens gets cloudy, like fog on your glasses, the image can't get through it clearly. This is called a *cataract,* and it may require surgery to replace your natural lens with a lens implant. If there is too much pressure in this whole front part of the eyeball, like overfilling a tire, the condition is called *glaucoma* and definitely requires medical treatment.

After passing through the lens for focusing, the image crosses through the eye's normal gel (the *vitreous*), whose purpose is to keep the eyeball spherical, like air in a soccer ball.

Finally, if all systems are working and all these layers are clear, the image is focused on the retina—but not just anywhere on the retina. The image needs to hit exactly on one tiny area called the *macula,* which is especially rich in nerves and is the spot that gives you focused vision. The rest of the retina, lining the whole back of the eye, is used only for peripheral vision—to allow you to see things "out of the corner of your eye." By far the most important spot is the macula. If the image reaches the macula unimpaired, you have good, focused vision; if not, you won't focus well.

What Happens in Diabetes?

You and your eye physician want most to avoid severe bleeding into the vitreous gel. As you can imagine, if blood pours into this part of the eye, no image will get through to the retina. But bleeding into the vitreous doesn't just happen: it is the end result of a buildup of diabetic retinopathy that occurs over many years.

The first sign of any diabetes in the eyes is almost always what is called *background retinopathy.* It usually starts after 5–10 years of diabetes, is extremely common in people with diabetes, and is usually not dangerous in itself. To determine whether you have background retinopathy, the doctor will dilate the pupil with drops (to use a common analogy, if the doctor doesn't dilate the pupil, he or she is trying to see a whole room through a keyhole, and it cannot be considered a complete diabetes eye exam). Background retinopathy is seen as little red spots on the retina called *microaneurysms,* larger smudges called *micro hemorrhages,* or yellowish deposits called *exudates.* Do not be alarmed if the doctor comments on some "spots" or "small hemorrhages," or "diabetes in the eye." Background retinopathy occurs in about 50% of people after 7 years of diabetes, and in 90% after 15 years.

The presence of background retinopathy alone is not a big concern. It does not cause any symptoms unless some fluid accumulates in that special area of focus called the macula (a condition called *macular edema*), in which case treatment would be considered. However, the main concern, and the primary reason background retinopathy should be watched closely, is that it can progress to the next stage, called *proliferative retinopathy.*

In proliferative retinopathy, tiny new blood vessels form, which are fragile and liable to break and bleed. These new blood vessels are the culprits that can lead to visual impairment by bleeding into the vitreous.

When a major vitreous bleed occurs, it causes loss of vision in that eye within a matter of hours as blood fills up the vitreous. Often the blood will drain out of the eye over a few weeks or months, and vision will return. The bleeding can recur, though, and scars and clots can form that will actually pull the retina out of place, off the back of the eyeball *(retinal detachment).*

Detecting Diabetic Eye Disease: The Eye Examination

We mentioned that early stages of diabetic eye involvement usually don't produce symptoms, but it is extremely important to follow diabetic eye disease so that treatment can be started at the right time. There is no way for you to know the status of your eyes unless a qualified eye doctor examines them. Two questions arise at this point, neither of them easy to answer: who is a qualified doctor? How often should you be examined?

A qualified doctor is one who does this often and is used to looking for the subtle changes of proliferative retinopathy that signal trouble. We mentioned that a good exam must be done with a dilated pupil (which is accomplished by putting in the drops that sting for a moment and make your vision blurred for several hours). Ophthalmologists (medical doctors who specialize in eye disease) are generally well trained to detect retinopathy and decide whether the eye has reached the stage where it requires laser photocoagulation (see below). Few other doctors, with the possible exception of diabetologists, are well qualified to detect diabetes in the eye.

Some optometrists (non-M.D.'s) are competent to examine a dilated eye for diabetic retinopathy, although their main work is assessing eyes for glasses or contact lenses. General internists and family practitioners are usually much less experienced at detecting retinopathy, and other medical specialists usually are not trained to do such exams.

How often should you be examined? The standard recommendation is annually for people who have had Type I diabetes for more than five years and for everyone with Type II diabetes, since the onset of Type II is less accurately dated.

A *fluorescein angiography* is used to detect any leaking vessels. The ophthalmologist (or assistant) injects a yellow dye into a vein in your arm and takes pictures of your retina in rapid sequence. The dye makes some people nauseous for a few minutes and always turns the urine a bright orange/yellow.

The key point to remember is that diabetic eye disease is treatable if caught at the right time. The whole point of having regular eye exams performed by an expert is to pick up the changes at a stage where diabetic retinopathy can be successfully treated, before major bleeding occurs.

Treating Diabetic Eye Disease

Photocoagulation

In laser photocoagulation, a laser beam is used to coagulate the fragile new vessels in the eye that cause vitreous bleeding. Laser beams are used because they can be very finely focused and accurately aimed. Since the early 1970s laser beams have been used to treat many types of eye problems, including those due to diabetes.

When laser therapy is done, the doctor dilates the pupil and numbs the surface of the eye with drops. A beam of light is then focused on a particular spot of the retina and the laser burn is placed using a foot pedal. The doctor then moves to another spot on the retina and does it again. Hundreds of little spots, or burns, are placed on the retina in one sitting, but even so you may need to come back for more.

There are generally two patterns of laser treatment for diabetic eye disease. In *pan-retinal photocoagulation,* the doctor places laser therapy in a pattern throughout most of the retina, *except for the macular area.* If you think about it, the macula (which is where the focused image comes) is the very spot that the ophthalmologist wants to *protect,* not touch with a laser burn. And indeed, the pattern of photocoagulation is applied with the goal of touching the rest of the retina, but not the macula. The second pattern of laser treatment is called *focal photocoagulation* and is used to touch up just a few leaking spots that have caused macular edema.

Does laser therapy hurt?   Most people report no pain or only minor discomfort with laser photocoagulation, although sometimes it does seem to "hit a nerve." If the procedure is painful, the doctor can put a local anesthetic in the back of the eye, much as a dentist uses Novocain. Fairly often, there will be some aching after the treatment.

How does laser therapy work?   Interestingly, the answer to this question is not all that clear. The first thought would be that the doctor is burning out the fragile little blood vessels that cause the bleeding, essentially clotting them off. But there seem to be other effects of laser photocoagulation that reduce new vessel formation.

Does laser therapy work? There is no doubt about the effectiveness of laser photocoagulation. Several large, well-conducted studies have shown that laser photocoagulation works and that its benefit is lasting. If done at the right time, the treatment will reduce the rate of severe visual loss by as much as 90% and possibly more. This treatment is worth taking advantage of, and it is the main reason why every person with diabetes should have eye exams as recommended.

Vitrectomy

Vitrectomy is a surgical procedure in which the gel of the eye (the vitreous) is removed and replaced with a clear solution. It is done only when there has been repeated bleeding in the vitreous and vision is cut off by scars or other debris that block transmission of the image though what should be clear gel.

Since it is only done after vitreous bleeding has occurred, vitrectomy should be thought of as a last-ditch effort to save vision in an eye that is not otherwise likely to be useful. Its success rate varies considerably depending on the amount of damage that has already occurred and whether vitreous bleeding recurs after the vitrectomy.

Prevention of Diabetic Eye Disease

The Diabetes Control and Complications Trial has been mentioned many times in this book. It is especially relevant to a discussion of eye disease, however, because the main point of the DCCT was to prevent retinopathy and the most significant finding was that intensive treatment of diabetes can in fact prevent retinopathy.

The DCCT showed that intensive control of diabetes reduces the incidence of new retinopathy both when none exists to begin with and when there is already some eye involvement at the start. This finding has practical implications. It means that treating diabetes well, keeping the blood sugar in a good range, is effective not only early in the course of diabetes but also later on. Even when you are diagnosed as having diabetic retinopathy, it is not too late. Your chances of maintaining good vision are considerably improved if you control your diabetes well.

There is evidence that stopping smoking and controlling blood pressure also improve your chances for avoiding visual loss. Finding out about and treating other eye conditions, particularly glaucoma, is very important to maintaining good vision.

There are two important steps you can take to prevent diabetic eye disease: control your blood sugar well throughout your life with diabetes and have regular eye exams performed by an expert in the field. With these two measures, there is every reason to think that there will be many, many fewer cases of visual impairment from diabetes.

Chapter 26

Diabetic Kidney Disease

- *"What's the relationship between the kidneys, high blood pressure, and swelling in the ankles?"*
- *"I was told that I have protein in my urine. What is the significance of that, and can I do something about it?"*
- *"What is involved with dialysis? Different people I've heard of seem to do it completely differently."*

The Diabetes Control and Complications Trial proved that intensive blood sugar control greatly reduces the incidence of diabetic kidney disease, as well as its progression in people who already have it. But most people with diabetes never develop diabetic kidney disease. No more than about one-third of people with Type I diabetes ever show a sign of kidney involvement, no matter how long they live, and a recent study even found that as few as 9% of Scandinavians with Type I diabetes developed kidney disease.

You may never face the problem of diabetic kidney disease, called *diabetic nephropathy,* but it is a possible long-term serious complication of diabetes. There are steps you can take to improve your chances of avoiding this complication or of controlling it if you already have it.

The Kidneys

A major role of the kidneys is to clean the blood of waste products. As the blood circulates through the body, it flows through the kidneys, which consist of millions of little filters, like the paper filters in a coffee machine. The filters clean the waste products from the "dirty" blood into the urine, with the "cleaned" blood circulating back into the bloodstream.

Another crucial role of the kidneys is to regulate the salt and water balance of the body. Our normal body fluids are just about as salty as seawater. We drink fresh water and we eat salt, and the kidneys have the job of making sure that our body fluids maintain just the right volume of water and concentration of salt. They either spill out excess salt and water or conserve them, to get the balance just right. Kidneys are especially sensitive to fluid volume. You can check this out for yourself: drink a big bottle of water very quickly, and presto! the kidneys will get rid of it by producing a large volume of diluted urine.

By controlling the water and salt content of the body, the kidneys also have a key role to play in regulating blood pressure. If a person retains salt and fluid, the blood vessels become overfilled, like the pressure in an overfilled balloon. This is called high blood pressure, or hypertension. On the other hand, when the vessels are seriously underfilled—for instance, when someone loses a lot of blood—blood pressure may fall dangerously low, and the person may go into shock. Well-functioning kidneys keep the fluid level and blood pressure normal.

What Goes Wrong with the Kidneys in Diabetes?

Kidney damage due to diabetes is classified along with diabetic eye disease as a *microvascular,* or small blood vessel, complication of diabetes. In diabetic nephropathy, the little filters of the kidneys (called *nephrons*) develop thickened borders and eventually clog up entirely. If this is going to happen, it probably starts within the first 10 years of getting diabetes. But we don't know about it until later because we can't see the kidneys as easily as we can see the retina of the eye. (To look at the filters of the kidneys under a microscope, it's necessary to perform a kidney biopsy, which is not a common procedure.)

The first clue that diabetic nephropathy is developing is usually the appearance of protein in the urine (called *proteinuria*). Proteinuria means that the kidneys' filtering system has become leaky. It's as if the same paper coffee filter has been used over and over again, eventually developing holes and letting the coffee grounds fall through. Instead of coffee grounds, however, the kidneys leak protein.

There are several different ways to test for protein in the urine (Table 16), all of them using a urine sample. The *least sensitive* but the *easiest* test is to dip a reagent stick into a urine sample. Significant protein in the urine will change the color of the stick. The *most sensitive* is a test for *microalbuminuria,* in which even tiny amounts of the protein albumin in urine can be measured. This can be done on a "random sample" (which means that you urinate into a cup without worrying about the time the urine was collected). The *most accurate* assessment is a timed sample. You collect in a bottle all the urine you make for

Table 16.   Tests for Protein in the Urine

Test Name	Sample Collection	Normal Values[a]
"Dipstick"	random urine sample	negative
Microalbumin	random urine sample	less than 20 mg/gm creatinine
24-hour microalbumin	24-hour urine collection	less than 30 mg/24 hours
24-hour protein	24-hour urine collection	less than 150 mg/24 hours
Creatinine clearance	14-hour urine collection	more than 100 cc/minute

[a]Normal values will be different for different laboratories. The figures used here are estimates.

some fixed period, usually 24 hours. The timed sample measures the total amount of albumin or the total amount of protein put out in the 24-hour period. This test also provides a very good idea of how the kidneys are working by measuring what is known as *creatinine clearance* (see below). Exercising during the period when a timed sample of urine is being collected may cause some protein to be jarred through the kidneys into the urine without any abnormality at all, so it's a good idea to avoid exercise during a timed sample.

Significant amounts of protein in the urine, on repeated measurement, are abnormal. To understand the meaning of a urine protein result, a few rules of thumb are helpful. If proteinuria is present on one sample but not on a repeat test, the finding may not be significant. The hallmark of diabetic nephropathy is *persistent proteinuria* (documented more than once), not just a single occurrence. A current bladder infection or a history of kidney disease independent of diabetes (some people have a condition called *nephritis* in childhood) may also cause elevated urinary protein. But when protein is found in the urine in two consecutive samples, and there is no other known cause, it usually does mean that diabetic nephropathy is occurring, and measures should be taken to slow or halt its progression.

Treating Diabetic Nephropathy

There are three general approaches to slowing the progress of nephropathy: blood pressure control, blood sugar control, and diet.

Blood Pressure Control

We mentioned that kidney problems can cause high blood pressure (hypertension). But the opposite can also happen: high blood pressure may worsen kidney problems. So the single most important thing you can do to slow the progress of kidney disease is to interrupt this vicious cycle of high blood pressure and kidney damage by controlling your blood pressure.

What is normal blood pressure? You would think, after all these years of study, that we would have an easy answer, but we don't. The usual figure quoted is under 140/80. (The first, higher, number in blood pressure is called *systolic,* and the second, lower, number is called *diastolic.* When taking a blood pressure reading, the systolic number is the reading when you begin to hear the pulse sounds; the diastolic reading is when you stop hearing them.) If your systolic pressure is under 140 mm and your diastolic pressure is under 80 mm, there's usually no need to worry.

Many people think that when it comes to blood pressure, the lower the better. In fact, the only concern about blood pressure being too low is if you become dizzy as you stand up or go about your regular daily activities. Called *orthostasis,* and sometimes caused by neuropathy, this is a condition when blood pressure may in fact be too low, with not enough blood getting to your head. Otherwise, if your systolic blood pressure is, say, 110–130 and your diastolic is 60–80, that's probably fine.

You may have heard about the *ACE inhibitors,* used to treat high blood pressure and kidney disease in diabetes. *ACE* stands for *angiotensin-converting enzyme.* There are several ACE inhibitors, each with different side effects and different durations of action. A common one, captopril, is taken three times daily (it often causes a dry cough); others, such as lisinopril and enalopril, are longer acting and can be taken once a day.

This class of medications blocks a key chemical reaction in the kidneys' control of blood pressure—a reaction that is often overactivated in diabetes, causing high blood pressure. A large research trial showed that if people with diabetes have proteinuria, they do better with ACE inhibitors than with other medications used to treat hypertension. In our practice, we recommend the use of ACE inhibitors as the first choice to treat high blood pressure, and we prescribe them when a person with diabetes has proteinuria even without hypertension. So far there's not enough evidence to indicate to us that they should be used when a person has neither hypertension nor proteinuria.

It is important to state that blood pressure, like blood sugar or heart rate, is not static: it doesn't just stay at one level minute to minute, hour to hour, day to day. As a person with diabetes, you are used to this concept, because you have seen your blood sugar levels bounce around. If you have hypertension, it makes sense to test it regularly, not to rely on one test at the doctor's office.

You've probably heard the term *white coat hypertension,* referring to the fact that a visit to your health care professional can temporarily raise your blood pressure. (We prefer to blame it on the traffic, but whatever . . .) White coat hypertension really does happen to some people, but sometimes it's just an excuse for ignoring high blood pressure. To find out, you have to check your blood pressure repeatedly at other times. Ask a nurse at your workplace or a well-trained family member. You may want to learn to do it yourself, possibly with an automatic device you can use at home. *Do not ignore high blood pressure,* especially if you have diabetic nephropathy.

Blood Sugar Control

Throughout this book, we have provided lots of reasons for controlling blood sugar. Avoiding or slowing diabetic kidney disease is another good reason. We aren't sure exactly how uncontrolled diabetes causes kidney damage—theories abound—but we are sure that it does. One study found that an average glycohemoglobin over 8% (when normal is under 6%) caused kidney disease, while under 8% was "safe." The DCCT found that the lower the average sugar, the better. It also showed that there was no special "danger" point. We believe that your blood sugar control should be as good as you can make it.

High blood sugar affects the kidneys, like other parts of the body, over a long period of time. There is no reason to think that occasional episodes of hyperglycemia will have a serious effect. Rather, you should work on the averages, keeping your glucose control on average in as good a range as possible.

Diet

A basic part of blood pressure control is to cut down the amount of salt you eat each day. If you do have high blood pressure, it is especially important to learn where salt occurs in your diet and to avoid foods that have a high salt content.

A surprising research finding over the past decade or so is that a high-protein diet, which used to be considered the secret to strong muscles, may in fact be a hazard to the kidneys (and of no use to the muscles). The evidence is not complete, but most specialists recommend a relatively low-protein diet when a person develops proteinuria. Protein usually makes up about 15% of total calories in a balanced diet, but when kidney involvement is found, we recommend restricting it to about 10%–12% or less.

Kidney Failure

The progress of kidney damage can be hard to follow and hard to predict, at least until it is quite severe. Proteinuria may precede kidney failure by as long as 10–15 years or more, especially if a person follows the treatment approaches described above, and especially if the proteinuria is picked up early, as microalbuminuria.

Until kidney damage is severe, it's impossible to predict how soon complete kidney failure (called "end stage renal disease") will occur. We believe that everyone should know about kidney involvement in diabetes. Although most often it eventually proceeds to complete kidney failure, we do not agree with the approach that gloomily attempts to predict exactly when someone will need dialysis. We really don't know.

A test called the *creatinine clearance,* which involves collecting urine over a 24-hour period, provides a rough indication of kidney function. A creatinine clearance result of 100 ml per minute or more is about normal. A creatinine clearance of 50 ml per minute suggests that the kidneys are functioning at about 50% of normal. Symptoms are not likely to until occur until the rate is below about 20–30 ml per minute, and dialysis or transplantation is usually necessary when kidney function falls below about 10–15 ml per minute.

Nephropathy is largely a "silent" problem—one that does not make you feel ill. Its symptoms, when they do occur, occur very late. The first symptom may be ankle swelling, but don't panic if you have some ankle swelling: there are many causes, and some, such as premenstrual fluid retention, have nothing to do with diabetes. When kidney function becomes seriously impaired, the person develops anemia and feels constantly tired. This will progress to severe fatigue, itching, nausea, vomiting, and eventually less urine production. In that case, the kidneys are no longer filtering out the toxins, which are building up to dangerous levels in the blood. The lab tests used to measure the waste products in the blood are *blood urea nitrogen* (BUN)—sometimes measured as *serum urea nitrogen* (SUN)—and *serum creatinine.*

People with failing kidneys should be told what is happening and what their options are well before their kidneys fail completely. They should have a chance to think over what is involved with each of the options. There are two options. When end-stage renal disease is reached—in other words, when the kidneys are essentially nonfunctional—only dialysis or kidney transplantation is possible. Otherwise, kidney failure is fatal. One comfort to the person facing end-stage kidney disease is that under current law the person automatically qualifies for Medicare, which will pay for dialysis and transplantation. Without such coverage, these extraordinarily expensive therapies would be out of financial reach for almost everyone.

Kidney Dialysis

Dialysis is a life-saving approach that takes over the functions of the failed kidneys. It was introduced some 30 years ago as a treatment that makes it possible for a person to live with end-stage kidney disease. There are two ways to do dialysis: *hemodialysis* and *peritoneal dialysis*.

People receiving hemodialysis either go to a dialysis center several times a week or learn to do it with proper equipment at home. Either way, they are hooked up to a machine that takes the blood as it flows through an arm, runs it through a filtering apparatus, and returns it to the arm through another line. To make it easier for the blood to be drawn out of the arm and returned to the arm, a "shunt" is surgically placed in the forearm before the first dialysis treatment. The shunt is a large tube running from an artery in the arm to a vein. Beneath the surgical scar, a U-shaped lump is visible, which has a vibration that can be felt as blood rushes through the shunt.

People undergoing hemodialysis are usually not uncomfortable during the procedure. They sit in a special chair, reading or watching television, for a few hours. But they may feel below par for a while before dialysis, when the waste products have built up in the blood, and afterward, because the fluid shifts have been so abrupt. Anyone using hemodialysis must get it without fail. This treatment (in fact, any dialysis) requires a major and faithfully given commitment of time.

Peritoneal dialysis is done very differently. To start it, a tube is surgically placed through the skin into the abdominal cavity. This access line into the abdomen has to be kept very clean to prevent infection. With *chronic ambulatory peritoneal dialysis* (CAPD), a large amount of liquid is made to flow through the tubing into the abdomen, swelling it up. A few hours later, the fluid is drained out, drawing with it the blood's waste products. A different approach, called *continuous cyclic peritoneal dialysis* (CCPD), is somewhat more automated. Either way, with peritoneal dialysis there is no need to go to the dialysis center because you can do it yourself. It is not painful, but it does take time and a great deal of equipment (tubes, fluids, and so forth) stored in your home.

Most people do well on dialysis, often for many years. Because of the inconvenience, the chance of crises such as infections, and side effects such as disequilibrium after dialysis, many people look on it as an interim stage, hoping for a kidney transplant to provide a better solution.

Kidney Transplantation

Kidney transplants are now done routinely at large medical centers, but it is major surgery that requires careful postoperative care. Unfortunately, there are not enough healthy kidneys donated to transplant into all the people who need them.

A kidney that is to be transplanted is called a *donor* kidney; the person getting the donor kidney is the *recipient.* Donor kidneys have to be "matched" to the recipient to reduce the chance that the recipient's body will reject the new kidney. Matching is done by a series of tests, starting with the blood group (A, B, AB, or O) of the donor and the recipient.

On the whole, chances are a bit better if the donor is a close relative. Another reason why the related donor may be the best option is that the transplantation surgery can be planned electively rather than being dependent on finding a suitable donor and rushing the kidney to the recipient. Donating one kidney will not affect the long-term health of a normal donor. Not every family member is suitable as a donor, however: the match may not be close enough or the donor candidate may have some kidney problem that makes it dangerous to give up a kidney and dangerous for the recipient to receive a potentially damaged kidney.

There are several other medical reasons, as well as social reasons, why a relative may not be available as a donor. In fact, most kidney transplant recipients do not have a suitable living related donor. Instead, the donor kidney is removed when someone, somewhere, has been pronounced brain-dead as a result of a sudden, catastrophic accident, such as a motor vehicle accident, or a medical event, such as a severe brain hemorrhage. Organs are taken for donation only when people have no chance of surviving and are essentially dead.

We want to clear up some common misconceptions by stating that you absolutely are not risking your life when you sign your approval as a potential organ donor (for instance, on your driver's license). There is no way your organs could ever be used if there were any chance at all that you would survive. On the contrary, agreeing to be an organ donor assures that, if an exceedingly unlikely tragedy ever strikes you, parts of your body can at least provide life for someone else. Until more people sign on to be potential organ donors, there won't be enough donated organs to fill the need.

The system for identifying, analyzing, and transporting the donor organs is well organized. Donor organs are computer-matched with people waiting for transplants. The person most in need—and with the best chance to make good use of the organ—gets the call. A dramatic set of events then unfolds rapidly. The donor kidney is removed from the donor, rushed to the recipient's hospital as the recipient is made ready, and the new organ is transplanted to the recipient.

After the transplant comes the process of circumventing the body's normal rejection mechanism. That is, a normal body recognizes when a foreign organ is put in and tries to reject it, so the recipient must take *immunosuppressive* drugs to suppress the body's normal immune defenses against the donor organ. Complications often arise in the posttransplant period, such as episodes of rejection or infections. But when the urine begins to flow again and the person can say goodbye to the dialysis staff, this is a thrilling moment.

Combined Kidney-Pancreas Transplantation

At the same time that a kidney is transplanted, or in a later operation, it may be possible to transplant a pancreas also. In this surgery, a donor pancreas is placed surgically in the lower abdomen, with drains into the bladder. Since the working pancreas delivers insulin automatically, the successful pancreas transplantation in essence cures the diabetes.

Why, you will ask, don't we recommend pancreas transplantation to everyone, as soon as diabetes is diagnosed, regardless of whether a kidney transplant is needed? The reason is actually quite simple: the surgery required, the postoperative risks, the need to suppress the recipient's immune system, and the chance that the pancreas will ultimately fail make pancreas transplantation, as currently done, a worse risk than controlling diabetes by other means. Organ availability is another factor: there are not nearly enough pancreases available each year to provide for everyone with diabetes.

We understand that this is very disappointing for anyone who gets diabetes and wants the quicker, easier fix by transplanting a pancreas. But it is a fact that pancreas transplantation, for all the good it does in selected cases, does *not* provide an easy, safe alternative to treating diabetes conventionally. With the current state of the art, this procedure should be reserved for people who also need a kidney and therefore need immunosuppressive therapy anyway.

The future of islet cell transplantation, in which only the islet cells are transplanted, rather than the whole pancreas, is discussed in Chapter 33.

Diabetic kidney disease, like so many of the long-term complications of diabetes, presents real challenges. The best news is that in most cases of diabetes it will never develop, and when it does its progress can be slowed significantly. Protein in the urine is the first sign. Control of blood pressure (preferably with ACE inhibitors), control of blood sugar, and restriction of dietary protein are the best ways to slow the progress of kidney insufficiency. But if the kidneys do fail, dialysis can keep you going and a successful kidney transplant can give you a new start.

Chapter 27

Diabetic Neuropathy

- *"My feet feel funny—that's the only way I can describe it—but my doctor says it's just my nerves."*

- *"I rarely get an erection any more, and if I do, it doesn't last. I'm afraid my wife thinks I'm not interested in her, but I am."*

- *"Sometimes everything I eat just seems to stay in my stomach. I get bloated really quickly, feel nauseated all the time, and vomit. Forget blood sugar control at times like this—it's impossible."*

Nerve damage from diabetes is called *diabetic neuropathy*. The nervous system itself is extremely complex, and the symptoms of diabetic neuropathy can be distressing and baffling. In this chapter, we want to help you understand how the nervous system works, what can go wrong with it in diabetes, and what can be done to prevent or treat the nerve damage.

Diabetic neuropathy is another long-term complication of poorly controlled diabetes. A person with newly discovered Type II diabetes may already have neuropathy, but if so, the diabetes has most likely existed undetected for some years before the diagnosis. Neuropathy rarely develops before 10 or so years after the start of diabetes and sometimes later than that. One exception is when the high blood sugar itself causes the nerves to act up immediately, and then the person will feel better as soon as the blood sugar improves, whether or not there is any permanent damage to the nerves. It's important to distinguish this *acute* complication of high blood sugar from the *long-term* complication of diabetic neuropathy, because the acute complication will go away quickly with proper control of the blood sugar.

As with most long-term complications of diabetes, there is a lot yet to be discovered about exactly what causes diabetic neuropathy and how to prevent or reverse it. But there are thought to be two basic causes, each producing a very different kind of neuropathy. The most common kind of neuropathy is a gradual deterioration of the longest nerves, due to years of high blood sugar. The less common kind is due to sudden loss of blood supply to a segment of the nerve, like a mini-stroke outside the brain.

The Nervous System

Think of the body's nervous system as a massive telephone system, with each nerve being an individual line, all eventually joining one single large cable (the spine) leading to a switchboard (the brain) that is immeasurably more complex than any telephone switchboard. Each individual nerve has a cell body with a nucleus, usually located in the spine or brain, and then grows a long *axon,* like a single thread, that can extend all the way from the spine to the toe.

Every one of the billions of nerves outside the brain is specifically assigned either to incoming messages (in the case of sensory nerves) or to outgoing messages (the motor nerves). The sensory nerves convey to the brain messages about body temperature, position of a limb, pain, and so on. The motor nerves deliver messages from the brain to the muscles. These messages may instruct muscles to make large, conscious movements, like "throw the ball" or "press the piano keys in sequence." Other motor nerves control completely unconscious, automatic actions, commanding the body to do such things as "speed up the heart rate," "widen the pupils," "move material through the intestines," or "breathe." These are called *autonomic motor* nerves.

The messages normally run quickly and smoothly along nerves, and to function properly everything has to work just right. Let's say the incoming lines carry the following message: "This is my right hand, and I feel warm; my second finger is especially warm and—OW! it suddenly hurts like the devil!" The brain doesn't even need to get involved when this alarm goes off. The message turns right around in the spinal cord, and your body receives a command to move fast and pull that finger off the top of the stove with lightning speed.

Think what happens if the part of the message signaling pain never arrives—if the nerve bringing the incoming signal, the sensory nerve, is damaged. Damage could be done to the finger without the person even knowing it. Think also what could happen if the autonomic motor nerves didn't work right: the person's bowels might be underactive (constipation), sexual function might be affected, or the stomach might not move the food along properly into the intestines. These sorts of nerve defects can be a big problem in diabetic neuropathy.

The nervous system, then, consists of a complicated, delicate set of incoming and outgoing signals. Most often, it is the incoming sensory nerves that are affected by diabetes. If they are irritated, it is like static on the telephone line, drawing attention away from normal conversation. If the nerve is nonfunctional, like telephone lines that have been cut down by a storm, the signal never gets through at all. Furthermore, once cut, nerves grow back only very slowly. So it makes far better sense to prevent nerve damage in the first place than to count on regrowing dead nerves.

Recognizing and Living with Diabetic Neuropathies

Peripheral Symmetrical Polyneuropathy

Peripheral symmetrical polyneuropathy, generally called *peripheral neuropathy,* is the common diabetic nerve damage that occurs to some extent in many, perhaps most, people who have had poorly controlled diabetes for many years. It can be very mild or quite severe, causing no problem or many problems.

There are various theories about what causes the nerve damage. It may be due to swelling of the nerve cell or axon, caused by the accumulation of the sugar sorbitol, or it may be due to the accumulation of glycation end products, which are proteins essentially gummed up by sugar. Research is under way to find out whether blocking sorbitol accumulation by using drugs called *aldose reductase inhibitors* will prevent or delay the onset of neuropathy, and studies are also looking at whether blocking the glycation end products will affect nerve damage.

Since gradual nerve damage first affects the nerves with the longest axons, its most common targets are the parts of the body farthest away from the spine: the toes. This is why it is called *peripheral* neuropathy. But the same process can also affect the nerves that carry messages to the automatic functions of the body (autonomic nerves), in which case it is called *autonomic neuropathy* (see below). All these forms of neuropathy develop slowly and are especially hard to reverse since, as noted, damaged nerves grow back only very slowly.

Symptoms.   Peripheral neuropathy usually starts as numbness or tingling in the toes, progressing very gradually, over the years, up the ankle and leg. Sometimes the symptoms are barely noticeable and sometimes they are bothersome. Everyone describes the feelings differently: some people say it's like wearing thick-soled shoes, some report that they don't feel the movement of toes as well as they should, while others say that their feet feel too sensitive. Some people aren't even aware of any symptoms and are surprised when the doctor finds that their reflexes are not normal. Others report that even the feel of the bedsheets bothers them at night. The constant features of peripheral neuropathy are the location (almost always the toes and feet), the gradual onset, and the symmetry, since it usually occurs at least to some extent in both legs.

When peripheral neuropathy is severe, people experience either a great deal of discomfort or numbness. The painful stage usually doesn't last, as the feet become more and more numb. It is a blessing that the pain goes away, but if the numb foot is not well taken care of, it can be in great danger. Let's consider some examples.

> *Cheryl is 68 years old and for 10 years has known that she has diabetes, although she suspects that she has had it for much longer, since she was diabetic during her last pregnancy, gained a lot of weight in her 50s, and was unusually thirsty for many years. She began having real discomfort in her feet. At night she could hardly sleep, the pain was so bad. Even the sheets on the bed bothered her. The pain never really went away, although a combination of analgesics helped a little bit. After suffering for a long time, Cheryl went to her doctor and received proper therapy.*

There are several approaches to treating painful peripheral neuropathy like Cheryl's. The most effective are the medications amitriptyline or desipramine, which are also used to treat depression. When prescribed for peripheral neuropathy, these medications actually affect the nerves. Neuropathy is the result of structural damage to the nerves; psychological problems, which are every bit as real and serious as neuropathy, are not caused by nerve damage.

To treat painful peripheral neuropathy, a relatively high dose of amitriptyline or desipramine is prescribed, often 50–150 mg per day. The most common side effects include dry mouth and some drowsiness. Other medications for pain, often either carbamazepine (Tegratol) or phenytoin (Dilantin), are sometimes prescribed along with these drugs. A cream or ointment called capsaicin, composed of the ingredient that makes chili peppers hot, has been recommended, but it is hard to demonstrate whether the stinging effect that gradually deadens the nerve endings is actually effective. Finally, as mentioned, several new drugs are under development, such as the aldose reductase inhibitors and a blocker of end glycation products called aminoguanidine.

James has had Type II diabetes for more than 20 years and never thought much about it. He went to his doctor every now and then but did not follow a diet or exercise regimen. He certainly never pricked himself to do blood sugar monitoring (although he did have his own meter, which he never took out of the box). He was always a water drinker. At one point James began to notice a lack of sensation in his feet, but again he didn't think much about it. Later, he was alarmed to find that after wearing a pair of new shoes, he had developed a large ulcer on his big toe. It didn't hurt, but the doctor told him that the ulcer was due to peripheral neuropathy and that he had better treat it with great care.

When peripheral neuropathy causes the toes or feet to be numb, the danger is that they will be injured without the person even knowing it. A new pair of shoes, a longer-than-usual hike, stepping on something while going barefoot: all these are common causes of the skin damage that can cause injury or an ulcer, which can become infected and ultimately even require an amputation. (Diabetic foot problems are considered in more detail in Chapter 28.)

Lack of sensation is a danger. The nerves to the foot are there for good reason: they warn you about the pinching shoe, the pebble in the sock, or the tack you stepped on. When the nerves are damaged and you do not get that warning signal, you have to be very careful to take good care of the feet. We recall a patient who arrived home after work, took off his shoes, and found that his sock was bloody. It turned out his son's tiny metal toy had fallen into his shoe. Another patient of ours, as he put his shoes back on after an exam in the office, found a comb inside the shoe and stated matter-of-factly, "Oh, here it is—I lost that two days ago." Numb feet can be dangerous!

Autonomic Neuropathies

As we noted above, the autonomic nerves control all those nerve functions that you don't have to think about: your heart rate, your stomach and bowel function, breathing, sweating when overheated, the opening of your pupils in response to low light levels, and, in men, erections. Just like the peripheral nerves, the long nerves that regulate these unconscious activities can be affected by diabetes. In fact, it is unusual for a person to have significant autonomic nerve problems without also having at least some evidence of peripheral neuropathy. When you consider the number of different functions the autonomic nerves control, it is not surprising that many different problems can arise if these nerves are affected by diabetes.

Impotence. Male impotence is the most common of the autonomic neuropathies resulting from long-term diabetes. In males, achieving and holding an erection requires a complex series of interactions of the nerves and the circulatory system, and these interactions can be easily disrupted. There are many causes of male impotence, but if none of the others exists, it may well be due to diabetes. After many years of having inadequately controlled diabetes, a man's sexual function can deteriorate. In women, the ability to have orgasms may be diminished by decreased sensation in the genital area, often called female impotence. (Male and female sexuality, including treatment options for problems with function, are discussed in Chapter 30.)

Intestinal involvement (enteropathy). People with diabetic involvement of their intestines generally alternate bouts of diarrhea with periods of constipation. The diarrhea may occur especially after eating a meal and may become watery. It is not bloody, does not cause severe abdominal pain, and usually responds to simple over-the-counter antidiarrheal medications. Likewise, the constipation is usually not disabling and responds to cathartics, such as prunes, or over-the-counter laxatives.

Urinary retention. Sometimes the nerves to the urinary bladder stop functioning as well as they used to, and people retain some urine in their bladder even after voiding. If this problem is severe, the urine can back up to the kidneys, damaging kidney function. Often, the condition causes no symptoms until it reaches the point where the person is not able to void at all. If you have significant neuropathies elsewhere and seem to be voiding only small amounts very frequently, you should be examined by a urologist. The urologist will use an ultrasound image to determine whether urine is left in the bladder after you have voided.

Stomach involvement (gastroparesis). Although it is an uncommon neuropathy, gastroparesis can be a real problem in long-term diabetes. In gastroparesis, autonomic nerves that are responsible for emptying the stomach by squeezing food along from the stomach into the intestine are not functioning normally, and the stomach becomes a slack, inert bag. Eating even a small meal leads to a bloated, full feeling that may last for hours or be relieved only by vomiting. Nausea is common. And because the stomach empties slowly and erratically, it is especially hard to predict what the blood sugar will do following a meal, so diabetic control is often poor. Fortunately, there are some effective treatments, including medications such as metachlopramide, which help restore the stomach's normal movements.

Dizziness upon arising (orthostasis). Autonomic nerves normally cause blood vessels in the lower body to constrict when you stand up, so that gravity doesn't pool all your blood into your legs. With autonomic neuropathy, though, this reflex may not happen. The result is that blood can pool in your lower body as you arise, causing you to feel dizzy because of a lack of blood in your head. There are medications that will cause your kidneys to hang on to more fluid, "filling up the tank" more, but this approach may not be advisable, especially if you have any tendency toward high blood pressure or heart failure. Usually, we just advise people to get up slowly if they have been sitting or lying for some time. Also we use specially designed stockings to keep the blood from pooling in the legs.

Sweating abnormalities. An unusual kind of autonomic neuropathy causes abnormal patterns of perspiration. Sometimes parts of the body do not perspire normally, causing other parts to perspire excessively. Occasionally, this occurs on only one side of the body.

Single Nerve Involvements (Mononeuropathies)

Mononeuropathy is caused by a sudden blood loss to a segment of the nerve, like pinching off one wire in a telephone line. The lack of blood supply is apparently like a mini-stroke to a peripheral nerve.

Symptoms. The symptoms are very different from those caused by the more common peripheral neuropathies. Mononeuropathies come on suddenly and do not affect the toes or feet symmetrically; instead they affect only one part of the body, supplied by a single nerve. The person may experience pain down the side of one leg or from one side of the back right around the flank to the front of the abdomen, or in any other spot on the body. Sensory nerves are affected more often than the motor nerves, but sometimes a cranial nerve can be affected, for example, causing an eyelid to droop.

Any number of conditions, from arthritis to sciatica, can cause sudden pain in one area, so diabetic mononeuropathy is usually diagnosed only after other problems have been excluded. It is very encouraging to know that mononeuropathies usually go away spontaneously within a period of several weeks to six months or so.

Bell's palsy. Bell's palsy is a cranial mononeuropathy that involves the cranial nerves that control the muscles on one side of the face. People develop Bell's palsy with or without diabetes, but it is more common in people with diabetes. Like the other mononeuropathies, this one usually resolves within weeks to months, although some people continue to have a droop on one side of the face for years.

Multiple single nerve involvement (mononeuropathy multiplex).
Mononeuropathy multiplex is an unusual condition with many names. As
this name implies, it occurs when single nerves—but more than one—are affected simultaneously. One classic if unusual example is when a whole series
of nerves at the base of the spine are affected, causing a person to develop
progressive weakness, especially of the hips and upper thighs, to the point
where the person cannot stand, climb stairs, or do physical work. Neurolo-
gists must be sure that some other disease or disk problem is not being
missed, but if the condition is really mononeuropathy multiplex, it will resolve just like other mononeuropathies, in a matter of six months to a year.
The improvement can be dramatic in a person whose muscles were becoming alarmingly weak.

The nervous system is so complex and sensitive that it is not surprising that
it can be severely affected by years of high blood sugar. The most common
form of nerve damage (neuropathy) affects the longest nerves, those running
to the feet. This peripheral neuropathy causes various degrees of discomfort,
progressing to numbness. It does not reverse with treatment, so people must
learn to accommodate to the lack of feeling in their feet by taking especially
good care of them. The take-home message with peripheral neuropathy,
then, is to "think for your feet" just as, if you have Type I diabetes, you "think
for your pancreas."

Autonomic neuropathy affects the automatic, unconscious nerve functions, causing such problems as impotence or gastrointestinal symptoms.
Like peripheral neuropathy, it occurs over many years and does not reverse
easily. Treatment of the symptoms, however, is usually effective.

The third main kind of neuropathy affects single nerves (mononeuropathy). It comes on relatively suddenly, affects only a limited nerve area,
causes symptoms such as a droop on one side of the face or a sudden strip of
pain, and reverses in weeks to months.

Chapter 28

Diabetes and the Foot

- *"My doctor keeps telling me to stop smoking to protect my feet. I know that smoking is bad, but what does that have to do with my feet?"*
- *"I'm young and I'm athletic. Is this foot care thing really that important?"*
- *"My feet feel like they're made of stone, and I feel like I'm walking on stones."*
- *"Now that I'm exercising regularly, the pain in my legs has gone away."*

Most people associate diabetes with foot problems, and for good reason. Lower extremity complications are among the most frequent causes of hospitalization for persons with diabetes. In addition, half of all nontraumatic amputations are reported among people with diabetes. These are sobering statistics, and yet amputations are not inevitable. We now know that 50%–70% of all amputations can be prevented with proper care.

In this chapter we will focus on why diabetes increases the risk of foot problems, emphasizing how to evaluate your personal risk. Then, we'll look in some detail at preventive foot care measures and treatment of specific problems. There's a big difference between *being at risk* for an amputation and actually *having* an amputation. A great many people develop some degree of neuropathy (see Chapter 27), but only a small fraction of them ever have an amputation. The whole purpose of this chapter is to help you limit foot problems, keeping them from ever leading to an amputation.

Why are foot problems associated with diabetes? There are two reasons: peripheral neuropathy and poor circulation.

Peripheral Neuropathy and Poor Circulation

Diabetic peripheral neuropathy is damage to the peripheral nerves as a result of diabetes. The symptoms are extremely variable and can range from tingling to mild or severe pain, from numbness to strange sensations such as feeling as if water is running over the feet when the feet aren't wet, or a hypersensitivity to bed linens.

Although the pain and other odd sensations can be particularly bothersome or disruptive to daily life, the real danger is not to feel anything at all. It is the numbness that gets people into trouble: if your foot is numb, you can't tell whether you've hurt it or not. We know a man who stepped on a golf tee and continued to play the entire game of golf, unaware that the tee had become imbedded in his foot. Believe it or not, we also know a man who played a round of golf with a golf ball in the toe of his shoe! If your feet are numb, you not only have trouble feeling serious trauma like that, but you can't even feel when your shoes are too tight, the bath water is too hot, or there is a warm, inflamed area on the foot.

The other cause of foot problems is decreased circulation, or *peripheral vascular disease*. Circulation is the flow of blood to and from the tissues of your body through the pipelines, the arteries and veins. The blood brings nutrients, oxygen, and infection-fighting cells to keep tissues healthy. If the rate of circulation is decreased by the narrowing of arteriosclerosis (see Chapter 24) and the effects of smoking, then the tissue gets less blood and it complains. When blood flow is diminished because of peripheral vascular disease, there is a risk that small infections will not heal well.

Together, neuropathy (numbness) and peripheral vascular disease (decreased circulation) hit the foot with a double whammy. Trauma can occur without your recognizing it, and infection can set in quickly. But you can compensate for this double whammy with attentive foot care, greatly reducing the chance that symptoms of neuropathy and decreased circulation will progress to a worse complication. A positive note: young, athletic people like the one quoted above probably don't have neuropathy or circulatory compromise and therefore are not really at risk for foot problems. We mention this because no one needs *additional* things to worry about—we can all find plenty as is. It's worth knowing your own risk status for foot complications.

What Is Your Risk?

Testing for Significant Neuropathy

The ability to feel trauma is probably the most important protection against serious foot problems. After all, that is a primary purpose of nerves: to alert the brain to a problem. But a person generally doesn't lose sensation suddenly. It's not a case of one day you feel it, the next day you don't. It is a gradual process. People with minimal changes may notice that they have to touch their feet a little harder in some spots to feel the touch. It may just be that you no longer have the increased sensitivity that used to bother you. More complete loss of sensation leads some of our patients to say that their feet feel as if they were made of stone. Poor sensation from the feet can also cause difficulty walking, leading to a staggering gait and increasing the risk of undetected injury.

Your doctor can determine whether your level of sensation is still "protective," that is, sensitive enough to detect trauma. This is sometimes tested by touching the toes very lightly. A more exact measure is the monofilament test, which is nothing more than a three-inch piece of stiff nylon filament (like fishing line). The filament is pressed against your toe, and you say if you feel it. If you cannot feel it, your risk of foot injury is definitely higher. Your doctor may also test for less specific evidence of neuropathy by checking your ankle reflexes with the reflex hammer or by testing your ability to feel the vibrations of a tuning fork.

Testing for Significant Circulatory Compromise

Circulation can be assessed in several ways. One crude measure is simply to feel the temperature of the feet. With a decrease in the flow of warm blood to the foot, one foot may feel colder than the other. Note that we said *one* foot, which would indicate that a specific artery may be partially blocked. Don't be upset if your toes stay cold at night or your feet feel damp and cool. These signs are so common and so nonspecific that we just don't put a lot of stock in them. While we are on the subject of unreliable signs, medical students are taught that a lack of hair on the lower legs is evidence of circulatory compromise. Wrong again! It's much more likely due to long-term use of calf-length socks.

A classic symptom of decreased blood flow to the legs is called *intermittent claudication*. In people with this condition, the calf gets sore or cramps when they walk briskly or uphill. The doctor will want to feel your foot pulses, to assess blood flow through your arteries at specific pulse points—a spot on top of your foot and a spot behind your ankle. Don't do a physical exam on yourself, however, since the pulses may be hard to find even when the circulation is flowing strong, and they may not be present even in perfectly normal people.

If there is reason to think that the circulation is poor, sophisticated tests can be done. One, called a Doppler test, magnifies the sound that comes from the pulses. If things get serious—in other words, if surgery is being considered to address the circulatory problem—then specialists may want to do an angiogram, running dye from the groin down through the leg arteries and taking X-rays to see exactly how much blockage there is.

Orthopedic Deformities

In assessing your risk, consider the shape of your foot. A normally shaped foot distributes weight evenly. Irregularity in bone structure can create atypical pressure areas and possible tissue breakdown. Prior injury or advanced neuropathy can create irregularities in the bone structure. Your doctor or a podiatrist can help you determine whether or not the shape of your foot is causing significant risk. The professional can also look for calluses or bunions that may cause problems.

High-Risk Habits

Harmful habits can contribute to your risk of foot problems. Smoking is the most important. Is there anyone who hasn't gotten the word that smoking causes lung cancer and contributes to the risk of arteriosclerosis? But how many people realize that smoking a single cigarette causes decreased blood flow with a corresponding change in temperature in the extremities for up to an hour afterward? If you smoke, maybe you can even feel, or at least imagine, the blood flow to your feet being squeezed off with each cigarette. Smoking and diabetes is a very dangerous combination. Another harmful habit is wearing too-tight shoes that cause pressure points on the foot.

High Cholesterol and Blood Sugar

Elevated blood cholesterol increases the risk of circulatory problems and thus foot trouble. Increases in the LDL cholesterol or decreases in HDL cholesterol are the main risks. High blood glucose levels also increase the risk of foot problems, first, by impairing the ability to fight infection and, second, by causing neuropathy.

What Are the Common Causes of Foot Injury to the Person at Risk?

Evidence has accumulated in recent years that the worst outcomes, amputations, are almost always preceded by some recognized or unrecognized break in the skin of the foot. To the high-risk foot, dangers are always lurking: injury, pressure, repetitive stress, infection.

A dangerous break in the skin can come when walking barefoot or with thin-soled shoes. We mentioned a penetrating wound, such as a tack poking through the shoe. Injuries from heat occur by stepping into a too-hot bath or onto a hot surface without first testing it with a sensitive area of the body or a thermometer. We know of a woman who burned the soles of her feet by walking on a beach on a sunny day, unaware of the intense heat of the sand. There have also been reports of heat injuries from the floors of motor vehicles on particularly long trips.

Sustained pressure concentrated on one spot on the foot can prevent blood flow to the area. Eventually, this lack of blood flow results in tissue breakdown or ulceration—a pressure sore. The most common cause of pressure sores is tight shoes, and the first tell-tale sign of a problem is a reddened area. If a person can't feel that the shoes are too tight, the fitting at the shoe store may have been wrong in the first place. We hope you are not so hung up on fashion trends that you put your feet in real danger. High-heeled shoes with pointed toes compress the foot into an unnatural shape (we have yet to see a foot actually shaped like an arrowhead), and the high heels concentrate the body weight toward the front of the foot.

Repetitive stress can create unnoticed inflammation in a vulnerable foot. Imagine that you are on vacation and sightseeing on foot. If your sensation is normal, you will notice if your feet get sore from too much walking, and you will rest or maybe choose a bus tour for the next day. If your feet are numb, however, you may continue to walk day after day, unaware of the inflammation and tissue breakdown that might be taking place. An early sign of too much stress is heat radiating from the inflamed area—heat that you can feel with your hand.

A final danger to feet is infection. It may not be dramatic—just some cracks caused by athlete's foot, for instance. But further invasion of bacteria can occur through an opening in the skin created by any cause, and infections increase the demand for blood (Figure 24). In people with intact circulation, the body with or without prescribed antibiotics will probably be able to fight off small infections. If the circulation is decreased, however, the

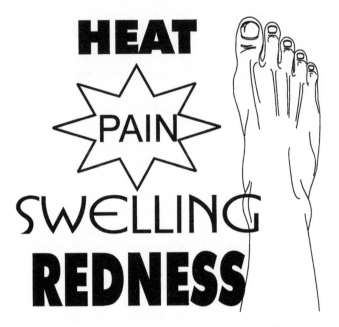

Figure 24. **Warning signs of infection** are heat, redness, swelling, and pain.

bacteria may win and more aggressive measures may be needed to keep the infection from spreading.

Osteomyelitis.   An infection in the bone, *osteomyelitis* is sometimes hard to diagnosis, since it doesn't always show up on X-rays. Some surgeons prefer to sample the inside of a bone with a needle, to get a culture of bacteria. We seldom find this useful. Once established, osteomyelitis is very hard to treat successfully, because antibiotics don't get into the bone well. It can usually be suppressed so that it doesn't flare up, even if it is not entirely cured. If it affects a relatively limited area, such as one small bone in the foot, it may be best to remove that bone, or that toe, to keep the infection from spreading.

Preventive Foot Care

Because the compromised foot is vulnerable to injury, pressure, stress, and infection, the key to avoiding serious problems is prevention. There are some very effective measures you can take to stay out of trouble. We ask our high-risk patients to treat their feet like fine china: wash them and dry them carefully, and give them the utmost protection. It's really not optional: if you have serious neuropathy or serious circulatory problems, you *must* practice prevention.

We'll look at each component of foot care separately. It may seem like an endless list. You may begin to feel as if you won't have time for anything but worrying about your feet, but that's not so. Foot care will become a simple habit once you do it consciously for a few days or weeks. Think about all the little things you do in a day to keep from bumping your head or pinching your finger. We're just asking you to take as good care of your feet as of the rest of your body.

Shoes

Shoes protect feet—shoes that have hard soles and fit well enough to give all parts of your foot, including bony prominences, enough room without squeezing. Shoes should not be too loose, either, because loose shoes can rub a blister or ulcer as they slide back and forth on your foot. We recommend that shoes be made of leather, which breathes better and takes on the shape of the foot more readily than manmade materials.

If you can't tell whether your shoes fit right, ask for assistance from a knowledgeable salesperson. Break in new shoes slowly, wearing them for only two to three hours at first and inspecting your feet for areas of redness. It is best to alternate between two or three pairs of shoes throughout the day, especially if you have new shoes.

You may not think of this, but things do get inside shoes—pebbles, pennies, buttons, a protruding nail, and the aforementioned assortment of children's toys, combs, and golf tees. In some parts of the Southwest, people routinely shake out their shoes before putting them on, to get rid of any spiders or scorpions! So before putting your shoes on, please give their insides a quick check.

The most important point about shoes is to wear them! *Never* go barefoot if your feet are the least bit numb. Obviously, you shouldn't walk barefoot on a lawn or beach. But can you guarantee that even in your own house, there won't be anything on the floor that could cause the catastrophic break in your skin? It's not worth the risk. Wear shoes or at least slippers.

Foot Hygiene

Daily bathing of the feet is an important measure in reducing the risk of infection. Wash them as carefully as you wash your hands. Just taking a shower and counting on some soap to drain over your feet is not good enough.

Dry carefully between the toes. Bacteria and fungi like moisture. Don't make it easy for them.

Trim your toenails by filing them straight across, even with the top of the toes. Round the edges slightly so that they don't dig into the next toe. The best time is after bathing, when your nails are soft and clean. Using scissors or clippers is not recommended, as any slip could cause a break in the skin and point of entry for bacteria.

Some people think of themselves as bathroom surgeons. They will get out razor blades or knives and try to whittle away at a callus or cut out an ingrown nail. Don't! It may not cause pain (if your foot is numb), but it *can* hurt: we've seen serious infections that have been started by callus trimming.

It also is not advisable to use chemical agents that promise to make a corn or callus disappear, since they can dissolve your healthy skin, too. If you need care beyond trimming your toenails, you should see a foot specialist: a podiatrist, a specially trained physical therapist, a nurse, or an orthopedist. A corn or callus is an indication of a high-pressure area that should be evaluated.

Sometimes dry skin is a problem. It can crack, creating an entry for bacteria. You can moisturize dry skin by applying a thin layer of lotion, petroleum jelly, or lanolin after bathing to seal in the moisture. It should not be put between the toes, as this can cause the skin to break down. Soaking the feet is not recommended, either. Ironically, soaking the feet actually causes the skin to become *more* dry, because it removes the natural protective oils from the skin. If you have sweaty feet, your feet may do better if you use a small amount of foot powder.

Make sure that your socks do not become a source of injury. Socks that are too loose and create wrinkles or socks with holes or seams can all cause sores. Socks should be clean, intact, smooth, nonbinding, and appropriate for the shoes being worn.

Inspect Your Feet

Daily foot inspection is most important. You can't rely on your feet to tell you that something is wrong. You have to use your (or somebody else's) eyes and hands to check for problems.

Go over your feet systematically: top, bottom, and between your toes. Check for areas of redness, openings, warm or hot spots, overgrown calluses, ingrown toenails, or discoloration. If you can't maneuver to see the bottom of your feet, use a mirror. It only takes a few seconds. Report any worrisome changes to your physician. It's better to treat small problems quickly, so they don't turn into big problems. Take off your shoes and socks as a gentle reminder to your doctor to inspect your feet at office visits; if you need to, *ask* your doctor to do this. It's important.

Be aware of what comes in contact with your feet. Test your bath water with a sensitive area on your wrist or a thermometer before stepping into it. Hot water can burn the feet, and very cold water can cause blood vessel constriction. If you have cold feet, wear socks. Heating pads and hot water bottles can cause burns.

Improving Circulation

Narrowing of the arteries is to some extent reversible. The quickest, and probably most effective, thing you can do is stop smoking. The next most effective is to exercise, which causes new blood vessels to grow, creating bypass routes around small blockages in the arteries. This is called *collateral circulation*, and it's a marvelous nonsurgical bypass phenomenon.

While massage feels good and may help you relax, it doesn't do anything to promote circulation. Neither does elevating the legs (although putting your feet up can reduce swelling). To encourage new blood vessel growth, you have to create a demand for more oxygen in the muscles by exercising vigorously. That means walking or cycling for a sustained period, stopping if you experience any painful sensation. (Some people whose circulation is seriously reduced won't be able to exercise vigorously.) With the development of collateral circulation, the pain of claudication will decrease or go away.

Finally, promote circulation by not squeezing it off. Tight bands at the top of socks or stockings will actually cause a mechanical constriction of the blood vessels. Circulation can even be temporarily reduced by crossing your legs or sitting on your leg. (The tingling sensation you get from the leg "falling asleep" is actually due to compression of a *nerve*, not an artery.)

Treatments for Foot Trouble

What do you do if you find a problem when you inspect your feet? It depends on the nature of the problem, its seriousness, and how fast-changing it is. Most people aren't in a very good position to tell how serious a problem is, so our recommendation is: *when you see a change that worries you, get professional help quickly.* Specifically, when you first see a foot ulcer, redness suggesting an infection, new loss of color, a significant break in skin, or any other sign of new change, go see your health care professional. Treatment will vary depending on what is wrong and how serious it is, but the following are the most commonly prescribed treatments.

Antibiotics

Antibiotics are used for the treatment of infection or inflammation (*cellulitis*) that has resulted from bacteria entering into the skin. They are most effective if used early, so at the earliest sign of infection (redness, warmth, swelling, streaks of redness, fever), be ready to start antibiotics—by mouth if the infection is not severe or intravenously in the hospital if it is a serious infection. Don't stop the course of antibiotics too soon, just because things look better. Discontinuing treatment too early can result in an immediate relapse.

Bed Rest and Elevation

This can be the most frustrating recommendation both to the patient, because it pretty much stops life in its tracks, and to the doctor, because patients don't take it seriously. But when trying to get an infection or ulcer to heal, staying off your feet may be the most important thing you can do. Usually the patient is allowed to walk to the bathroom, but without question, staying off the foot helps it heal.

Debridement

Debridement is the removal of dead (*necrotic*) tissue from around the edge of an infected or ulcerated area. It eliminates a breeding ground for bacteria. In superficial infections, this can be accomplished quite easily. In deep infections, debridement may take place under anesthesia in an operating room. It cleans up a wound, allowing healing to occur, and may have to be done several times.

Casting

Most of us think of casts only for broken bones. But they are also used very successfully in the treatment of foot ulcers. The rationale is to protect the area from external stress. The cast spreads the pressure and stress around. And because there's no mechanical jarring when moving the foot, the ulcer has a chance to grow new tissue and skin. Casts are put on in various ways. Usually they are walking casts, and sometimes they are bivalved (meaning that they are in two pieces, held together with a dressing, and are taken off at night). Just be sure you are dealing with someone who is experienced in treating foot ulcers with casting, because a poorly applied cast can do more harm than good.

Special Shoes

Your doctor may have suggested special shoes, called *orthotics,* usually with extra depth. The extra room in the shoe is to accommodate an interior that can be molded to the exact shape of the foot. When the shoe makes full contact with the sole of your foot, weight is more evenly distributed, decreasing the risk of pressure areas with repetitive stress and skin breakdown. Sometimes, a shoe with a "rocker bottom" is also prescribed, to take some of the stress off the forefoot as a result of normal walking movement. Orthotic shoes are expensive. Be sure your insurance provider understands the medical necessity, and get a prescription from your doctor.

Vascular Surgery

In cases where the circulation is severely limited and the foot is not getting enough nutrients, vascular surgery may be needed to prevent tissue destruction. The angiogram is the first step and is used to determine which blood vessel is involved, whether the blockage can be corrected, and whether the other vessels seem to be reasonably open. Often in people with long-term diabetes many arteries are affected, rather than just one. This limits the surgeon's ability to correct the problem. As with so many of these treatment options, finding an experienced physician is essential to successful treatment.

Orthopedic Surgery

Orthopedic surgery may be considered if you have a bone irregularity that is causing a projection vulnerable to skin breakdown. The goal is to make the foot as even as possible so that weight is more evenly distributed. This may involve removal of bony projections and correction of deformities.

Hyperbaric Oxygen

Some medical centers have used a procedure called *hyperbaric oxygen* to treat various nonhealing wounds, particularly of the feet, in people with diabetes. The treatment amounts to being enclosed in a chamber that has a high oxygen concentration at a high pressure. Each treatment takes 90 minutes, and often 20–30 treatment sessions are used. There are certain unusual conditions in which hyperbaric oxygen is a proven therapy, but its use in treating difficult wounds in diabetes is controversial. We are not convinced that it does any good.

Amputation

Probably since you first heard that you had diabetes, you worried about amputations. This chapter has emphasized preventive approaches that will greatly improve your chances of avoiding amputations. But amputations still happen, especially to older people with long-term diabetes that hasn't been well taken care of over the years. If doctors have talked to you about the possible need for an amputation, it is important for you to have some background and understanding of what it all means and what the options are. We also believe that an understanding of the facts is less scary than worrying about the unknown.

Types of Amputations

There are many kinds of amputations and many surgical approaches. Some are minor, some major. They are always done under either general or local anesthesia, so the procedure itself doesn't hurt. Amputations may involve only one toe or even part of one toe, the full toe and its connecting bone in the foot, half the foot *(transmetatarsal amputation),* sometimes the whole foot *(below the knee amputation,* or *BKA),* or the foot and lower leg *(above the knee amputation,* or *AKA).*

The amount of disability that will occur is related to what is removed. This is important to understand, because the very word *amputation* may be so frightening that its actual significance is blown out of proportion. The amputation of a toe, for example, rarely leaves any disability at all. Far better to lose a toe than have the significant risk of a toe infection spreading to the entire foot.

When Is an Amputation Considered?

There are two general situations: when an infection is out of control or has no likelihood of healing and when gangrene has set in. Sometimes infections can be aggressive, showing signs of spreading despite repeated debridement (see above) and intravenous antibiotics. Sometimes the infection is not so aggressive but still is not curable. In this case, there is more time to consider the options, but one option may be to remove the bone, as mentioned above.

Gangrene occurs when tissues die. The area becomes black, lacks feeling, and cannot "come to life again." Gangrene can also be a breeding ground for infection. Sometimes, a gangrenous toe can just be left to *autoamputate,* just as a deadened fingernail will eventually drop off. More often, surgeons need to amputate a gangrenous digit or even the foot. They may want to wait until it *demarcates,* meaning that a clear border is established between dead and live tissue.

Will One Amputation Lead to Another?

This is a real concern, for the patient and doctor alike. Depending on the seriousness of the underlying problem, there is always the chance that a particular operation will not heal and that further amputation will be needed later. The importance of having an experienced surgeon cannot be overemphasized. The object is to remove *all* the diseased tissue, to the point where healthy tissue remains that can heal over the wound.

There is really no way for us to generalize about the chances that one amputation will be followed by another, since it depends so much on the specific situation. You should talk to your surgeon, get his or her opinion, and remember that no one can be absolutely sure.

Rehabilitation and Life after an Amputation

Without being overly optimistic, we do want to emphasize that life will go on and that life can actually be very good indeed despite an amputation. When there has been only a small amputation—for example, a toe—the scars are psychological more than physical. Normal activities probably won't be affected at all. And with more extensive amputations, the opportunities for rehabilitation—with an artificial limb, for example—are really extraordinary these days. People may learn to walk virtually normally, so that people around them may be completely unaware that they have an artificial limb. Some patients suffer from *phantom limb pain,* in which the nerves continue to give signals that make the brain think there is still a limb there when it has actually been removed. This is relatively unusual and generally decreases or goes away over time.

So amputations are definitely not the end of the line. We believe that patients and their families should consider the facts of a situation very carefully, talk about it, think about it, even pray about it. The right answer will usually become clear. If, for example, it becomes evident that a toe or a foot is just not going to get better and is never going to cause anything but pain and more risk, then there is not much sense in delaying the inevitable. Better to move on to rehabilitation and the rest of your life.

Diabetes increases the risk of foot problems, but with good self-care, amputations are certainly not inevitable. The underlying problem is that neuropathy can make the foot numb, increasing the chance of undetected trauma, and decreased circulation can slow healing and promote infection. If you have neuropathy and poor circulation, then attentive foot care is essential for prevention. You may be used to thinking *on* your feet, but we recommend that you get into the habit of thinking *for* your feet.

The object is to prevent any breakdown in the skin that could initiate a nonhealing wound. Early detection of problems is critically important, so that aggressive treatment measures can be taken to prevent progression. Remember, numb feet won't give you the early warning that a foot problem is starting. You have to be vigilant. When you see a problem, get it taken care of quickly—by your health care professional or even an emergency room. Prevention and early treatment are the keys to staying on your feet!

Chapter 29

Diabetes and the Skin

- *"What are those bumps where I take my insulin?"*
- *"Now that my blood sugars are down, my skin feels better—less itchy and less of those awful fungal infections."*
- *"My skin gives me fits. Are all my problems due to diabetes?"*

If your skin looks just the way you want it to and doesn't hurt or itch, you probably don't think about it very much. For most people, however, the skin doesn't look or feel just right. And for people with diabetes, it's often difficult to know which skin problems are due to diabetes and which are due to completely unrelated factors. In this chapter, we take a closer look at the skin. If you have a skin problem that's not mentioned in the following pages, you should see your family doctor or a dermatologist.

Skin Changes Due to Insulin Injections

Christine has noticed a few things about her skin. At age 55, after 22 years of multiple daily insulin injections, she occasionally gets a bruise where she injects, but that doesn't bother her. She has also noticed, though, that she has a fairly distinct band of fat just below her belly button, extending about 10 inches across her abdomen. As much out of curiosity as vanity, Christine wonders why she's fat in just this one spot. She also wonders why the skin at the top of her arm, where she used to take her insulin every day, is so tough and has areas of actual depression.

Christine is noticing some of the most common skin consequences of taking insulin by injection. The occasional little bruises, insulin hypertrophy, and insulin lipoatrophy are all worth discussing here.

Bruising

Regularly injecting insulin sometimes causes a small bruise at the site of injection. This is due to a tiny blood vessel being nicked by the needle in the skin. It really isn't a significant problem unless some of the insulin injected enters right into the bloodstream through the nicked vein, in which case it will have a quicker-than-usual effect on blood sugar. The bruise will heal before long, and the whole problem is avoidable by looking to see if a drop of blood shows up at the site of injection. If so, apply some pressure right over the site, to keep the blood from spreading in the skin, causing the bruise. Taking a blood thinner, such as Coumadin, or even daily aspirin may increase your tendency to bruise. but again it usually is not a major problem.

Insulin Hypertrophy

Insulin hypertrophy is the accumulation of fatty tissue where you inject. The cause is presumed to be the normal action of insulin in stimulating growth of fatty tissue. It may be a fairly large area, measured in inches; it's soft and doesn't hurt at all. Insulin hypertrophy may not be present at all, may be barely noticeable, or occasionally becomes very obvious if you look for it. Usually, insulin hypertrophy can be avoided just by moving around the sites of injection, and usually it is of no consequence. At worst, it causes some unwanted fat in part of the skin.

Lipoatrophy

Lipoatrophy is the opposite of insulin hypertrophy: it is the loss of the normal fat under the skin due to insulin injections. It appear as a slightly depressed area of skin, with a firm or fibrous feel to it. There is some evidence that lipoatrophy may be an immunologic response to the insulin, but most observers think of it as the result of repeated trauma to the skin in one spot. Some people have treated it by injecting insulin, or insulin with a small amount of steroid added to the bottle, directly into the middle of the area. In our experience, though, it is rarely even noticeable. Insulin injected directly into an atrophic area is erratically absorbed, so our advice is to find other absorption sites.

There is a very unusual form of diabetes called *lipoatrophic diabetes* in which the whole body is lacking in fat tissue. People with this form of diabetes look very muscular, but this is just because they have no fat smoothing out the muscle. They may require very high doses of insulin.

Dry Skin

Dry skin is usually not caused by diabetes, although it may be made worse by high blood sugars if dehydration is chronic. It can also be caused by decreased sweat gland activity as a sign of autonomic nerve damage.

Whatever the cause, dry skin can pose a danger because it is susceptible to cracking or breaking, which opens the door for infection. So, especially if you have neuropathy or circulatory compromise in your feet, you will want to take care that the skin of your feet and other areas does not become too dry. We suggest the use of lotions and lip protection, as well as superfatted soaps, such as Dove or Lever 2000.

Fungal Infections

Dewayne called, worried about athlete's foot. He is a 17-year-old high school student and was concerned about what he's heard about foot infections and diabetes. He takes good care of his blood sugars, though, and we were able to reassure him that athlete's foot is responsive to over-the-counter medications, such as Tinactin, and that if properly taken care of, it does not pose a threat to his feet.

A fungus infection of the skin can appear as a red, itchy rash. But even more commonly, it will develop under the nails or between the toes. These infections occur more often in people with diabetes simply because fungus needs sugar to grow and multiply. Fungus also likes moisture and for that reason is more typically found in skin folds, such as under the breast and in the armpits, in the genital area, and in between the toes. Preventing and treating fungal infections means making the environment less hospitable for them by lowering blood sugars and washing and drying carefully. We further recommend wearing only all-cotton underwear, since it "breathes" better. Women should avoid using vaginal douches or feminine hygiene sprays unless specifically prescribed, since they can alter the pH balance of the vagina and set the stage for increased fungal growth.

As noted in Dewayne's story, superficial fungal infections, such as athlete's foot, that occur between the toes respond very well to over-the-counter medications. If not treated, however, they can become chronic and more difficult to eradicate. Sometimes small invisible fissures occur in the skin, serving as an entrance port for bacteria that can then infect the body elsewhere.

Fungal infections that lodge beneath the skin or under a toenail are very hard to get rid of. They have even been implicated in passing infection to other parts of the body. When in doubt, talk to a dermatologist.

Vitiligo

Vitiligo is a patchy depigmentation of the skin. Areas with vitiligo look completely white and do not get the least bit tanned. Vitiligo is most probably an immune problem of the skin, just the way Type I diabetes is an immune process involving the pancreas. It's not a coincidence that vitiligo is more common in people with Type I diabetes than in those without it. There is presently nothing that can be done to alter its course, though staying out of the sun (so the unaffected skin doesn't get even darker in contrast) and using body makeup can help conceal the problem. It is especially important to have a doctor make this diagnosis, since vitiligo can be confused with fungal infections.

If you have vitiligo, you should be sure to cover the depigmented area carefully with a sun block. Lacking the normal pigmentation, that part the skin is extremely sensitive to sunlight.

Necrobiosis Lipoidica Diabeticorum (NLD)

Necrobiosis lipoidica diabeticorum (NLD) is a skin condition that is characteristic of diabetes, usually Type I. It has a very characteristic appearance: usually located on the shins or ankles, though sometimes on the feet, it is a patch anywhere from $\frac{1}{2}$ inch to 3–4 inches in diameter of purple to violet skin, with clearly demarcated edges. It comes on gradually over weeks, often in people who have had Type I diabetes for only a few to several years (for that reason it is not classified as a long-term complication).

NLD does not itch and is usually not a serious problem, although some people are bothered by its appearance. Occasionally the skin may become so thin that an ulcer forms. There is no specific treatment for NLD, although many dermatologists believe that taking an aspirin daily can help, and some doctors try injecting steroids into the NLD or applying a steroid cream. Usually NLD stabilizes spontaneously and becomes a slightly depressed, brownish area.

Shin Spots

People with diabetes tend to have pigmented spots, about half an inch or less in diameter, on their shins. These spots aren't as big as the NLD described above, and they do not go through a phase of being purple. It may be that shin spots simply represent slow healing of bruises. They are usually of no real concern.

Xanthelasma

Xanthelasma is the name for the small, yellow plaque-like marks some people develop on the eyelids or at the corner of the eyes by the nose. It's a condition that runs in families. Xanthelasma may indicate high blood cholesterol, so if you notice these spots, be sure to have your cholesterol checked. On the other hand, most people with xanthelasma have perfectly normal cholesterol levels.

Loss of Hair on the Head (Alopecia)

The condition doctors call *alopecia* is what most people know as simple hair loss, occurring abnormally and often in clumps. It is different from normal male balding. It is seen occasionally in Type I diabetes or in diabetes out of control and as a result of other significant stresses. The cause of alopecia is not clear, and there is little to be done about it. But the kind associated with diabetes is usually mild and self-limited.

Waxy Skin and Stiff Joints and Other Musculoskeletal Problems

There is a skin and joint condition that consists of thinning of the skin at the fingers and stiff joints, especially in the fingers. It has been likened to the disease called scleroderma and in fact is called *pseudo-scleroderma*. But this condition is not progressive or serious, as scleroderma can be. Its cause is not known, and there is no particular treatment.

There are also certain musculoskeletal problems that are more common in people with diabetes than in the general population. We will mention them here even if they are not, strictly speaking, skin conditions. The most frequent is tendon contractures of the hands. This consists of painless stiffening and shortening of the tendons in the palms of the hands, causing difficulty straightening out the fingers. Depending on its severity and on how extensively you use your hands in work, it may not require treatment or it may require tendon surgery.

Bursitis is also more common in people with diabetes. It usually involves shoulder joints and sometimes elbows, knees, or hips. The symptoms include limitation of movement by pain, for example, when you raise your arm above your head or try to scratch your own back. Bursitis is managed in the same way whether or not you have diabetes, except that if a cortisone injection is used, you should expect your blood glucose to increase considerably for a day or a few days. Be ready to increase your insulin dose if you are on insulin.

Acanthosis Nigricans

Acanthosis nigricans is a skin condition that occurs particularly in people of African descent with Type II diabetes. It is a velvety-feeling increase in pigmentation (a darkening of the skin), located most often around the back of the neck and in the armpits. Acanthosis nigricans can indicate a high level of insulin resistance, which, you will recall, is associated with Type II diabetes. People with severe forms of insulin resistance may need unusually high insulin doses to control their diabetes. The acanthosis nigricans, though, does not in itself cause any problem or require any treatment.

The skin can be considered our most vulnerable as well as our most visible organ. It can be damaged by almost anything, from sunlight to trauma. Because skin is our physical interface with the outside world, we are always sensitive to the slightest imperfections in it. Luckily, the skin is not often or seriously affected by diabetes. The specific complications of insulin injections, such as insulin hypertrophy or lipoatrophy, are rarely significant cosmetic problems, and fungal infections, though persistent, are generally controllable. Even the skin complication most specific to diabetes, necrobiosis, usually goes away by itself. The most common skin conditions, such as acne and simple sunburn, occur equally in people with or without diabetes.

Part V
Sexuality, Pregnancy, and Genetics

At one of our first Johns Hopkins Diabetes Center self-management programs in 1986, there was a newly diagnosed, newly married 22-year-old man sitting next to a 55-year-old man who had had diabetes for 35 years. The 22-year-old was, quite naturally, panicked. He had heard on the street that people with diabetes couldn't have children. Luckily, the man he sat next to had eight children and six, going on seven, grandchildren. So much for rumors about diabetes and fertility!

There is so much emotion, as well as good and bad information, swirling around reproduction and heredity, that we decided it deserves a section of its own in this book. People beyond their child-bearing years won't be so interested in the fine points of managing diabetes during pregnancy, but older people are at least as concerned about the genetics of diabetes: what chance their children, and their children's children, have of getting it.

Part V deals with many aspects of sexuality, pregnancy, and genetics. We try to distinguish fact from rumor, we are realistic, and we are optimistic.

Chapter 30

Diabetes and Sexuality

- *"Sex is just not what it used to be. I hardly ever get excited any more, and even when I do, I almost never have an orgasm."*
- *"When I became impotent it really shook me up. Sometimes I wonder if life's worth living."*
- *"I haven't had an erection in four years, but my wife and I have learned there's more to sex than intercourse."*

Diabetes can affect a person's interest in sex, called the libido, as well as his or her physical ability to carry out sexual activity. What's more, out-of-control diabetes can make this situation much worse. Emotional problems, physical problems, lack of energy, or even just not feeling well from diabetes can also take a toll on your sex life.

Psychological factors are most important in having an acceptable sex life, and we know that high blood sugars can activate depression (see Chapter 18). Sexual activity is one of the most vulnerable areas when a person with diabetes is depressed. Some studies show that depressed people with or without diabetes tend to have similar symptoms *except* when it comes to interest in sex. In that one area, depressed people with diabetes report more problems than those without it. Of course, depression also takes its toll on energy level, which makes it difficult to work up much enthusiasm for sex.

The physical symptoms of diabetes, whether acute (such as vaginal infections) or long term (such as trouble holding an erection) can also take a toll on sexual pleasure. And, as we have also seen, high blood sugars make you feel dragged out generally, not a condition that enhances interest in sex. Fortunately, there are things you can do to improve your sexual experiences by paying attention to both the psychological and physical aspects.

Most people think about their sex life a lot but talk about it rarely, even with their partner. Some people find it hard even to bring up the subject with a doctor or nurse. Sexual experiences are very important but very personal. We hope this chapter faces the issues squarely and helps you understand how diabetes might be affecting your sexual experience, as well as putting you in a position to pursue available remedies.

About Women

Physical Consequences of Poorly Controlled Diabetes

As we've seen throughout this book, for people with diabetes there are direct, immediate effects of high blood sugar. When it comes to the area of sexual functioning, many of these symptoms can get in the way. The immediate effects of high blood sugar usually play out, for women as well as for men, as generalized fatigue, lack of energy, and feelings of whole-body exhaustion. It doesn't help the mood when a person has to urinate every few minutes and is constantly thirsty.

There are other problems for women with diabetes. For one thing, the dryness in a woman's mouth is often matched by vaginal dryness. In addition, when diabetes is out of control, a woman is very likely to develop vaginal infections (specifically moniliasis and candidiasis). The itching and discomfort caused by these infections naturally makes sex less appealing. But these symptoms will all improve when she gets her sugar into control (usually when less than 200 mg/dl).

Poor blood sugar control over months to years may lower a woman's estrogen levels, and this will cause inadequate vaginal lubrication. Diabetes isn't the only thing that can do this. All women have low estrogen levels following menopause or surgical removal of their ovaries (unless they receive hormone replacement therapy), and these women also suffer from reduced vaginal lubrication. A woman can use topical ointments to improve lubrication or estrogen replacement in the form of pills, patches, or vaginal creams. Internal lubricants, such as Replens, may help maintain a favorable pH balance in the vagina, but they are expensive. An alternative is to use a water-based gel on the outside or, for severe dryness, a vaginal suppository, which she can insert before she has intercourse.

Poor control can also cause menstrual irregularity or even absence of menstrual periods. Improving the blood sugar control is the best way to remedy this, although artificial cycling with birth control pills may also be prescribed.

Usually, the physical problems that lessen sexual enjoyment in diabetes are due to these acute, immediate effects of high blood sugar and will resolve when the diabetes is in better control. This is just another reason to get in control of diabetes. The only long-term complication of diabetes that can occasionally affect sexual function in women is neuropathy, which can affect the genital region. In women, this condition may prevent adequate lubrication and orgasm.

Psychological Factors

To enjoy sex, it's important to feel sexually attractive. For many women who have Type II diabetes (and for some who have Type I), being overweight can be a barrier to sexual enjoyment, even when it's much more of a self-image problem than a lack of desirability in her partner's eyes.

We mentioned depression and its potentially devastating effect on one's sex life. Don't ignore the signs. Even mild depression may be playing a role.

What Women Can Do

If you are not satisfied with your level of interest or performance in sex, the first thing to do is recognize that your sexual problems may be related to your diabetes. Knowing this may help right away, because you'll be relieved to know that it's not you, it's your diabetes. And once again, if it is your diabetes, chances are it's the blood sugar at the time and not some permanent problem. The solution is to improve your blood sugar control. We know that's difficult, but now you have another reason to try.

Even if you're embarrassed, try to bring up the subject in talking with those who can help. If you are in a relationship, you should talk to your partner. He may have been feeling that it was all his fault. Talk with your health care provider. You will probably have to bring up the topic yourself, especially if your physician is a man. A survey of physicians (both male and female) showed that 85% of the doctors regularly asked their male patients about sex, but only 33% regularly asked their female patients the same question.

If you are depressed, counseling, possibly combined with antidepressant medication, may help. You should also ask yourself whether your sexual dissatisfaction could be related to fears of pregnancy. If you think this might be the case, then the next chapter, on pregnancy and diabetes, may be helpful.

Finally, if you, your partner, and your diabetes health care provider have addressed the emotional and physical components of sex and things still aren't going well, we advise you to seek help from a mental health professional who is specially trained in dealing with sexual problems. It's always important to get a referral from your doctor or the local teaching or community hospital and to find out about the counselor's background and experience. Many counselors will send you detailed printed information about these matters if you request it, so that you can be an informed consumer before you make an appointment. Use your common sense and be wary. There are excellent, experienced sex counselors available; there are also charlatans out there ready to take advantage of the unwary.

About Men

Some of the emotional and physical problems caused by diabetes can decrease libido in men, just as they can in women. But for men, sexual problems are often more obvious because of the ability or inability to have an erection. Some men link having an erection to their image of what it means to be "a real man." Others take it much more in stride, as just another part of the anatomy. But there's no getting around it: a common long-term complication of poorly controlled diabetes is deterioration of potency—the inability to have or keep an erection.

Although it's difficult to say what proportion of men with diabetes will have difficulty with potency, we do know that the odds increase with duration of diabetes, poor level of control, and the presence of other neuropathies. Let's consider some facts.

Having and maintaining an erection is a complex process, involving psychological, hormonal, vascular, and nervous systems. To have an erection, *all* systems must be functioning well. Like most diabetes-related problems, interest in sex is affected by recent blood sugar control. Good control is generally associated with high levels of libido and well-being, sexual and otherwise.

Impotence can be permanent or temporary. Temporary impotence can be caused by exhaustion, overconsumption of alcohol, ingestion of some prescription drugs, and worry, especially the worry that you might be impotent.

If you are impotent, you have to determine whether the cause is physical or psychological. Don't shy away from the possibility that it is "all in your head." The strongest, toughest men get just as stressed, depressed, and anxious as anyone else. You can start to find the answer by asking yourself these questions:

—Did the impotence begin suddenly?
—Is the impotence on and off, sometimes or in some situations being complete and in other situations being no problem at all?

—Do you get an erection when you masturbate?

—Do you have erections during the night, when you wake up, or when you are especially sleepy or bored?

If your answer to any of these questions is yes, then psychological factors are almost certainly at least a part of your problem. This is good to know, because counseling and recognition of the psychological roots may lead to their correction. If you essentially never have erections (at night, when bored or sleepy, when fantasizing or masturbating), then there is a physical problem.

Tests can confirm whether impotence is primarily psychological or physical. One test to determine whether you do have erections is relatively simple. You place a device called a snap gauge around your penis before you go to sleep at night. With each erection, the gauge will snap. Normally, a man will have an average of four erections each night, each lasting 15 to 45 minutes. If you want to try the test yourself without buying a snap gauge, you can substitute postage stamps. Wrap the stamps around your penis and seal them. If the stamps break at night, you've had an erection. Try this for several nights to be sure.

If diagnostic tests performed by your physician indicate that there is a physical cause for your impotence, your physician can arrange for other tests to determine whether hormone, blood vessel, or nerve problems are involved. Low blood testosterone (the primary male hormone) is usually not the cause, but if the doctor picks up signs or symptoms that are suggestive, it can be measured.

Causes of Impotence in Diabetes

Most men who experience impotence want to know why. "It's the diabetes" or "It's psychological" usually aren't good enough answers. So let's look more specifically at the causes of impotence in diabetes.

As noted above, emotional distress can cause or contribute to impotence. We suspect that every man, and we do mean every man, has at one time or another questioned his ability to achieve or maintain an erection. Men with diabetes, however, may have more than their share of questions about their ability, and they may find it particularly difficult to let themselves go sexually instead of constantly monitoring the state of their penis. This "performance anxiety" can, and often does, contribute to impotence.

More general psychological factors, such as anxiety or depression, may also lead to impotence. Estimates of how often impotence in diabetes is caused by psychological factors vary widely. We see figures ranging from 10% to 67%. One reason is that psychological factors can *contribute* to impotence even when they are not the sole cause.

Neuropathy is the most common *physical* cause of impotence. The autonomic neuropathy that is discussed in Chapter 27 is usually associated with peripheral neuropathy and is a long-term complication of high blood sugar. The impotence is partial at first, causing difficulty in maintaining an erection. It may fluctuate to some degree but is not related so much to the situation: you may be very interested and aroused, but "the flesh just isn't willing." Over the years, it can progress to complete inability to achieve an erection.

Vascular problems that interrupt blood flow to the penis also contribute to impotence. They occur more often in older men with diabetes, especially those with heart disease or evidence of poor circulation to their feet. Hardening of the arteries blocks blood flow to the penis and prevents it from becoming erect and firm. Smoking is a major contributor to this problem.

You should also be aware that many prescription medications can contribute to impotence, including blood pressure drugs such as beta blockers and diuretics, some antidepressants, ulcer medications, and drugs to prevent vomiting. Be sure to talk to your physician about the possibility that these medications (or others) might be contributing to your impotence.

A decrease in the male hormone testosterone may also cause impotence, though this is a less common cause. Most men don't have a problem with their hormones, but this is something that your doctor can easily check with a blood test.

What You Can Do

There are several successful approaches to treating impotence. Some primary care physicians can explain the options and make recommendations, or you may want to consult a urologist. To some extent the treatment can be based on understanding the specific cause; in other cases, it may be worth just trying a given therapy to see if it works.

One of the more common and successful approaches is to inject a medication directly into the base of the penis. Several medications have been used, and new ones are coming out. It may sound odd and unpleasant, but it works very well for many men, causing a normal erection that lasts for a half hour or so. Side effects can include bruising and priapism (erections that take a long time to go away.) The medication should be prescribed, and you should receive careful instruction on its use.

If your impotence is caused primarily by inadequate blood flow, you could take an oral medication called yohimbine. This drug works for some people, but it can aggravate high blood pressure. Remember that smoking may be the most important contributor to vascular impotence. So if you smoke, please stop. While impotence is only one of many good reasons to quit smoking, maybe it's the one that will finally inspire you. Also be aware that while alcohol and illicit drugs sometimes increase desire, they almost always decrease performance.

Finally, there are several mechanical devices you can use to produce an erection. One kind looks like a large, solid condom. The penis is inserted, and this device generates a vacuum to draw blood into the penis, with a band to prevent the blood from flowing out again until the ring is removed. The only problem with these devices is that they can cause tissue damage if the band is left on too long.

For some men a surgical penile implant is the best solution, since they're always ready, at any time, with no worries about having external devices nearby when the mood strikes. We recommend this approach, though, only if the problem of impotence is disturbing your life.

Penile implants come in two types: inflatable and semirigid. Inflatable implants are much more expensive than semirigid ones. Neither device interferes with intercourse, orgasm, or ejaculation. Still, if you have nerve damage due to diabetes, neither device will restore any sensation you have lost.

Inflatable implants provide the most natural-appearing and naturally functioning organ. They consist of a reservoir with fluid (implanted in the abdomen), a pump to move the fluid (implanted in the scrotum), and cylinders (implanted in the corpora cavernosa of the penis). (The *corpora cavernosa* fill with blood to create an erection in men who aren't impotent.) With the inflatable implant, the man squeezes the pump and fluid fills the penis, making it erect.

Semirigid implants are simpler. By a relatively simple procedure, a custom-fitted silicone rod is inserted surgically into the penis. The newest models are flexible and bendable and thus easier to conceal. But none of them is really easy to conceal.

Feeling good about yourself is important, whether or not you have diabetes. Feeling happy and confident sexually may be an important part of feeling good about yourself. We noted that there are many causes of impotence in men and unsatisfactory sex life for women with diabetes. It is just as true that people's response to less sexual activity varies enormously. So in your own thinking, be honest and know the facts. Your sex life does not define you as a person, does not make you one bit more or less of a man or a woman. If is important to you to have an active sex life, think of the things we have discussed in this chapter, talk over the issue with the appropriate person, and take action.

Chapter 31

Diabetes and Pregnancy

- *"I never even thought of diabetes until now. But here I am, 32 years old, 8 months pregnant, and now I have diabetes too."*
- *"Some people say you shouldn't get pregnant if you have diabetes, others say it's no big deal. I just want to know if the baby will be okay."*
- *"Will having a baby make my complications worse?"*
- *"I'll tell you what pregnancy with diabetes is like—it's as if the doctors want me to have a nine-month insulin reaction."*
- *"I think the 3 A.M. blood sugar check they make you do is just to get you ready for middle-of-the-night feedings."*

To any woman, the very idea of pregnancy is both exhilarating and frightening. There is more worry, though, if that pregnancy is complicated by diabetes. In this chapter, we want to help you understand what is involved. We will give you and your mate the right information, so you can make informed decisions and take action to improve your odds. We'll say it again: every pregnancy is both scary and beautiful. We wouldn't dream of taking the wonder out of pregnancy, even if we could.

We also recognize that the pregnant woman isn't the only person who is anxious in a pregnancy: the father is too (not to mention the grandparents-to-be). This chapter focuses on the *mother,* however. Although a father with diabetes may affect, to some degree, the chance of the child eventually developing diabetes (see Chapter 32), the father's diabetes has no effect on the pregnancy itself.

We start this chapter with a general description of how diabetes and pregnancy interact, summarizing the reasons for treating diabetes in pregnancy intensively. Then we'll discuss more specifically what you can expect, what goals to set, and how to take care of yourself. Our overriding message is this: *you control the diabetes well and see your doctors regularly during pregnancy for two good reasons, your developing baby and yourself.*

First, some definitions are in order. *Gestational diabetes mellitus* (GDM) is diabetes diagnosed first during pregnancy. It is usually a signal that Type II diabetes may develop later in the woman's life. *Pregestational diabetes mellitus,* on the other hand, refers to diabetes that exists before pregnancy—in other words, when a woman with known diabetes becomes pregnant. Since most diabetes in young people is Type I, pregestational diabetes usually means the woman has Type I diabetes. Now let's take a closer look at these different kinds of diabetes in pregnancy.

Gestational Diabetes Mellitus

Gestational diabetes mellitus usually comes on in the last half of pregnancy, when the fetus is growing larger. Testing for GDM has become routine in the health professional's office, not only by looking for sugar in the urine with a urinalysis but also by doing a screening test with an oral glucose challenge, usually in weeks 24–28 of pregnancy. Urine glucose is a very poor test for diabetes in pregnancy, since many women with no diabetes show some glucose in their urine during pregnancy. Glucose in the urine may serve as a reminder, though, that all women should have the glucose challenge test as a screen during pregnancy. The challenge test uses a smaller amount of glucose (50 grams) than a full oral glucose tolerance test (OGTT), and only a single blood glucose is drawn one hour later. The test does not have to be done while fasting; it can be done at any time during the day. If the blood glucose is 140 mg/dl or more an hour after this challenge, it is recommended that a full OGTT be done.

Gestational diabetes mellitus is by far the most common form of diabetes in pregnancy: between 2% and 5% of all pregnant women in the United States develop it. GDM is usually a shock to the woman who gets it, though, since it comes "out of the blue," in the middle of pregnancy.

Why Is GDM So Common?

In this book, when we talk about Type II diabetes, we stress that insulin resistance is the crux of the problem: that the body refuses to respond normally to normal amounts of insulin in the bloodstream. Obesity is perhaps the most common cause of insulin resistance, but pregnancy is another. In the case of pregnancy, the hormones made by the placenta counteract insulin, causing the resistance.

The same sequence that can lead to diabetes with obesity can cause it during pregnancy. If your pancreas is strong enough to step up its insulin output, it overcomes the resistance and you do not develop diabetes, but if the capability of your pancreas is limited, if it is not able to increase its insulin production in response to the hormones produced during pregnancy, then you may develop diabetes at that time.

The good news about developing diabetes during pregnancy is that the cause of the insulin resistance, the pregnancy, ultimately goes away (with delivery). In three out of four cases of GDM, the diabetes disappears at the end of pregnancy. GDM, therefore, is one of the few kinds of diabetes that is often temporary. The not-so-good news is that the reason why GDM develops in the first place is that the pancreas is not as strong as normal. This is a signal that a woman is at high risk to develop diabetes later in life. This information should provide a special incentive for her to try to maintain normal body weight, so that the insulin resistance caused by obesity does not tip over into diabetes. It also, of course, means that there is a high risk of developing diabetes with subsequent pregnancies.

How GDM Affects Pregnancy

Gestational diabetes mellitus increases the risks of miscarriage or neonatal complications to the baby (this is discussed in more detail below). It should be taken seriously and should be treated quickly and effectively. The usual medications for Type II diabetes (oral hypoglycemic agents) are not used to treat diabetes in pregnancy, for fear of damaging the fetus. So you will have to check your sugar often to see if diet and exercise are working. If not, you will have to start injecting insulin.

Pregestational Diabetes Mellitus

Not all women with Type I diabetes enter into a pregnancy on an equal footing. If you have diabetes and are thinking about becoming pregnant, there are some important questions you should ask yourself. You will want to consider these questions with your loved one and with your doctor:

—How long have I had diabetes?
—What is my complication status?

—Am I prepared for the hard work involved in being pregnant with diabetes?

Dr. Priscilla White, one of the first practitioners to specialize in the field of diabetic pregnancy, developed a classification of complications and noted that in general the more long-term complications of diabetes a woman has at the start of pregnancy, the less the chance of a successful outcome. Her finding makes sense. If your kidneys are significantly affected by diabetes (nephropathy) at the start of pregnancy, there is an increased chance of hypertension and toxemia. If you have severe retinopathy, hemorrhages may occur during pregnancy at an increased rate. If you have a weak heart, it may become overburdened by pregnancy. Established long-term diabetes complications sometimes worsen during pregnancy. The evidence, however, indicates that the downturn, if any, reverses after the pregnancy is completed, so pregnancy does *not* actually cause a *worsening* of long-term complications. Similarly, pregnancy does not cause new long-term complications where none existed. But if you already have significant or severe long-term complications, even the transient damage done during pregnancy (such as a major retinal bleed or serious toxemia of pregnancy) could affect your long-term health.

Our advice generally is that if you have late-stage diabetic complications, you need to consider carefully whether starting a pregnancy is really a risk you want to take. We know women who have successfully completed pregnancies despite serious long-term complications of diabetes, but it can be dangerous to the mother. If you are generally healthy despite your diabetes, then pregnancy is a perfectly viable option.

Healthy Baby, Healthy Mother

There's not much question about what you want out of pregnancy, is there? A happy, healthy baby. It's also important for *you* to stay healthy, so that you can raise your child and enjoy your grandchildren. These are not trivial matters.

We mentioned above that every woman is anxious about pregnancy: will I carry the pregnancy to term, or will I miscarry? Will the delivery be normal? And, most important of all, will the baby be normal? No person, and certainly no health care professional, can guarantee a normal pregnancy. But we can talk about your chances. To a considerable extent, we can work together to improve the odds (the specifics of self-care during pregnancy are discussed later in this chapter). Good health care, after all, is about improving your chances and your baby's chances.

No one can ever know the exact odds of having a healthy baby, since so many factors contribute. Some people don't want to know much at all; they accept the mystery of pregnancy and are happy to take the chance, whatever it is. Others want to know all the facts. Our own approach to healthy living with diabetes is that the more you know, the better off you'll be. Here, then, are some guidelines.

Spontaneous Miscarriage

About 16% of apparently normal pregnancies (without diabetes) are lost through spontaneous miscarriages. Many miscarriages occur early in pregnancy, often before the woman knows she is pregnant, and in most cases the fetus had a lethal abnormality, meaning that the abnormality was not compatible with life. It's encouraging to know that in well-controlled pregestational diabetes, the spontaneous miscarriage rate does not seem to be any higher than in women without diabetes. (GDM doesn't occur until the middle of pregnancy, when the risk of miscarriage is lower.) The risks of losing a pregnancy are much greater if you do not control the diabetes very closely throughout pregnancy and if you do not get good regular prenatal care. As we discuss below, the chance of carrying a pregnancy successfully with diabetes increases directly with good blood sugar control.

Congenital Malformations

The other serious issue is whether the child will be born with any malformations, called *congenital anomalies*. These are divided into major and minor anomalies. In the minor category would be small skin discolorations or a webbed toe that can be easily corrected. Minor congenital malformations do not require major surgery and have no long-term impact on the baby. Major congenital anomalies, in contrast, can include such important medical problems as heart abnormalities, spina bifida, or severe cleft lip and cleft palate.

The chance of major congenital abnormalities is in the range of 2%–3% without diabetes but increases to as much as 7%–13% with poorly cared-for pregestational diabetes. Most studies show that good diabetes care before conception reduces the chance of major congenital malformations to a range of 1%–5%. We want to emphasize once again that such estimates of odds are very inexact and may not apply to a particular individual.

Macrosomia

Macrosomia is the technical term for an abnormally large, fat baby. What does abnormally large mean? To some extent it depends on the size of the parents: big parents will normally have big babies. It also depends on whether the delivery is premature. But generally speaking, a baby who weighs more than 10 pounds at birth is considered large. For generations, macrosomia has been known to be a complication of diabetic pregnancy. Now we not only know that it happens and what complications it can cause but we also know *why* it happens.

When a mother's blood glucose is high during pregnancy, that sugar passes through the placenta to the developing fetus. Any insulin that the mother takes does *not* pass well through the placenta to the baby. Because the fetus is continuously bathed in high glucose blood, its own developing pancreas is continually stimulated to produce more and more insulin (which stays on the fetal side of the placenta, not passing through to the mother). The high levels of glucose and insulin in the fetal blood cause fat to develop. Thus, the baby is born large. More specifically, it is *fat;* other than the fat tissue, the baby's organs are not large or overmature, and they may be undermature. But if the mother's diabetes is well controlled, this cycle never occurs, and the baby can be born with normal body weight.

Complications during Delivery and in the Neonatal Period

The complication rate is increased in deliveries of a large baby, especially to a small mother. Sometimes the labor is more difficult. Sometimes it takes longer for the actual birthing. And sometimes the baby is just too large to be delivered vaginally, requiring a cesarean section.

There are also more complications than normal in the first few days and weeks of life. These fall into two categories: neonatal hypoglycemia and complications of prematurity. The hypoglycemia results from the baby's extra-strong pancreas, which has been producing large amounts of insulin to try to correct the high blood glucose environment that he or she lived in throughout gestation. On the outside of the womb, this pumped-up pancreas can well cause hypoglycemia before it readjusts to the baby's own normal blood glucose levels. Again, it shouldn't be a problem if the mother's diabetes was well controlled during pregnancy, and even if neonatal hypoglycemia does occur it can be managed in a modern newborn nursery.

It's often surprising when complications of prematurity develop in a baby born of the poorly controlled mother with diabetes, since the baby appears to be large, healthy, and anything but premature. As mentioned above, though, this is not a mature baby, it is a fat baby. The internal organs may actually be underdeveloped and underfunctioning at birth.

The Mother's Blood Glucose Control throughout Pregnancy

Very early in the pregnancy (in the first four to eight weeks), as the baby's vital organs are developing, there is good reason to think that high blood sugars increase the chances of these organs developing abnormally. Even though the evidence is not quite airtight that poor control early in pregnancy causes an increased rate of major congenital malformations, the major study of the issue found a relationship between distinctly poor control and congenital malformations. So it is certainly prudent to strive for good blood glucose control as the fetus's organs are developing and to start this effort even before conception, since the fetal organs develop very early, often before you know you are pregnant. The recommendation, then, is to *establish excellent blood sugar control before attempting pregnancy.*

In middle and late pregnancy (from three to nine months), the mother's blood glucose control has a direct effect on the *size* of the developing fetus. Obstetricians are generally zealous in recommending that the diabetes be very well controlled during this period, and we agree. We have seen too many large-baby complications develop from poorly controlled diabetes during pregnancy.

The encouraging thing about all this is that the chain can be broken simply by controlling the mother's blood glucose to start with. True, it's anything but simple to control diabetes during pregnancy (see below). So let us say that the *concept* of control is simple: control the mother's blood glucose in pregnancy and avoid the abnormally large baby with all the associated risks. Good control is also good for the mother.

The Healthy Mother

We have described the "odds" of having a successful pregnancy in diabetes. But to any individual woman, the only statistic that matters is her specific pregnancy. There is no doubt that pregnancy can be successful despite diabetes; the odds, overall, are about 95% in your favor. For some couples, especially if the woman has severe long-term complications of diabetes or if other options, such as adoption, are attractive, trying for a pregnancy may seem ill advised. To many others, if long-term complications are not established and if the woman is willing to work hard on blood glucose control, pregnancy is not only possible but is likely to work out well.

Caring for the mother before conception of the fetus, called *preconception care,* is important for all women—but for women with diabetes, it is crucial. Plan a pregnancy, establish good blood glucose control *before* pregnancy, and recognize the pregnancy as soon as possible. Then, once you've conceived, prenatal care—caring for the mother and fetus during pregnancy—begins.

We know it's a tough road, demanding even more attention to diabetes than you ever thought possible. But the successful pregnancy and the healthy child is about as great a reward as we can think of. So let's get on with it: let's discuss what to expect, what goals to set, and how to achieve them.

What to Expect in a Pregnancy with Diabetes

Nine months can seem like an eternity when you are going through it: just imagine 2,160 blood sugar tests, 840 snacks, 25 doctor visits, sonograms, cravings, fatigue, and nausea. (Pity the mother elephant's two-year pregnancy, even without the tests and office visits!) But when you stop to consider what happens during that time, it's amazing that it doesn't take longer. In only nine months, a whole baby is being built in your uterus—from two little cells that came together at conception to a baby boy or girl.

There will be profound physical changes in your body to support it all. Obviously, your pregnancy will be apparent in your waistline, your breasts, and your enlarged uterus. There will be an increase in your blood volume (this can sometimes stress your heart, if it is weak to begin with). And there will be an increase in your body's fat stores, which is nature's adaptation meant to protect the baby if a period of starvation should occur during pregnancy.

Huge hormonal changes also take place in pregnancy, regulating the growth of the new body inside your womb and keeping a supply of glucose available for you and your baby. A direct effect of these hormones of pregnancy, however, is the predictable increase in your insulin requirement (if you take insulin) late in pregnancy. (More on this later.)

Finally, pregnancy puts a stress on your body as a whole. Pregnancy can change your complications status: retinopathy may worsen (usually temporarily), and hypertension or toxemia can develop, especially if you had protein in the urine before pregnancy.

Blood Glucose Goals in Pregnancy

All the usual prenatal care steps apply to pregnant women with diabetes: regular health professional visits, a healthful diet, vitamins, and so on. But with diabetes, you have another area of concern: controlling your blood glucose as much as possible. Having very specific control goals can help in this effort.

The ultimate blood glucose goal, of course, amounts to nothing short of perfection: the same sugar levels as found in a pregnant woman who doesn't have diabetes (these levels are actually lower than normal blood sugars in the nonpregnant state). Here are the targets:

—Before breakfast: 60–90 mg/dl
—Before lunch, supper, and bedtime snack: 60–105 mg/dl
—After meals: less than 140 mg/dl
—2 A.M. to 6 A.M.: 60–100 mg/dl

If you have gestational diabetes, you may be able to achieve these targets on a fairly regular basis. This is because GDM, like Type II diabetes, is intrinsically easier to manage, since the pancreas can still make insulin and blood sugars are relatively stable. But if you have pregestational diabetes—in other words, if you had Type I diabetes before the pregnancy—you may be thinking that these targets are impossible. Our answer is that these are *targets,* not levels that are required for every successful pregnancy. In fact, brief elevations of blood glucose are unlikely to cause you to lose a pregnancy. Also, tolerance to insulin reactions is better during the second and third trimesters of pregnancy, so tight blood sugar control is that much more doable. As with all parts of diabetes self-care, we suggest that you do the very best you can.

Avoiding high ketones is also important during pregnancy. Recall that ketones are a by-product of fat breakdown. They increase in the blood and spill into the urine in two situations: when you are not eating enough calories and when you have a seriously inadequate amount of insulin in your body. Pregnancy has been described as a condition of "accelerated starvation," so not eating enough (fasting) causes ketones to show up in the urine more quickly in pregnancy. There is debate about whether these "ketones of fasting" pose a danger in pregnancies complicated by diabetes, but the answer is probably not. However, spilling ketones in the urine because of inadequate insulin treatment—in other words, as a result of poor diabetic control (high blood sugar)—is a serious risk. Actual ketoacidosis (see Chapter

23) during pregnancy, when ketones not only increase but accumulate in the blood to the point of acid build-up, is associated with a high rate of loss of the pregnancy.

So keep an eye on your ketones by checking your urine daily. If they are positive, figure out why: if you are not eating enough calories (and have good blood sugar control), you should increase your dietary intake; if your blood sugar control is poor, you need to improve it, quickly.

Prenatal Care with Diabetes

The largest and best conducted study of blood glucose control in pregnancy made a surprising discovery: early in pregnancy, the mother's blood sugars themselves did not have as important an effect as just *getting good medical supervision.* This doesn't mean that blood sugars don't matter, it just means that the whole package of good prenatal care is most important. Good prenatal care improves the chance of a successful pregnancy.

Having a good health care team is always the best way to ensure good diabetes care. During pregnancy, however, the team is even more important. There is no way you can handle diabetes and pregnancy by yourself. You will need professional help—to understand diabetes care if you just developed GDM and to fine tune your regimen if you have preexisting Type I diabetes.

You need to be sure that someone is "quarterbacking" the health care process, checking to be sure that you have the appropriate eye exams, urine tests for protein, and so on. Your blood sugar management may be handled by your obstetrician or by your primary care doctor, endocrinologist, or nurse educator team, in conjunction with your obstetrician.

Let's consider the role of the new member on the health care team, the obstetrician. Although many women are well served during pregnancy and delivery by midwives and other health care professionals who are not physicians, for a woman who has diabetes complicating her pregnancy, close involvement of an obstetrician is essential. The medical issues are more complex, unpredictable, and dangerous than in an uncomplicated pregnancy. A primary role of the obstetrician will be to monitor your baby's progress during pregnancy. At regular intervals, she or he will probably be measuring the size of your abdomen, listening to the heartbeat, and recommending such tests as the sonogram, amniocentesis, alphafetoprotein, and the contraction stress test. Let's consider each of these commonly done assessments.

The sonogram.   The *sonogram* is a harmless and painless procedure. It amounts to sending sound waves through your skin and picking up their echo, like a depth finder used in boats. A picture of the fetus is obtained (it generally does not look much like the full-term infant you have in mind). Sonograms are used to estimate fetal size in comparison to fetal age and to inspect for malformations. Your doctor may also order a special sonogram called an *echocardiogram* to inspect the baby's heart more closely for defects. Like all tests, the sonogram is helpful but not perfect; some abnormalities cannot be picked up by a sonogram or any other test.

Alphafetoprotein. Th *alphafetoprotein* test is done at 16 weeks' gestation with a simple blood sample drawn from the arm. But the idea of the alphafetoprotein test may be scary and emotionally upsetting, because its aim is to screen for defects in the baby's spinal column. In some cases, the blood test will be positive even in the absence of any defect. If it is positive, an amniocentesis is recommended to confirm or refute the presence of an abnormality in the developing fetus.

Amniocentesis. Doing an *amniocentesis* involves sampling the fluid surrounding the developing fetus (the *amniotic fluid*) and cells from the fetus that float around in this fluid. It is done with a needle that looks formidably long, but it is usually not a particularly uncomfortable procedure. By examining the fluid and the cells, doctors can determine a number of things: whether there is evidence of Down syndrome or other chromosomal abnormalities, whether the baby is a boy or a girl, and, near the end of pregnancy, whether the baby's lungs are ready for delivery. You may want to ask your obstetrician if having an amniocentesis would be a good idea; if the obstetrician suggests this test, of course, you will want to know why. In any case, you choose which of the available results you want to know, including knowing the sex of the baby before birth.

Contraction stress test and nonstress test. The *contraction stress* and *nonstress* tests are done to assess whether the baby is developing normally and would respond normally to labor. The contraction stress test measures the changes in the baby's heart rate during spontaneous or induced mild contractions of the uterus. It is a painless procedure done by attaching an electronic fetal monitor to your abdomen with a belt. The nonstress test is similar to the contraction stress test except that the baby's heart rate is measured in response to his or her own movements, rather than to contractions of the uterus. Other tests are available to help the obstetrician decide whether a fetus is ready for delivery.

Timing of Delivery

The timing of delivery is the obstetrician's call. Many factors go into the decision, but the general preference is to let pregnancy continue to term or near term. The old practice was to deliver the baby early when the mother has diabetes, in order to avoid a late-in-pregnancy death of the fetus. In recent years, however, it has become clear that this practice was misguided—that more problems arose from delivering too early than from letting the pregnancy progress.

Tests of fetal maturity are now quite sophisticated, and obstetricians can determine pretty well when a fetus is ready to be born. Unless an emergency develops, it would be unusual for a pregnancy to be prematurely delivered just because the mother has diabetes; if elective delivery is recommended (either by inducing labor or by cesarean section), tests are usually done to be sure the baby is ready for birth. (The rate of cesarean section to deliver women with diabetes is three to five times greater than in women without diabetes.) Again, the decision on the timing of delivery is best left up to the obstetrician.

Common Problems in the Management of Diabetes in Pregnancy

Morning sickness, that "Will I make it to the bathroom before I throw up?" feeling that is common in early pregnancy, can present a challenge to the woman who has Type I diabetes and is trying to maintain her meal plan and control her blood sugar. (Recall that gestational diabetes usually doesn't show up until later in pregnancy.) The nausea may be worsened by low blood sugar or may *cause* low blood sugar. Eating crackers or dry toast seems to help. Avoiding spicy and greasy food and eating smaller, more frequent meals may also be helpful.

Constipation plagues many women during pregnancy, whether or not diabetes is present. Your intestinal muscles are more relaxed, and your baby will press on your intestines with increasing intensity as the pregnancy progresses. Increasing your fiber intake along with your fluid intake often takes care of the problem. Gentle, regular exercise helps too.

In later pregnancy, your baby will be taking up so much room in your abdomen that he or she will compress the volume of the stomach, forcing some of the acids into your esophagus. The result is a burning sensation in the stomach or throat (heartburn). Again, taking smaller, more frequent meals helps, along with avoiding high-fat foods.

Achieving Tight Blood Glucose Control in Pregnancy

Any attempt at tight blood glucose control is hopeless without close self-monitoring of blood glucose, and this is especially true during pregnancy. For starters, you never really know where your blood sugar is if you don't test. Also, you will have to know when during the day you are too close to low, so you can adjust your regimen to avoid hypoglycemia. Most health care professionals suggest that women test their blood sugar much more often during pregnancy—usually before and after meals, at bedtime, and at 3 A.M. We even advise a test before driving as well, because walking the line of tight control increases the risk of a serious low blood sugar at any time.

There are other ways than self-monitoring to test for your average blood sugar control: specifically, hemoglobin A1c (glycated or glycosylated hemoglobin) and fructosamine assays. Remember that the hemoglobin A1c assesses blood sugar control for a period of 8–12 weeks, which is too long in pregnancy to make the right corrections in treatment. The fructosamine assays may be used to get a better indication of what has happened over the previous two weeks or so. In the end, though, self-monitoring of blood glucose is the way to know up to the minute, day in and day out.

If you find your sugars increasing in a certain pattern—for instance, always high before breakfast—call your health care professional and adjust your regimen. If the sugars are very high (and by this we mean, in pregnancy, over about 180–200 mg/dl), take corrective action right away. You don't want to go on long with inadequate diabetic control, and you certainly don't want to slip into ketoacidosis. Ketoacidosis may occur during pregnancy with blood sugars not much over 200 mg/dl.

Diet

A healthful diet in pregnancy is one that meets your nutritional needs, helps keep your blood sugars stable, *and* provides for the growth of your baby. The total weight gain and pattern of weight gain are important measures of the adequacy of diet, but they are not the only measures.

Calories and weight gain. You will need sufficient calories to support the growth of the baby and maintain nutrient stores in your own body. This means weight gain—about 30 pounds, more or less. Specific weight goals are individualized, depending on whether you are underweight, at ideal weight, or overweight before pregnancy. Set a target with your obstetrician.

Weight gain is usually minimal at first, peaks mid-pregnancy at about a pound a week, and is a little slower thereafter. Generally, underweight women should gain the most, as they will need to add nutrient stores in the form of fat, and overweight women will not need to gain as much, since they may have sufficient fat stores before pregnancy.

In deciding how to control your weight gain, consider that your caloric requirements increase by an average of about 300 calories per day. However, actual intake needed will vary considerably depending on activity, resting metabolic rate, and prepregnancy weight. Your doctor and dietitian will help you estimate caloric requirements for your pregnancy, given your usual intake and activity.

Bear in mind that pregnancy is not the time to lose weight. Some people, especially when confronted with the need to keep their diabetes under especially good control, mistakenly restrict their calorie intake too much, endangering the pregnancy. Although weight loss may be a goal in the treatment of obesity, it is never a goal during pregnancy. Calories must be sufficient to meet the glucose demands of the growing baby. Measuring urinary ketones in the morning is a good way to determine whether calorie intake is sufficient to prevent the breakdown of fat. Your urine should be free of ketones.

Changing nutrient requirements during pregnancy.   Protein and micronutrient needs increase during pregnancy. You should increase the protein in your diet to include an extra 10 grams per day. This amounts to just an extra ounce and a half of meat (cooked) per day.

Pregnancy significantly increases the requirements for the micronutrients iron, folic acid, and calcium. Iron is needed for the increase in blood production during pregnancy and for the production of the baby's blood. It is difficult to meet this need from food alone, so most doctors prescribe an iron supplement.

Folic acid is needed for rapid cell division during pregnancy. It prevents some birth defects. Dark-green leafy vegetables like kale, dried beans, and whole wheat products are good sources. You will need extra calcium for bone development as well. A daily intake of at least 1,200 mg is recommended. That's equal to a quart of milk or the equivalent in other milk products. You'll also need vitamin D, to promote calcium absorption. Milk is usually fortified with vitamin D, or you can get enough through exposure of the skin to sunlight. To be sure you get sufficient amounts of the proper nutrients, your doctor may prescribe a vitamin and mineral supplement. Please don't self-prescribe megadoses of vitamins and minerals, though. They could be harmful to you and your developing baby.

Timing of meals.   Your baby will be drawing glucose from you at the same time that your hormones are working to make sure that glucose is available. In the end, it will be a balancing act to provide carbohydrate to keep your blood sugar up but not so much at any one time so that your blood sugar goes too high. Eating small, frequent meals often makes this easier to accomplish, especially since large meals may be unappetizing when you are nauseous in early pregnancy and distended in late pregnancy.

You should be especially alert to the composition of breakfast. In many women, glucose is hardest to control just after breakfast, especially if you have not given Regular insulin time to be absorbed and start acting. So breakfast is usually not a good time to load up with carbohydrates. Instead, spreading the carbohydrates out with a smaller breakfast meal and a mid-morning snack will often keep the blood sugar from spiking up.

A bedtime snack should be part of your meal plan. Because the baby will continue to take glucose from you through the night, low blood sugar and ketones are a risk if you do not have a snack. Your dietitian will probably have you take some protein along with the carbohydrate, to provide a slower release of glucose through the night. Cornstarch has been used for this purpose. Some women may need to have a snack in the middle of the night as well.

Exercise

Activity during pregnancy has real benefits: relaxation, improved fitness, good overall body image, a sense of well-being, and also relief of constipation. But stabilizing blood sugar may be the most significant feature of exercise in pregnancies complicated by diabetes.

We have heard it all: some women have run marathons during pregnancy (though not at our suggestion!), and others have taken up residence in an easy chair for the duration, despite normal health (the nineteenth-century model). What's best? Ideally, you should engage in safe exercise in moderation. As usual, individualization is the key. There are conditions, such as premature labor or mid-pregnancy spotting, that specifically rule out any exercise whatsoever, and there are some women whose level of fitness is perfectly compatible with heavy exercise remarkably long into pregnancy.

In general, safe exercise is any type of activity that gets you moving but prevents injury to your baby and your changing body structure. Injury can come in the form of direct trauma, from falling down, or straining ligaments and joints. Whatever your self-image, pregnancy does change the center of gravity and may make you more likely to tumble. It may be best to avoid water skiing or snow skiing, for example, since a fall at high speed could be harmful to you and your baby. Activities that involve twists and turns, such as racquetball, volleyball, and basketball, can also damage ligaments and joints that are loosened up in preparation for childbirth. Jogging, up to a certain point in your pregnancy, may be okay if you're already used to it before pregnancy. Swimming or water aerobics is, on the whole, a safe activity during pregnancy, as the buoyancy eases the strain on joints. Walking should be safe as well.

Moderation is recommended. If you were not used to exercising beforehand, pregnancy is not the time to start a strenuous activity regimen. If you were a regular exerciser before, you may be able to continue.

There are further precautions for pregnant women with diabetes. First, as with activity at any time, hypoglycemia is a danger. Test your blood sugar before you exercise. Prepare for exercise by eating an appropriate snack, and carry a source of quick-acting carbohydrate. Skip the exercise altogether if your sugar is very high—over 200, for example—since exercise at this time can raise the blood sugar higher, rather than lower it, if not enough insulin is circulating. Treat the high blood sugar right away, preferably with insulin rather than by not eating or by exercising, as you might if you weren't pregnant.

We are often asked whether repeated insulin reactions (hypoglycemia) can harm the developing fetus—a natural question, since the very tight control we are talking about in pregnancy often causes more hypoglycemic reactions. The fetus can grow normally in a relatively low glucose environment, and there is evidence that the placenta maintains a certain glucose level even when the mother's blood glucose is very low. So the answer is no. No studies have shown that hypoglycemia damages the fetus. But that does not minimize the effect on the mother, who is, after all, the carrier of the baby. It does not help the pregnancy if the mother has repeated dangerous insulin reactions.

A final concern with exercise during pregnancy has to do with complications. Some types of exercise can exacerbate unstable retinopathy—for example, weight training. Don't get us wrong: we're all for exercise. But when you're pregnant, you have to be a little more careful. Seek the guidance of your health care team.

Insulin and Oral Hypoglycemic Agents

Let's start with oral hypoglycemic agents: forget it. They aren't used in pregnancy and aren't even approved for use in pregnancy. Their potential for doing damage is not well established, but neither is their safety. Therefore, as with so many other drugs during pregnancy, do not take oral agents when you are pregnant.

There are limited options for treating diabetes in pregnancy: diet, exercise, and insulin. Given that the blood sugars have a strong tendency to rise as pregnancy progresses and that you definitely want to control blood sugar closely in pregnancy, many, probably most, women with diabetes in pregnancy are well advised to use insulin shots, so don't be upset if this is the recommendation. Keep telling yourself that it's for the good of that beautiful creature growing inside you. Remind yourself that if you didn't need insulin before pregnancy, the chances are good that you won't need it afterward. But using insulin can be a tricky thing in pregnancy, whether or not you used it before.

Insulin treatment during pregnancy usually means an intensive regimen, generally three or four shots a day, although two may be adequate if you have gestational diabetes. First, you want to have adequate insulin circulating throughout the 24-hour day to avoid uncovered gaps of insulin in your blood. Second, you want to cover carbohydrates ingested and to provide for rapid correction of high blood sugar. (Refer to Chapters 12 and 13 if you are unclear about specific insulins, their duration of action, and so on.)

Twice-a-day regimens. In a basic twice-a-day regimen of mixed NPH and Regular insulin, a problem may arise. The NPH can wear off before the next injection is given, resulting in high sugars at bedtime, overnight, or in the morning. You will know that just increasing the amount of NPH doesn't work if you get *hypoglycemic* as the NPH peaks but still get *hyperglycemic* later. In other words, an insulin reaction in the afternoon or the middle of the night, while still finding high blood sugars at suppertime or before breakfast, means that the twice-a-day schedule just isn't working for you: there are still uncovered times during the day, and you'd better move to at least three doses a day.

Three- or four-dose regimens. We have found that adding an injection of Regular insulin at lunchtime is often effective in covering afternoon highs, if that is the problem. (Obviously, if afternoon *lows* are the problem, lunchtime insulin isn't the answer.) More classically, you can take Regular insulin before supper to cover that meal after the morning NPH has worn off, with NPH at bedtime to cover overnight. Some health care professionals prefer the use of Ultralente insulin instead of NPH, with the Regular to cover meals.

Let's be clear that the object of these intensified insulin regimens is to mimic the normal pancreas's output of a little insulin all through the day and night (basal insulin) and to provide a brisk increase in insulin level at meal-time (bolus). Contrary to popular belief, health care professionals are *not* just trying to make life more complicated or get you stuck more times every day.

Insulin pumps in pregnancy.   Our practice is to discuss the use of external insulin pumps with anyone who requires three or four shots of insulin a day, since on the whole we find pumps to be a more stable, more effective, and much more convenient approach to intensive insulin delivery (see Chapter 14). They are especially useful in pregnancy, when intensive regimens are more common and blood sugar goals are tighter. One cautionary note is the danger of ketoacidosis if an interruption in the flow of insulin from the pump occurs, since only short-acting insulin is used in the pumps. When appropriate, then, we use insulin pumps during pregnancy, but we prefer to start the therapy before pregnancy so that the woman becomes experienced in problem solving and can effectively prevent ketones from appearing in the blood or urine.

Matching your insulin to your intake.   This is especially important in pregnancy, when your intake may vary because you may not feel like eating if you are experiencing nausea. The thing to remember is that insulin is needed to cover the carbohydrate ingested. Adjusting the insulin not only to blood sugar but also to actual grams of carbohydrate is the most precise way to accomplish this match. Remember that because the carbohydrate will raise your blood sugar faster than the insulin can work to lower it, you will need to inject the insulin a good 30–45 minutes before eating. Your physician and nurse educator team will assist you in insulin dosing.

Correcting the highs.   The final element of the day-to-day insulin regimen will be relatively quick correction of the highs and lows. Your team should advise you on what adjustments of your insulin doses are reasonable for a given blood sugar. For example, you may learn to inject 1 unit of insulin for every 40 mg/dl of blood sugar above 100 premeal and 1 unit for every 80 mg/dl above 100 after meals.

The pattern of blood sugar and insulin during pregnancy.   There is a pattern of blood sugar that is predictable during pregnancy. In early pregnancy (around 8–12 weeks after conception), there is a tendency to have more hypoglycemic reactions and require *less* insulin. This may be just because nausea can reduce appetite so that a woman eats less or because she and her health care professionals are working so hard to obtain tight control. But there is also evidence that hormonal changes are involved. For whatever reason, women with pregestational diabetes are well advised to be alert to a possible decrease in insulin requirement during this phase of pregnancy.

From about week 12 to the end of pregnancy, the insulin requirement marches steadily upward. By the last weeks of pregnancy, the insulin requirements, on average, double in women with Type I diabetes and may even triple in pregestational Type II diabetes. To maintain good control, you can count on requiring more insulin.

One warning: this very much increased insulin requirement by the end of pregnancy will drop right back to the prepregnancy level as soon as the baby is delivered. The insulin requirement is purely a function of the pregnancy. Consider, for example, the case of Laura:

> Laura is a 32-year-old woman who has had diabetes since the age of 14. She always did pretty well caring for her diabetes and has very few long-term complications: the ophthalmologist mentioned just a few spots on the retina but was very pleased with how minor the retinopathy was. Laura and her husband decide to have a child. She is referred to an obstetrician experienced in managing high-risk pregnancies and is told to establish very tight control of her blood sugar even before discontinuing contraceptive methods. This is difficult, but Laura is reasonably successful, and she becomes pregnant. Her usual insulin requirement is 42 units per day, split into three doses of NPH and Regular insulin. Unfortunately, she has serious problems with nausea and vomiting in the first trimester and trouble in keeping her food down. She learns to compensate with her insulin dose, which falls to 28 units per day total. At week 15, Laura feels like a new person. Her amniocentesis and blood tests are all fine, her nausea is subdued, and her abdomen is starting to bulge. To keep blood glucose in range, though, requires more and more insulin. By the last month of pregnancy, she is astounded by the fact that she takes 80 units of insulin a day, 24 units of it in the morning—much more than she ever took in her life. Laura's delivery is vaginal, with labor induced after her obstetrician determines that the baby is ready. Delivering a beautiful baby girl on a Friday, she is a little surprised to be sent home on Saturday morning. Her doctor is away for the weekend and the covering doctor hasn't made rounds yet. Laura, not thinking much about it, takes 24 units of insulin that morning. All afternoon, as family gathers to see the new arrival, Laura is fighting serious insulin reactions.

The bottom line.   Excellent blood sugar control is the day-to-day goal in pregnancy. If you can demonstrate, to yourself first and your health care provider next, that your sugars are really in the range you want on a simple regimen, more power to you. Remember, though: if you aren't checking often, you don't know what the sugars are running. Usually it is hard to maintain tight control during pregnancy without a more intensive insulin regimen, especially if you have preexisting Type I diabetes.

Delivery and Postpartum

When the time comes, you will deliver your baby in one of three ways: *spontaneous vaginal* (through the vagina after labor has started spontaneously), *induced vaginal* (through the vagina after labor was started by the administration of medication), and planned or emergency *cesarean section*. As we said, your doctor will keep you updated on your and your baby's progress during pregnancy and will make a decision that is safest for both of you. Factors to consider will be the baby's health (is the baby still surviving well in your uterus?) and your health (are your blood sugar and blood pressure well controlled, and are there any changes in complications status?).

Blood sugar control during labor and delivery, regardless of the method chosen, will be important in controlling the baby's blood sugar as well. If your blood sugar goes too high, then the baby will overproduce insulin and have a low blood sugar immediately after delivery. If your sugar is too low or if you don't get enough glucose, then your body could start to produce ketones. So the balance is delicate. Although practice trends vary, a method commonly used is an intravenous infusion of insulin and glucose along with frequent blood glucose monitoring. The intravenous route has the advantage of acting immediately. But be sure to alert your doctor if you took long-acting insulin during the day of delivery.

During labor, insulin needs may be dramatically *decreased,* presumably due at least in part to the extreme exertion of labor. Upon delivery, as mentioned, you will have an almost immediate return to the prepregnancy insulin requirements. Most women with GDM will see the diabetes disappear altogether, at least for the time being. Not reducing your insulin dose even the day after delivery can cause serious hypoglycemia, as we saw in Laura's case, above.

Breastfeeding is good for your baby, and women with diabetes are encouraged to breastfeed if possible. Breast milk has all the nutrients that your baby needs, is prepackaged at just the right temperature, and has antibodies that fight certain infections. Best of all is the closeness that you will feel with your baby. Your and your baby's nutrient needs for breastfeeding can usually be met by your prepregnancy diet, provided it is adequate in calcium, fluids, and protein. If you have Type I diabetes, however, you may need to rearrange your calories and insulin regimen to compensate for the lowering of blood glucose that can occur as the baby takes glucose from you. Middle-of-the-night feedings may require an extra snack at that time or before retiring.

In the immediate postpartum period, you're likely to be exhausted. Seek out and accept help from those who can be genuinely supportive of your and your baby's needs. Preparing a meal, changing a diaper, helping you give your baby a bath: all these kinds of assistance can give you the support you need to recuperate.

It is well recognized that some women have bouts of depression after childbirth. With diabetes in the picture, you may feel especially down. Do not feel you are alone, do not feel ashamed. Be candid with your doctor about any blue feeling that persists day after day, any difficulties with sleep (besides feeding the baby), or any feeling of bringing harm to yourself. If it becomes a significant problem, seek professional help. Sometimes a change in thyroid function can be involved.

From the instant your baby is born, you and your partner become parents and have the responsibility and joy of meeting your child's every need. In some ways, having had diabetes, you are better prepared than most parents. The discipline and perseverance required to get through a pregnancy with diabetes will serve you well in dealing with middle-of-the-night feedings and figuring out a crying baby's needs, not to mention dealing with all the joys—and, yes, traumas—of parenthood to come.

Becoming pregnant when you have pregestational diabetes, or developing gestational diabetes when you are pregnant, is traumatic. You will be pushed by your health care provider and by your own conscience to test blood sugars frequently and to keep them as close to normal as possible. All this is an effort to improve the chances that you will have a normal pregnancy and a healthy child.

If you have diabetes, think carefully about whether you want to become pregnant. If so, get your diabetes under control, preferably before conception. Enter into good prenatal care immediately, and stay in close touch with your health care team throughout the pregnancy. You will probably have to use insulin, and if you've already been using it you will probably have to intensify your regimen. Requirements will increase late in pregnancy. But you can do it.

One final word: for nine months you've focused on taking good care of your health. Maybe you were able to sustain the motivation because of the baby. Don't let it stop. Continue it for your own good, and remember that your baby is still dependent on your health. If you are sick a lot or develop complications of diabetes, it will be difficult for you to care for your child.

As you take good care of yourself, give yourself a big round of applause. You have set a wonderful example for your child to see.

Chapter 32

The Genetics of Diabetes

- *"My family is shot through with diabetes. What are my chances?"*
- *"I couldn't believe that my child would get diabetes. They say it's genetic, but there is absolutely no history of diabetes on either side of our family. I just don't understand it."*
- *"Naturally, my first thought when I learned that one of my children had diabetes was, Will his brothers get it too?"*
- *"I love my boyfriend John, and I have no problem whatever with his diabetes. But frankly, I'm worried about whether any children we might have would get diabetes. Should I be worried about that?"*

We live at the beginning of a revolution in human genetics. Genes are the basic pieces of DNA that determine all of a person's genetic characteristics, and every day now genes are being identified, analyzed, and even *sequenced* (a process that defines their exact structure). But in terms of practical knowledge, we are really just at the beginning. If you think of the effort to understand all the human genes as being like mapmaking, then genetic research is about at the stage of the seventeenth-century explorers groping their way down the coast of Maine in the fog. We have a long way to go. We have a lot to discover, and genetics will be profoundly important in understanding and ultimately curing diabetes.

What do genes have to do with diabetes? We already know that it is to some extent inherited, but there are still many, many questions we can't answer. We can talk about the *chances*—that is, the risk—of getting diabetes, but we can't tell you whether you or your child *will* get diabetes, and we can't even tell you why one person gets it while another does not. When the genes that cause diabetes are discovered (and there will probably be several or even many of them), not only will scientists be able to predict diabetes but also they will be in a position to discover how to modify or correct the gene abnormality responsible for diabetes. This might prevent diabetes altogether.

At the moment we have only the most general notions about the genetics of diabetes. One of these observations is that Type I and Type II diabetes are two different diseases, not only clinically (as discussed in Chapter 2) but also genetically. It is clear that these two major kinds of diabetes run through families independently. If there are a large number of people with Type II diabetes in the family, that doesn't increase the chance of Type I diabetes occurring, and families with individuals with Type I won't necessarily have family members with Type II. We will therefore consider the genetics of Type I and Type II diabetes separately.

Type I Diabetes

Is Type I diabetes caused by your genetic make-up or by something in your environment? The answer is both. Some people start off with a genetic predisposition to Type I diabetes. If they meet up with the environmental trigger, they get diabetes; if they don't meet up with the causative factor in the environment, they never get diabetes.

By analogy, you could think of the tendency to get badly sunburned. If the person has dark skin genetically, bad sunburn may never be a problem. But even if the person is genetically susceptible to sunburn by having very fair skin, the sunburn will happen only if the skin is exposed to the environmental trigger (the sun). So sunburn is the result of both a genetic predisposition and an environmental exposure.

The trouble is, unlike sunburn (which obviously occurs more in genetically fair-skinned people and is triggered by an overdose of sun), very little is known about the genetic predisposition to Type I diabetes, and almost nothing is known about the environmental trigger. Certain genetic characteristics, called *haplotypes* or *HLA types,* are known to be associated with a greater or lesser chance of developing Type I diabetes, but little else is known about the actual genetic abnormality for Type I. Likewise, it has long been speculated that the environmental trigger is a virus, but this remains unproven. We do know that an illness or stress that occurs shortly before the diagnosis of Type I diabetes brings it out, but these stresses are *not* likely to be the cause, since evidence of the autoimmune process can be seen years before the onset of Type I diabetes.

As more of the basic genetics is understood, we think it will be possible not only to predict who will get diabetes but also to replace genes or prevent environmental exposures or take other approaches to prevent diabetes from developing. In the meantime, we have to rely on relatively crude information, such as that derived from twin studies.

Twin Studies

Identical twins have exactly the same genes; nonidentical (fraternal) twins have just a partial sharing of genes, like brothers or sisters who are not twins. If a characteristic is entirely determined by genetics, then both individuals in a pair of identical twins will be identical for that characteristic. Eye color is an example of this: both twins in identical twins always have the same eye color. If something is not genetic, then it will not be identical in both twins— for example, identical twins won't both break their arms at the same time (unless they fall out of the same tree at the same time).

When one identical twin has Type I diabetes, there is about a 35% chance that the other will develop it too, although the onset may be many years apart. This simple number tells a lot: it shows that there is a strong genetic component to Type I diabetes (or else the second twin would not have nearly such a high chance of getting diabetes), but it also shows that heredity is not the whole story, since about 65% of identical twins whose twin has Type I diabetes never do develop the disease. There is also a strong nongenetic component, whether viral or something else. If the disease were entirely genetic, like eye color, the second identical twin would always have it if the first one did.

That's why we say that Type I diabetes is both genetic and environmental. But where does this leave you, personally, in terms of planning for yourself and your family?

What Are the Odds?

As discussed in Chapter 2, there are laboratory tests available, called *islet cell antibodies* or *GAD antibodies,* that can detect, years before any apparent illness, that a person is undergoing the immune destruction of the beta cells and will probably get clinical Type I diabetes. But these tests are not always positive in people who do get Type I diabetes (false negatives), and sometimes they are also mistaken in predicting who will get it (false positives). Furthermore, the tests never turn positive until the diabetic process is already under way, so they cannot be used to predict who will ultimately get Type I diabetes before any damage is done.

Since we cannot predict with certainty who will get diabetes, we can only talk about the odds, or risk. Odds, as any card player will tell you, don't tell you what *is* going to happen, they just tell you what is *more or less likely* to happen. And sometimes the odds (or relative risk, as it is called) can be deceiving.

As an example of calculating the odds, consider that if you live on a farm instead of a city, there may be a much greater *relative risk* of your being hit by a bale of hay falling from a silo. But hay falling from a silo is not very common, so the *actual risk* is still very small. Similarly, the chance of Type I diabetes recurring in a family that already has one case is greater than if no one in the family has it. But the chance is still small.

So what exactly are the odds of getting diabetes if you have it in the family? If one parent has Type I diabetes, the chance that a given child will get it is about 2%–6% (actually about 1% higher if the father has diabetes than if the mother has it). If one child (but neither parent) has Type I diabetes, the chance that a brother or sister will get it is about 5%–10%. These odds are true over the whole population, but there are certain unusual families that have Type I diabetes much more frequently, often associated with other endocrine deficiencies, such as thyroid disease or adrenal insufficiency. If you have this sort of family, you probably know it, because there are a lot of cases of diabetes.

On the whole, these are pretty good odds. They also explain why in most cases Type I diabetes seems to come out of the blue, with no family history. That does not mean it isn't inherited, it just means that the gene never *showed itself* in living memory (wasn't "expressed," the geneticists would say). Someone in the family probably carried the gene but didn't develop the disease.

What Can I Do to Tip the Odds in My Favor?

Unfortunately, with Type I diabetes, there is very little a person can do to tip the odds in his or her favor. Unlike Type II diabetes, which is so closely related to body weight, there is nothing we know about in diet, exercise, or any other activity that changes a person's chance of getting Type I diabetes. The amount of sugar in a child's diet may cause dental cavities, but it has nothing to do with causing diabetes. One group of researchers has proposed that exposure to cow's milk at a young age (as opposed to breastfeeding) is a major factor in causing Type I diabetes, but this theory so far lacks independent confirmation.

We have mentioned the laboratory tests that can tell when Type I diabetes is developing. But unless we can do something to interrupt that progress—and so far we cannot—the information is not of much use. The Diabetes Prevention Trial, Type I, sponsored by the National Institutes of Health, is trying to find a way to prevent Type I diabetes. If one of the interventions being used in this study is shown to prevent Type I diabetes successfully, then a great deal more effort will be made to identify people who are in a prediabetic phase, because then we will be able to influence the odds in their favor.

Type II Diabetes

Type II diabetes is much more strongly determined by genetics than is Type I. The results of identical twin studies strikingly prove this point. If one identical twin has Type II diabetes, then there is a very high chance, perhaps 90% or more, that the other twin will get it as well.

In studies of the genetics of Type II diabetes, the majority of clues have come from certain very high-risk populations. About half of the Pima Indians of Arizona develop diabetes, for instance, and up to 80% of people over age 55 in the Nauruan tribes in the South Pacific have diabetes. Type II diabetes is also more common in African Americans and Hispanic Americans, compared to Caucasians. By studying individuals and families with these backgrounds, investigators are slowly piecing together "candidate genes" that may explain the inheritance of Type II diabetes.

An interesting line of research has emphasized the role that the environment, particularly the diet, plays in bringing out Type II diabetes in susceptible individuals. Investigators followed groups of people as they moved from one lifestyle to another. Natives of Japan who move to the United States, for example, with all the changes in diet, activity, and stress that such a move demands, are much more likely to develop Type II diabetes than are Japanese people who remain in Japan—so there clearly is an environmental effect. Similar studies have been done as other groups of people, whether Native American, Pacific islanders, or Arabian peninsula nomads, are introduced to Western civilization.

With less exercise and more food, obesity is more likely to occur, and obesity is the factor that is most closely related to Type II diabetes. Any way you look at it—whether in the whole population of a nation or a single individual—the more fat you carry, the more likely it is that you will get Type II diabetes.

If we put all these factors together, we find that the individual at highest risk of developing Type II diabetes is a middle-aged woman of Native American, African American, or Hispanic descent whose family has many cases of Type II diabetes and who is overweight and has a history of diabetes during pregnancy.

What are the Odds?

The odds are difficult to calculate, because they depend so heavily on *how many* of the risk factors a person has. But considering family members alone, if one parent has Type II diabetes, the chance is about 10%–15% that a child will ever develop it (usually in adulthood, of course). If both parents have it, the chance goes up.

What Can I Do to Tip the Odds in My Favor?

The most important thing you can do to tip the odds in your favor is *maintain normal body weight*. There is some evidence that reducing your dietary fat intake will help, even if you don't reduce your body weight. Exercise appears to be another effective preventive approach.

The Diabetes Prevention Program, funded by the National Institutes of Health, is investigating whether Type II diabetes can be prevented and, if so, how. People at very high risk for Type II diabetes are enrolled in the study and are assigned randomly to one of several study treatments. We hope to find out, for example, whether intensive counseling on how to improve lifestyle (by diet and exercise) is more or less effective than taking certain medications. The results of this research may be available by the year 2002 or so.

The genetics of diabetes is extraordinarily complex. One of the few certainties is that Type I diabetes and Type II diabetes are inherited independently—having one type in the family doesn't increase the chances of having the other type. In Type I diabetes, there is often no family history of diabetes, because even in families where one member has it, the chance that another person will develop Type I diabetes is about 1 in 50. There is no way to predict accurately who will get Type I diabetes unless the immune process that destroys the pancreas is already under way; attempts to prevent Type I are still in an early research phase.

Type II diabetes, on the other hand, is more strongly influenced by heredity, with family history usually revealing multiple cases. There are clear features that mark someone as being at especially high risk of Type II diabetes: obesity (especially abdominal), certain minority ethnic heritages, and a history of diabetes during pregnancy. Maintaining normal body weight is the best thing you can do to prevent Type II diabetes, at least until we know the outcome of the Diabetes Prevention Program trial, which may identify other approaches to prevention.

Part VI

The Future of Care

Recognizing that no one knows for sure what the future care of diabetes will be like, there are three certainties: it will be different, it will be better, and it will depend on research. In Part VI we try to describe what the future of diabetes care may be like. We don't describe diabetes research just to satisfy your curiosity or to solicit your support for a good cause. We write about diabetes research because it is exciting, it is fascinating, and it is ultimately the only way that diabetes and its complications will be stamped out.

Browse through the topics in research that we talk about, and use the resources we mention to stay abreast of new work. There is a strong link between the research being done now and the prognosis for people with diabetes: the more and faster the research, the better the outlook.

Chapter 33

Diabetes Research

- *"I don't understand research at all. I don't want to know what goes on in some test tube. What does it mean for me?"*
- *"What I want is an islet cell transplant."*
- *"I need a glucose monitor that doesn't require a finger stick."*
- *"I want to know how I can help: I believe in my heart that research is the way to go, but it's beyond me how I can get involved."*
- *"You won't catch me being a human guinea pig! What if I should get the placebo pill?"*
- *"I'm fortunate to have the ability to contribute money, but I want to know how to get it in the right hands."*
- *"Do you have any new experimental studies I can take part in?"*

Diabetes research is such an enormous topic that we could easily fill an entire book in discussing it. But since we have to limit ourselves to a single chapter, we will start with a general discussion of the research process, make some suggestions about how to read and interpret accounts of research in the lay press, and then give specific examples of diabetes research and how you can get involved.

The Research Process

First, the researcher asks a question. The question has to be a good one—one that's important and one to which the answer isn't already known. Saying that it has to be important is not to say that its importance has to be obvious to everyone at first glance. But to people in the field, the question should have significance.

The research question also must be *answerable* within the time frame and the budget of the proposed study. If it would take 1,000 people in a 5-year study to answer a particular question, then there's no point in starting if you can only afford to enroll 100 people for 1 year. How technical, how difficult to understand must research be? The best researchers are often also the best communicators, able to explain complex ideas in straightforward terms. But Albert Einstein once said that "a scientific question should be made as simple as possible . . . and no simpler." Much of modern research is complex. Full-time investigators are highly trained and must meet rigorous intellectual and ethical standards. Competition is tough if you want to make a career doing research. It is not a part-time hobby. Young people go through many years of education and training, with long apprenticeships, to become independent researchers.

Broad Areas of Diabetes Research

Basic Research

When we think of *basic research* we think of test tubes and lab benches. It is a fact that basic research usually does take place in a laboratory, but the location is not what defines the process. Rather, what distinguishes basic investigation is the kind of question asked. The questions are not "Does this treatment work?" or "How do I apply this new computer chip to treating diabetes?" but "How does the cell respond to insulin?" or "What genes cause fat cells to multiply?" If the answers to these basic questions eventually lead to a specific treatment, all the better, but the first step is to understand the process.

A good example of basic understanding leading to treatment is the discovery of insulin itself, described in Chapter 12. Each step in the discovery process was built on the understanding gained by the previous step. First the pancreas was discovered to have some antidiabetic factor. Then it was discovered that the factor resides in the islets of Langerhans. Finally, the technique was worked out to extract the islets from a pancreas without damaging them. To the public, insulin was "discovered" by this last step, but to those who understood the process, it was the climactic conclusion of a long chain of discoveries.

In the same logical way, the reality of human insulin started with basic research. DNA was found to be the genetic material that regulates all proteins made in a cell. The methods were developed to cut up DNA, splicing codes known to make cells produce insulin into cells, like bacteria, that don't normally make insulin. With this basic understanding of how insulin is made and the ability to splice insulin-producing DNA into bacteria, pharmaceutical companies could *apply* this basic research to insulin production.

Applied Research

Applied research is the effort to bring together what is known and apply it to a defined need. It is based on, and builds on, basic research. We can illustrate applied research with the story of implanted insulin infusion pumps, developed at Johns Hopkins.

In the early 1980s NASA had made huge strides in various technologies related to spacecraft. It had pioneered in miniaturization, since the payload had to be as small and light as possible. The computer microchip, an essential part of implantable insulin pumps, was in its formative stages. NASA had perfected remote communication, a development that led to remote controllers for televisions and garage doors, as well as to implantable insulin pumps. And NASA had pioneered in quality control, since you really couldn't afford to have things break down once they were launched into space at a cost of millions of dollars. Systems that promoted reliability were obviously essential for medical devices, such as pumps. Finally, NASA happened to have developed a small pump for the purpose of delivering tiny pulses of culture medium onto samples of the surface of Mars, to see if anything would grow. This little pump turned out to be just right for our needs.

All the elements were there for development of an implantable insulin pump. It took a major effort in applied diabetes research, though, to make the system a reality. A sophisticated engineering team was assembled at the Johns Hopkins University Applied Physics Laboratory, involving collaboration of mechanical and electrical engineers, software experts, telemetry specialists, insulin chemists, and diabetologists. A prototype device was fabricated, and in 1982 it was ready for four years of testing in dogs with diabetes.

Use of animals in medical research. We are well aware that people have very strong opinions about this subject, and they have a perfect right to their opinions. It is a complex subject, ethically and practically. We would say, first, that the ethical use of animals in diabetes research has allowed innumerable advances in the treatment of humans. The very fact that something in the pancreas (insulin) could prevent diabetes was discovered in dogs. Every treatment advance you can think of required testing in animals before use in humans. It is impossible to imagine how backward our treatment of diabetes would be today, how many people who are living and well today would be dead or dying, without animal research.

We also want to emphasize that there are now well-established standards and review processes to ensure that animals are ethically cared for in research, just as human research subjects are. We support the ethical use of animals in diabetes research. It is absolutely essential.

Using well-cared-for, happy, and healthy dogs with diabetes treated by implanted insulin pumps, we were ready for humans by 1986. The clinical research trials could begin.

Clinical Research

Clinical research is done in people. It may be treatment-oriented, as was the case with our pump and with any pill, device, or procedure; it may be psychosocial; it may be epidemiological (that is, involving the study of large groups of people); or it may ask questions about disease in humans that are not specifically tied to a treatment. We give examples of clinical research later in this chapter, but it is important first to understand the safeguards that protect human subjects.

Participation in human clinical trials isn't forced on anyone. The trials are definitely not done without participants' full knowledge and consent. They are highly regulated, governed by a carefully developed set of rules and ethical considerations. If a scientist wants to do a research project involving people, the proposal is subjected to a detailed scientific and ethical review to be sure that it is sound and that it is in the proposed research subjects' best interest to take part.

The institutional review board (IRB) is the basis of this review process. Made up of independent scientists, ethicists, lawyers, and community members, the IRB is designed to look out for the rights and safety of the research subjects, making sure the project is as safe as possible, with a reasonable *risk/benefit ratio*. In other words, a study that puts the subjects at more risk must have a correspondingly greater potential to benefit them. A minimal-risk project, such as just drawing a tube of blood, does not have to give much benefit. Issues of compensation are considered carefully. People may be offered monetary or other compensation (such as free medical evaluations). But there should not be such a high rate of compensation that people are induced to undergo what would otherwise not be in their interest.

Most of all, the IRB makes sure that a potential research subject knows what he or she is getting into. You are asked beforehand if you are interested in taking part; all aspects of the study are explained to you in understandable language; you have a chance to ask questions before or during your participation; and you sign a consent form. Only after all these steps are you ready to take part. This series of safeguards ensures that your rights are protected.

We discuss the benefits of taking part in research studies later in this chapter.

Understanding Diabetes Research from the Outside

Whether they take part in clinical research or not, people are often confused and even misled by reports they may read in the newspaper or see on television. Even scientists active in the field have trouble keeping up with the articles published in many journals devoted to medical research. If you are not trained in diabetes research but are eager to follow what's happening, it can be a problem. There is no easy answer to how to keep up with diabetes research, but responses to some frequently asked questions may help:

Where do I go for information?   There are several reliable sources of information, designed specifically to describe diabetes research to the public. The American Diabetes Association's *Diabetes Forecast,* the Juvenile Diabetes Foundation's *Research Report,* and publications from the National Institutes of Health's National Institute of Diabetes, Digestive and Kidney Diseases (NIDDK) come to mind.

We are strongly supportive of having diabetes researchers from a local academic institution speak at clubs, fraternal organizations, religious groups, or other meetings to give overviews of their research and diabetes research in general. Researchers are more and more eager to take part in these outreach programs, recognizing that public support is fostered by public understanding of research. So ask a researcher to talk with your group, and get it straight from the horse's mouth.

What sources of information are less reliable?   Paid advertisements are usually not objective reports of research findings, especially the kind that are direct mailings to you describing "breakthroughs." There is no control over what they claim or what they charge for unproven remedies. Company press conferences or press releases may not be quite what they appear. Mergers, new directions of research, new ideas announced from corporate headquarters may take years to translate into actual therapies.

Short television or newspaper reports are often technically accurate but may be hard to interpret. Such reports are usually based on new studies in reputable journals, but are often taken out of context. Longer articles by established medical reporters may provide far more reliable perspective than you get from a single brief news report. Comments by established experts can hint at the true importance of a study. "Dr. X commented that the findings are interesting but need confirmation or further study" means that Dr. X doesn't believe the results. "Dr. X commented that the findings are very important" means that Dr. X does believe the results. But remember that Dr. X does not want to give a negative picture of research and does not want to be a nay-sayer.

What will this finding mean to my diabetes?   We suggest that you try to figure out what stage the research is in. Is it just an idea that may or may not ever be practical? Is it a basic research finding that may translate into therapy years down the road? Is it a finding in lower animals or a human research trial?

You may have to ask your health care professional, but we do caution you, first, that the press usually gets journals before the practitioner, so there could be a lapse of time before the health care professional sees an article. We also caution you that no professional can read or understand all the articles, and it is unrealistic to expect an expert opinion on every research finding reported in the press.

The bottom line.   Valid research is necessary to test whether any given treatment works. We run into claims that all sorts of treatment, from seaweed to herbal teas, will cure (or reverse) diabetes. Most claims are simply untrue, based on testimonials but backed by no real evidence. At the risk of sounding too conventional, we emphasize that you and your health care professionals should make your decisions based on valid clinical research, published in the regular medical journals. Lots of treatments can *sound* good, but in reality they will range from useless to harmful.

So get your information from well-established sources, figure out where each research advance fits into the larger picture of diabetes, and take advantage of the long-range improvements in care options.

Active Diabetes Research

You may be wondering what areas are "hot" in diabetes research. Ask any researcher, and you will hear about his or her own work, of course. Indeed, if we all knew and agreed on exactly what research would prove most fruitful in the long run, that would be the only research done. But we can only guess. Here are our thoughts on some areas of diabetes research that are especially active and could be especially important. It is by no means a complete list and is intended only to give an idea of how broad the field of diabetes research really is.

Basic Research

Insulin action.   There is still mystery surrounding how insulin really acts on the cell, allowing glucose in and affecting so many of the cell's crucial actions. If the process always worked perfectly, then maybe it would be less important to understand in detail. But, as you know from reading about Type II diabetes, insulin resistance—when cells do not respond normally to insulin—is a fundamental part of that very common and very serious kind of diabetes.

We know that insulin resistance is closely linked to obesity, but we don't know why. We know that insulin receptors on the surface of the cell seem to be present in adequate numbers and that once they do their job the biochemical pathways inside the cell do not respond normally. If insulin action and insulin resistance are fully understood, it is likely that treatments will be developed that can reverse that resistance. The benefits in controlling Type II diabetes would be enormous. Basic research into insulin action is extremely active and important.

Genetics of diabetes.   Studying the genetics of diabetes goes way beyond drawing family trees. Genes have been recognized since the 1950s as the central determinant of how an organism develops; in humans, genes determine height, hair and eye color, and many of the diseases to which the person is susceptible. In Chapter 32 we described a "genetic revolution," and it is true that scientists' understanding of genetics is progressing very quickly. In the research laboratory, this means identifying and examining genes that make people susceptible to diabetes, either Type I or Type II. It means looking at how these genes are "expressed," that is, how they function.

The problem is made far more difficult by the fact that there is almost certainly no *single* gene responsible for causing either Type I or Type II diabetes. Both kinds of diabetes undoubtedly involve multiple genes as well as important nongenetic factors, such as the amount of food a person eats or exposure to particular viruses. Still, there are specific genetic factors with very practical implications. A new field of basic research has been studying obesity genes.

There is a kind of mouse, called the ObOb mouse, that gets enormously fat and, like overweight people, develops a disease very much like Type II diabetes. Obesity in these mice is an entirely inherited trait. In 1994–95, some investigators found the gene that goes awry in these mice and described the problem that gene has in making its protein, called *leptin*. Furthermore, the same gene and the same protein, leptin, are present in humans. Before anyone concludes that "the obesity gene" solves all human weight problems, it must be pointed out that most of the genes a mouse has are also found in humans, and they may or may not play important roles in human disease. While the ObOb mouse's problem is entirely genetic and is inherited in a straightforward way, human obesity is anything but straightforward. And human Type II diabetes involves factors other than obesity.

But this discovery of an obesity gene in the mid-1990s illustrates the power of medical genetics. Over the coming years, at the pace genetic research is moving, it is likely that new insights into diabetes-related genes will be forthcoming.

The dream is that a major gene defect could be identified that would be modifiable or correctable. Gene therapy has already had some success for certain unusual diseases caused by relatively simple, single-gene defects. It will be much harder to apply gene therapy to a disease like diabetes. But genetic research may ultimately find the cure.

Immunology of Type I diabetes.   In describing the causes of Type I diabetes earlier in this book, we referred to the fact that the insulin-producing pancreatic islet cells are destroyed by an immune process in which the body's defense mechanisms turn against its own beta cells. Immunology as a science has progressed rapidly in recent years, but it is fair to say that the immune process that attacks the pancreas in Type I diabetes remains poorly understood.

If the cause of the immune attack on the beta cells were known, it would be possible to try to block that response. For example, if there were an antibody identified that was causing the damage, scientists could work on a "blocking antibody" to neutralize the offender. Our basic understanding of just how this immune process works is still inadequate, and jumping to clinical trials before building the basic knowledge base is rarely productive.

Basic research into the immune processes causing Type I diabetes is an important area of basic research today, one that could lead to the prevention or cure of Type I diabetes.

Psychosocial Research

Psychosocial research is finally coming into its own. People are realizing that certain approaches to inducing behavioral change work better than others, that certain educational approaches are more effective, that there are even some predictors of who is ready for change. There have been various important areas of psychosocial research that continue to contribute to clinical care.

The concept of "locus of control," for example, was especially popular in the 1970s and 1980s. It tried to define whether a set of people considered *themselves* in control of their own behavior, their own destiny, or whether they felt that they were more strongly controlled by *outside* influences—their doctor, their disease, their environment. Like many concepts used to explain human behavior, "locus of control" made a contribution without being the last word.

Currently, there is an emphasis in psychosocial research on readiness for change and how to take best advantage of that moment. It is increasingly recognized that if someone is not ready, if the individual does not feel the need or have the personal drive to change, then that person is very unlikely to change, regardless of the amount of information or coaxing provided by a health care professional. Researchers in human behavior are looking into the characteristics that identify when a person is ready for change. A better understanding of readiness could make people's use of health care resources much more effective.

Cognitive function is a specific area of psychosocial support that has always been of interest in diabetes. Anyone who has seen a person fall into hypoglycemic coma and then be immediately aroused when they receive sugar has to wonder whether brain cells were lost, whether the episode caused any lessened intellectual function. Parents are naturally concerned about this when their children have even mild insulin reactions. Careful testing has, on the whole, found no loss of intellectual capability whatsoever from even recurrent hypoglycemia in the setting of diabetes therapy. It may be that the brain simply overcomes any loss of brain cells or that our methods of measuring intelligence are not quite sensitive enough. But the reassuring fact is that intelligence, as best we can measure it, is not affected by the number of hypoglycemic reactions a person has.

Another example of behavioral research is the study of social support. What does it mean to have supportive companions when a person is trying to make behavioral changes? When is it necessary for the supporting people to be undergoing the same stresses, as exemplified by classic support groups for alcoholism, weight reduction, or diabetes? When is a supportive family best? What substitutes can be effective? The questions are many, and it is safe to predict that research into human behavior will keep investigators busy for decades to come.

Approaches to Normal Blood Glucose

An underlying theme of this book is that the maintenance of normal blood glucose would eliminate the complications of diabetes, in effect making it a nondisease, since there would no longer be any ill effects of diabetes. So it is not surprising that a huge amount of research is directed toward investigating various ways to normalize blood glucose. Psychosocial research is part of this general effort, since having the right frame of mind puts people in a position to do better for themselves at controlling their diabetes. This section will describe some of the other directions being taken to facilitate blood glucose control.

New oral hypoglycemic agents.   As described in Chapter 11, 1995 and 1996 were landmark years in the availability of oral hypoglycemic agents. Two new types of antidiabetes pills became available in the United States: metformin and acarbose.

Metformin's development for the U.S. market was an interesting story, since it is not, in fact, a new drug at all, having been used in Europe for decades. In the 1970s it had been disapproved by the FDA because of its similarity to the drug called phenformin that was known to have occasional life-threatening side effects (lactic acidosis). To obtain FDA approval of metformin, the pharmaceutical manufacturer had to complete an entirely new clinical trial in the United States, even though the drug was in common use around the world. This large, multicenter trial showed that metformin is safe and effective (which, it can be argued, the rest of the world already knew). At any rate, the results were published, and metformin was approved by the FDA.

The so-called alpha glucosidase inhibitors, such as acarbose, represent an entirely new class of drugs that slow the digestion and absorption of dietary carbohydrates. The research that led to their discovery depended on knowing in detail the mechanism of carbohydrate digestion and absorption, then targeting the specific enzymes involved.

Troglitazone is another promising oral hypoglycemic agent. Research studies indicate that it specifically improves insulin's action at the cellular level (decreasing insulin resistance). A large body of clinical research has accumulated in support of its safety and efficacy.

New insulins.   Building on the advances in basic science, it has become possible to make new kinds of insulin. If bacteria can be "programmed" to make insulin that is exactly like human insulin, they can also be programmed to make insulin that is slightly different and has slightly different absorption characteristics. The latest development in this area is the availability of lispro insulin, which is absorbed through the skin more quickly. Other modifications of insulin may be developed that will make the insulin be absorbed more slowly and more consistently. It is possible that over the next few years a series of insulins will come out that have very specific times of action, more reliably than has been the case since NPH and Ultralente insulins were introduced close to half a century ago.

Mechanical insulin delivery systems. External insulin infusion pumps became a real option for intensive insulin delivery in the early 1980s (see Chapter 14). The research that led to implantable insulin infusion pumps was described earlier in this chapter. At this point, the current models have been used in research studies by over 500 people with diabetes.

Roughly the size of a hockey puck, implantable insulin pumps are surgically inserted under the skin of the abdomen. The pump's edges are seen under the skin to a variable degree—in heavier men and most women, they are not noticeable; in thin men, they are more visible with the shirt off. The pump is electronically controlled by using an external radiotelemetry device, like a television remote control. Between meals and overnight, the pump delivers a basal rate of insulin continuously; then, before each meal, the person tests the blood glucose and sends a signal to the pump to deliver the right amount of insulin for the situation. Every one to three months, the pump is refilled with a brief, painless procedure that involves putting a needle through the skin into the pump.

There are at least two companies conducting clinical trials of implantable insulin pumps, MiniMed Technologies Inc. and Strato-Infusaid Inc. Problems remain to be solved, particularly in avoiding blockage of the catheter in the abdomen and in having a stable, reliable insulin for pump use. But some great advantages have been demonstrated, starting with the ability to deliver insulin in a consistent, regular pattern without injections or an external pump and needle to worry about. Among the specific additional findings are that the chance of hypoglycemia seems to be markedly lessened with the implants.

The clinical trials are relatively far along. Application will be made to the FDA for general marketing, and if approved, implanted insulin pumps may be generally available within a few years. A next, very large step would be to link such a delivery device to an automatic measure of the blood glucose, allowing it to deliver just the right amount of insulin automatically. This advance awaits perfection of a glucose sensor.

Glucose sensing. We'll bet there is not a person with diabetes today who wouldn't love to be able to measure blood glucose without a finger stick.

There would be lots of uses: to sound an alarm if blood glucose went dangerously high or low; to feed information into the kind of delivery system described above; to monitor glucose during an unstable time in the hospital; to determine the effects of particular foods, exercise, or stress; and more. There would be any number of ways such information could be displayed: as a digital display whenever you wanted to know, as a continuous line showing the highs and lows each day, as averages at certain times of day, and so on.

The big problem is that it can't be done yet. We do not have the technology to continuously monitor blood glucose in a reliable and practical system, unless we have a constant blood withdrawal system. There are two general approaches undergoing intensive research. One is based on the enzyme glucose oxidase, the other on a light beam.

The glucose oxidase sensors would be put on the end of a needle or small catheter. The needle would be put into the skin much as the catheter from an external insulin pump is put into the skin and changed every few days or possibly weeks. Considerable work has gone into glucose oxidase sensors in recent decades, and it is possible that one could be ready for use in the not too distant future. These enzyme sensors have the advantage of being very specific for measuring glucose, but they have not yet been perfected.

The light beam proposed is a near-infrared beam. The idea is that shining a beam of light through some part of the body, usually the fingertip, the web next to the thumb, or an earlobe, will yield a spectrum that can be analyzed to find the amount of glucose in the blood. The concept was first presented at scientific meetings in about 1990. Thus far no practical system has been forthcoming. If it were to work, this near-infrared would be wonderful in that it would not require a needle to be kept in place. But it is unclear at this time whether the light beam/spectrum approach will ultimately work.

Islet cell transplantation.   The notion of pancreas transplantation is hardly new; Frederick Banting, the discoverer of insulin, wanted to try it within two weeks of demonstrating that his extract of dog pancreas lowered blood glucose. Transplantation of whole pancreases is now a generally available procedure for people who need a transplanted kidney (see Chapter 26). But much less extensive surgery would be required if the specific insulin-producing cells, the beta cells of the islets of Langerhans, could be separated and transplanted without the rest of the pancreas. This islet cell transplantation has been the object of extensive research over the last twenty years or so but has been successfully done only a few times so far.

The barriers to islet cell transplantation are formidable. To begin with, a great many islets must be gathered without damaging their viability or their sterility. This generally involves non-human sources. When the islets are implanted, they must survive in sufficient quantity to secrete enough insulin. The cross-species origin of the islets poses a particularly difficult rejection problem. Nevertheless, techniques have been developed to harvest large numbers of islets from pig pancreases and elsewhere, and by using modern immunosuppressive medications to prevent rejection, some cases of successful islet cell transplantation have been reported. The work has led to another research approach called the biohybrid artificial pancreas.

Biohybrid artificial pancreas.   Since a major problem in transplanting pancreatic islets is that they are so vulnerable to immune rejection, some investigators have come up with the interesting idea of putting live islets into a device that allows them exposure to the blood glucose and allows them to secrete their insulin into the bloodstream, but does not allow the immune response that would destroy the islets. The islets are put inside a tube or a bag that is made of a highly selective membrane. The membrane has pores that are the right size to keep the islet cells inside, allow the blood glucose to equilibrate in, and allow the insulin to flow out, but to keep out the cells and antibodies that make up the body's immune response to foreign tissue. Once the islets are inside this tubing, several designs have been developed to put it inside the body and into the flow of the blood. Hybrid artificial pancreases are essentially a protected islet cell transplant.

Like other approaches to establishing better, simpler insulin delivery, hybrid artificial pancreases have potential advantages as well as problems. Their biggest plus is that they would function in a "closed loop" fashion, with insulin being delivered in response to increasing blood glucose and turning off when the sugar gets low. But the technical problems are significant, too. Most important, they require a large number of islets to remain alive and well for quite awhile (although it might be possible to replace the islets occasionally).

Hybrid artificial pancreases have been used successfully in dog experiments and are said to be about to be tried experimentally in humans.

Approaches to the Prevention of Diabetes

The best approach to diabetes is to prevent it, but it is not yet clear how that could be done. We have said that understanding the basic causes of a disease, the mechanisms, is crucial to rationally approaching a treatment. One of the central understandings of diabetes is that Type I diabetes and Type II diabetes are quite different diseases. The approaches to prevention, then, must be different. Two large, government-sponsored trials are under way, one trying to prevent Type I diabetes and the other working on prevention of Type II diabetes.

Prevention of Type I diabetes. Since Type I diabetes is caused by the body's immune destruction of its own pancreatic beta cells, the first step would be to prevent this immune response. To do that, we would have to know when and in whom the beta cell destruction is happening. If a single virus or a single toxin were found to be the cause of Type I diabetes, then it might be possible to develop a vaccine for that virus or a way to avoid that toxin. But there is little evidence at this point that such a single cause is likely to be found.

In the 1980s a series of studies were done using the immunosuppressive drug cyclosporine to knock down the person's immune response as soon as the person showed signs of Type I diabetes, within weeks of the first presentation, during the "honeymoon period." But these studies had limited success, both because the drug has serious side effects and probably because the disease had already damaged the islet cells irreparably by the time diabetes was apparent.

The test of circulating antibodies against the pancreas has allowed this research to enter a new phase. The antibodies are rare in the population as a whole but common in people who are about to get Type I diabetes. This opens the window of opportunity for prevention before diabetes is actually manifest. The current large clinical trial called the "Diabetes Prevention Trial, Type 1" is screening large numbers of high-risk people (mainly first- and young second-degree relatives of people with Type I diabetes) to discover those with positive antibodies who are likely to develop Type I diabetes.

Once an individual is identified as in the process of getting Type I diabetes, several prevention approaches are being tested. One is to use low doses of insulin given by injection (although the person does not yet actually have diabetes). One theory is that, in this way, the beta cell can be "put to rest," meaning that, since insulin is being given by injection, the normal pancreas beta cells are not secreting so much insulin. Another theory is that this insulin is changing the immune response of the normal beta cells. There is background evidence, in animals, at any rate, that if the cells are not so active, they are less susceptible to destruction. The trial will probably not be completed until at least the turn of the century.

Prevention of Type II diabetes. Type II diabetes is very different from Type I, so the approach to its prevention is very different. The large trial now getting under way to prevent Type II diabetes is called the Diabetes Prevention Program. It will identify people at high risk for Type II diabetes and will test approaches that are likely to be effective in preventing insulin resistance. One group will be intensively counseled in diet and exercise, and other groups will be given metformin or troglitazone or a placebo. They will have glucose tolerance tests annually, and we will hope to find which approach to prevention of Type II diabetes works best. As with the Type I diabetes prevention trial, the results will probably not be known until at least the year 2002.

Treatment of Complications

There are so many advances in the treatment of complications that describing this field of clinical research would take far more than a few paragraphs, so a couple of examples will have to suffice. We'll start with a large ophthalmology trial called the Early Treatment of Diabetic Retinopathy Study. A previous study had proven that laser therapy is highly effective in slowing the progression of severe retinopathy, so this study asked whether treatment at earlier stages would be even more beneficial. In the course of the trial it was found that a condition called macular edema should be treated early, but that otherwise laser therapy at early stages of retinopathy gave no additional benefit.

A second example of research into the management of diabetic complications is a study of coronary bypass surgery compared to angioplasty. This study found that the bypass surgery gave a better long-term result in treating certain stages of coronary heart disease.

How You Can Help

Most people understand that diabetes research is the key to progress in treating and ultimately curing diabetes. But to many people it seems like another world, one that's technical, remote, and inaccessible. Researchers sometimes don't do a good job of bridging this gap, explaining in plain language what they're up to and helping people take part. We want to show you how to get involved, how to do whatever you can to advance diabetes research. There are three broad areas that need your help: personal participation in research trials, financial support, and advocacy. Each takes some explaining.

Participating in Research Trials

Clinical research requires research subjects, people who volunteer to take part. We think of the people enrolling in our research as partners, as well as heroes, in the advancement of medicine. They may benefit personally by getting a new treatment before anyone else, or they may benefit just from the knowledge that they are helping others. Their participation may be quite simple (one of us was a research subject, by taking a pill every morning for 12 years) or very demanding, requiring multiple visits or rigorous training. Being a research subject, of course, is not for everyone, but many people find it a thoroughly rewarding experience.

When we talk to people about taking part as a subject in clinical research, the following issues often come up.

What does it mean to say that I will be "randomized" to one treatment or another?   *Randomization* refers to the assignment of research subjects, as if by flip of a coin, to one of the treatments being tested. Randomization may be crucial in a study because if a person is consciously assigned to one group or the other, bias may creep in. For example, if the investigator really wants experimental pill A to seem to work better than pill B, he or she could consciously or unconsciously see to it that the least sick people were assigned to pill A.

What does it mean to use placebos?   A placebo is an inactive treatment; if it's a pill, it is made to look like the active pill. Placebos are used in order to have a comparison group. If pill A is active and pill B is placebo, the study compares pill A to pill B. If pill A, being active, were known to be safe and effective, the research trial would not be worth doing. It is very possible that pill A *won't* work, or will have some side effects that are worse than any benefit, so it has to be compared against the inactive pill. You may ask, why not just compare pill A to taking nothing? The answer is that pill A may seem to work but actually only provide a "placebo effect." Most people feel better if they are taking a pill, any pill, even a placebo. The point of a trial that uses a placebo comparison is to see if the active drug is really effective, not just by a placebo effect.

What does "double blind" mean, and why is it part of a study?   *Double blind,* or *double masked,* means that neither the subject nor the researcher knows what pill the subject is taking. Sound strange? Of course there *are* people who know which pill it is, and in an emergency it is always possible to find out. But double blinding is another important part of answering a research question fairly. If the doctor or nurse who sees you is unmasked (knows that you are on, let's say, pill A, the active pill) and is really hopeful about pill A, bias can creep in: the professional may consciously or unconsciously let you know that he or she expects you to be feeling better on pill A and that those taking pill B (placebo) aren't feeling better. Body language, winks of the eye, even the phrasing of questions can make all the difference:

"You're feeling better today on those pills, aren't you, Mrs. Jones?" "Not noticing much difference on those pills today, Mrs. Jones?" Double masking keeps the investigator from influencing the results unfairly.

How can I be sure I am getting the treatment that works? The answer is, you can't. A principle of clinical investigation is that *no one* knows if the treatment works. If the answer is known, it's unethical to do the study. Sometimes, in fact, a research study should *not* be done. For example, in 1922, when the new insulin extracts were shown for the first time to save children dying of diabetes in Toronto, no one then and no one now would suggest that there should have been a large clinical study giving insulin to only half the dying children on that ward. The answer was obvious, the material worked, and the question immediately turned to how more insulin could be produced. But results are seldom that spectacular. If a study is being done, it is because the answer to the question is simply not known.

Looking at all drug trials, we see that the majority of experimental drugs are never proven safe and effective; either they don't work or they have side effects that are worse than the benefits. So whichever pill you take, A or B, active or placebo, you're doing good for people with diabetes by helping find out which is best.

How long will the study go on, and when will I know the results? In principle, the study goes on until an answer is found or it is clear that an answer won't ever be found by this study. For instance, if it turns out that pill A is dramatically better than pill B, when this becomes clear, the study will be stopped. Most often, studies are planned for a period of time—six months, two years, or whatever—so that any difference should be found within that time. Usually, the results of the study are not revealed to the investigators or the subjects until the study is over and the results completely analyzed. This is often a frustration for everyone involved, since they naturally want to know as soon as possible how it turned out.

How to Become Involved as a Research Subject

Becoming a subject in a research study may not be as easy as you would expect. ("Leaving my body to research" usually refers to the use of cadavers for training of medical students and is very different from signing an organ donor card. The widespread use of organ donation cards is absolutely essential to organ availability for transplantation and is recommended for everyone.)

There are several barriers to getting involved as a research subject. First of all, studies take place in a limited number of settings—often at universities or in specialists' offices. Second, in order to have a relatively comparable group of people in the study, investigators have to set up a very specific set of *exclusion criteria*. There may be an age range (such as 20–60 years old), a certain kind of diabetes (for example, Type II diabetes) may be required, maybe anyone taking insulin is excluded, and so on. The sad part to investigators and potential subjects alike is that many people have to be excluded who would be terrific participants in all respects and are eager to take part. All we can say is, "Keep up the interest, don't feel rejected or sad. Keep in touch. Maybe you'll be right for the next study."

How do you find out what studies are available in your area? You may want to ask the American Diabetes Association or call your local medical center. Read the papers and look for advertisements.

In summary, it can be rewarding and satisfying to take part in diabetes research. It can keep you in touch with the latest advances, provide some good contacts for you, and even offer personal benefit from trying a new approach to diabetes care. It can also be rewarding to support research financially.

Supporting Diabetes Research Financially

In our opinion, there is no more noble, effective, or satisfying place to put your charitable donations than into diabetes research and education. If you are fortunate enough to have substantial assets, you will find associations and university groups especially eager to demonstrate the need. But small donations, annual giving, planned giving, and even in-kind support, such as helping organize fundraisers, all make important contributions.

You may want to give, but you may be unsure how and to whom you should give. It is reasonable to ask questions, to want assurance that your money goes exactly where you want it to go. Here are some guidelines:

—The two large, national, volunteer-driven diabetes organizations, the *American Diabetes Association* (ADA) and the *Juvenile Diabetes Foundation International* (JDF), are rock solid. Organizations such as the *Lions Club International* and the *Shriners* also donate generously to diabetes research. Each group has its own distinct characteristics and priorities, as well as its own fund-raising campaigns. But you can be sure that contributions given to the ADA, the JDF, the Lions Club, or the Shriners, and earmarked for research, will be used to extremely good purpose.

—*Established universities and nonprofit medical centers* usually have diabetes research projects that represent excellent opportunities if you are eager to contribute to a local activity. Call the development office or the people involved in diabetes research.

—*Various private foundations* and even medical practices accept donations for diabetes research. These may be perfectly good choices, but you would be wise to check into them carefully.

Planned giving (your written decision to donate some portion of your assets to diabetes research upon your death) is a popular approach these days. All varieties of tax-saving mechanisms can be explained to you by experts from the larger organizations and universities. This is strongly recommended.

In sum, diabetes research needs individual charitable giving, and many families with diabetes in their midst, or even people who just understand the need, are willing and eager to give. The established nonprofit organizations, such as the ADA, the JDF, or universities, are ready and eager to receive donations and manage them responsibly. They have the experience and mechanisms to see that the money is well spent. There really is no reason to go outside these established routes when you consider charitable giving.

Being an Advocate for Diabetes Research

Most funding for diabetes research comes from the federal National Institutes of Health (NIH), particularly through the National Institute of Diabetes, Digestive and Kidney Diseases. Hundreds of millions of dollars are devoted to diabetes research each year, but this is not enough. Fewer than one in four approved grant applications from qualified investigators receives funding. The competition for NIH grants is fierce.

One way to increase diabetes research is to keep up the pressure for funding at the federal level. This is what we call advocacy, and it works. The Diabetes Research and Training Centers around the country and the NIDDK were founded, and the Diabetes Control and Complications Trial and many other important studies were funded, as a result of effective advocacy.

The ADA and the JDF both organize specific, targeted public campaigns to advocate for diabetes research. Through them, you can target your letters or your visits to the right people at just the right time. But it is up to you. We do live in a democracy, and both federal and state governments respond to pressure. Rest assured that if you don't put on the heat for biomedical research, whatever funding is available will go to other types of projects.

The world of diabetes research is vast and exciting. It stretches all the way from laboratory attempts to understand the most fundamental questions of insulin action to psychosocial research on how to get whole populations to lead a healthier life. There's no way to tell for sure which research approaches—for instance, islet cell transplantation, mechanical insulin delivery systems, or prevention trials—are the best way to go. A broad-based, well-balanced, and well-funded research effort is necessary to optimize our chances for improving the life of people with diabetes today and ultimately curing the disease.

You can make a difference. It is enormously important to the effort as a whole for you to understand the process and support it. You may be able to promote diabetes research through a letter to the editor of a newspaper or to a member of Congress. You may meet someone tomorrow who can give substantially. You may get more involved yourself. We believe that an educated, supportive population is the key to a healthy, strong diabetes research effort. And only through such a research effort will the future of diabetes be as bright as we think it can be.

Chapter 34

The Prognosis

- *"I'm really worried about my future. I hear all these things about diabetes, and I've seen plenty to make me think they're true."*
- *"I don't understand why things seem to move so slowly. People say we're making progress, but I don't see it. Will it help me in my lifetime?"*
- *"Every day, I look in the paper for a breakthrough in diabetes. When something hits the news, though, I usually don't understand it."*

This book is full of explanations, suggestions, and factual information about how to live life to the fullest with diabetes. We didn't write it for the perfect patient—that would be too small a market, since we haven't yet met him or her. Nor did we write it for hopeless cases, because we don't think anyone's hopeless, and if they do exist we suppose they don't buy such books. The fact is, this book was not written for a *patient* at all, but for a *person*. A person with diabetes. *You*. You will take from it what you need, use what you can, and leave aside what does not apply to you now.

The *prognosis*, or outlook, for people with diabetes is excellent. That is not just wishful thinking, it's a scientific fact. Using what is available today, using your best understanding of diabetes and controlling it to the best of your ability, there is every reason to think that you can avoid long-term complications and lead a long and healthy life.

"How good do I have to be?" you're probably asking. We don't know the answer, but we like to quote the army ads and say, "Be all that you can be." We know that in the bad old days blood glucose levels for most people were routinely in what we would now consider a poor range, say chronically in the 200s and 300s. We know that the Diabetes Control and Complications Trial, mentioned many times in this book, did remarkably well in preventing and slowing complications by maintaining blood glucose with averages of about 155 mg/dl. So it is doable.

Several themes recur throughout this book, reflecting our own beliefs and our thoughts about how to help you improve your own prognosis. First, we don't believe in perfection. We believe in frailty, human nature, original sin, or whatever you want to call it. But we also strongly believe in people's *ability to get back on track,* and this is one of the most important skills you will learn. An occasional deviation from the straight-and-narrow won't kill you, but the failure to get back on track might. Whether it is watching your diet, exercising, visiting your health care professionals, or even taking your medication, think hard about how to get yourself back on track if you have strayed. It will help your prognosis immensely.

We believe in *knowledge.* We believe that it's vitally important for you to understand what you are being asked to do and why. Ask questions of your doctor and nurse educator. Discuss things with them. Be sure they hear you and you hear them. It is much easier to live with diabetes when you understand why you should be doing certain things and not doing others.

You need to be able to *separate the more important things from the less important.* Let's say that in thinking about how to improve the circulation to your feet, you read that you should try to walk upstairs at work to improve activity, quit smoking, and try not to cross your legs when you sit. Which of these is most important? We'll give you a hint—it's not uncrossing your legs. Or let's say you live alone and are getting hypoglycemic reactions. It's most important to make note of the timing. Feeling a little low before lunch, when you can readily take a snack if lunch is delayed, pales in comparison to the seriousness of having significant hypoglycemia in the middle of the night and waking up confused. Understanding your diabetes will help you in more ways than you can imagine.

We believe in *communication.* Your health care visits can be more productive if you communicate well. So can your interactions with friends and family. Communicating well about diabetes shows a comfort level, an acceptance of diabetes as part of you. You'll learn your own balance between hiding the diabetes and wearing it on your sleeve. You can put the diabetes in the proper perspective, not ignoring it but not letting it dominate you. *Remember: diabetes is just a part of you, like being tall or short, having brown eyes or blue eyes.* Diabetes is not the whole you.

We also believe in the *gradual* cure of diabetes. Does this sound odd? Do you like to think that a day will dawn when diabetes is just—poof!—gone? We'd all like to think that, but it may not happen quite that way. It may be more like cancer cures: certain cancers that used to be incurable are now fully curable, some have much improved survival rates, and some remain incurable. Therapies may develop for diabetes that make the disease more and more "forgettable," requiring less and less of your own input to achieve good control. Various approaches to the various kinds of diabetes will move at differing rates.

We have emphasized that the real challenge is not so much to eliminate the diabetes as to eliminate the personal burden it places on people, and, of course, to eliminate the complications. If you could have one procedure, whether it's a gene transfer or a transplant or a pump, and never again have to think about diabetes, that would be tantamount to a cure. But it may come gradually, not as a single flash of glory.

Finally, we believe in *taking advantage of what is available to you.* This book describes many ways to help control your diabetes today. If we had written it just 20 years ago, this would have been a very different book. The same will be true if we revise it several years from now. So it is up to you to stay on top of things, to follow the advances, not just in research or theory but in practical, available tools that can help you manage your own diabetes.

Diabetes care is not a fixed, static set of rules, but a wave that moves steadily forward. Care has advanced, is advancing, and will advance. If you ride the wave, taking advantage of what is available as you go along, you put yourself in the best possible position to be strong and healthy when diabetes is ultimately cured. That is the promise of having diabetes today. That is what makes the prognosis excellent.

Index

acanthosis nigricans, 346
acarbose, 148, 149, 152, 157, 158
ACE inhibitors, 312, 318
acesulfame K, 91
acetohexamide, 154
acromegaly, 32
actuary, 266
adrenaline, 67
adult onset diabetes. *See* Type II diabetes
adverse selection, 266
air hunger, 291
alcohol, 92–93, 108; and chlorpropamide, 154; and hypoglycemia, 71, 92–93
aldose reductase inhibitors, 321, 322
allergies: to insulin, 168, 169; to sulfa drugs, 150, 155–56. *See also* food allergies
alopecia, 345
alphafetoprotein test, 367
alpha-glycosidase inhibitors, 157, 398
alprazolam, 239
Amaryl, 154
American Diabetes Association, 253–54, 393, 406, 407
Americans with Disabilities Act, 271
amino acids, 84, 121
aminoguanidine, 322
amitriptyline, 237, 322
amniocentesis, 367
amputation: and foot problems, 331, 338–40; rehabilitation from, 339–40; types of, 338
anaphylactic reactions, 132
anemia, as side effect of sulfonylureas, 155
anger, 213–15
angina pectoris, 144, 298–99
angioplasty, 300

angiotensin-converting-enzyme inhibitors. *See* ACE inhibitors
anorexia nervosa, 239
antibiotics, for foot problems, 336
antidepressants, 237
antioxidants, 86–87
anxiety disorder, 237–39; clinical, 238; medication for, 239
arbamazepine, 322
arteriosclerosis, 249–301; and cerebrovascular disease, 300–301; and heart disease, 298–99; and peripheral vascular disease, 300; risk factors for, 294–98
aspartame, 91
Ativan, 239
autoamputation, 339
autonomic motor nerves, 320
autonomic neuropathies, 321, 323–25, 326

background retinopathy, 304
Banting, Frederick, 19, 159, 160, 400
basal rate, 192, 193, 199, 202
behavior modification: research on, 396–97; for weight control, 116
Bell's palsy, 325
Best, Charles A., 19, 159, 160
beta cells, 19, 24, 159
BIDS therapy (bedtime insulin, daytime sulfonylureas), 151, 183
bill of rights, patient's, 256–58
birth defects, 361
Bliss, Michael, 19, 159
blood glucose. *See* blood sugar; blood sugar monitoring
blood glucose awareness training (BGAT), 73

Library of Congress Cataloging-in-Publication Data

Saudek, Christopher D.
The Johns Hopkins guide to diabetes : for today and tomorrow / Christopher D. Saudek, Richard
R. Rubin, Cynthia S. Shump.
    p.   cm. — (A Johns Hopkins Press health book)
    Includes index.
    ISBN 0-8018-5580-2 (alk. paper). — ISBN 0-8018-5581-0 (pbk. : alk. paper)
    1. Diabetes—Popular works.   I. Rubin, Richard R.   II. Shump, Cynthia S.   III. Title.
IV. Series: Johns Hopkins health book.
RC660.4.S28   1997
616.4'62—dc21

                                                                                        96-49161
                                                                                             CIP